CHIROPRACTIC TECHNIC

WRYNECK

The Neck Has Gone Awry

TORTICOLLIS

Its Analysis
and Correction In
Infants/Children/Adults
And
Selected Adjustments,
Subluxations, and Papers

Vol. IX
by

F. H. Barge
1998

First Edition

ISBN: 1-885048-12-2 softcover
1-885048-11-4 hardcover

Library of Congress: 98-093092

Printed in the United States of America
by Palmer Publications, Inc.
318 North Main Street
Amherst, WI 54406

DEDICATION

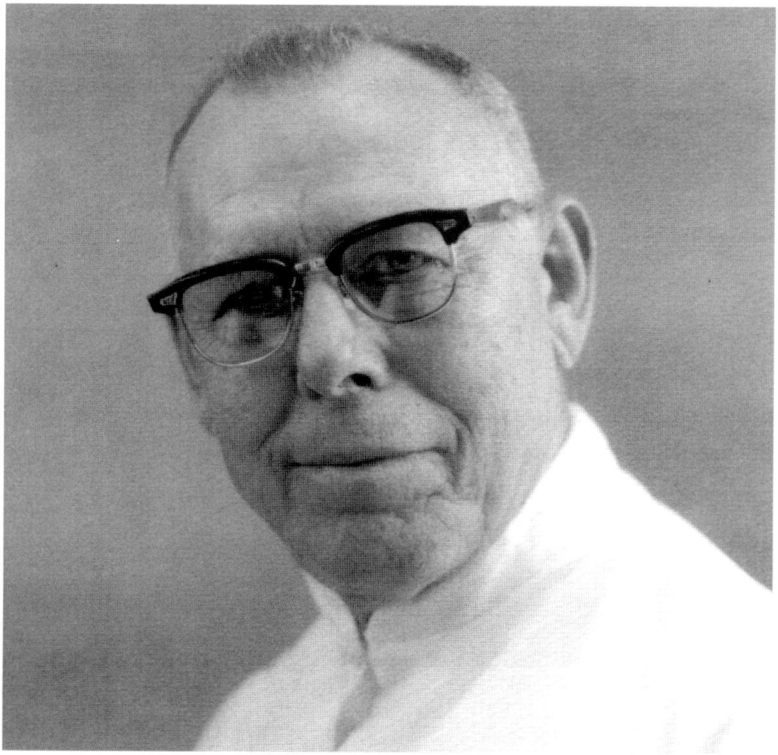

To my father, Henry A. Barge, D.C., who graduated from The Palmer School of Chiropractic in 1923. His lessons in vertebral adjusting guided me in my early efforts with this subluxation. He was a chiropractic pioneer extraordinaire. Paralyzed by a cerebral hemorrhage when only 38 years old, he fought back against the ravages of his stroke under the chiropractic care of his sister, Dr. Alma Stauff, R.N., D.C. After two years with this serious handicap, he returned to practice adjusting with only one hand and rebuilt his flourishing practice. Only death separated him from his profession.

He strove valiantly in life,
he knew no other way.
And with him, death too,
battled for its day.

FHB

About The Author
1998

A second generation chiropractor, Dr. Fred H. Barge was number nine in the Barge family to pursue the chiropractic profession; today he can count fifteen D.C. family members. He graduated from the Palmer School of Chiropractic in 1954, underwent postgraduate studies at the Logan Basic College of Chiropractic in 1955, he then interned with Dr. Clarence Gonstead and his father, Dr. Henry Barge. He received his philosopher's degree in chiropractic (Ph.C.) from Palmer College in 1965, and among his most prestigious awards are included the D.D. Palmer Scientific Award and the Life Chiropractic College Science Award. Dr. Barge is a Distinguished Fellow of the International Chiropractors Association, and a fellow in the Palmer Academy of Chiropractic. An international lecturer and author, Dr. Barge has served the graduate education faculties of thirteen chiropractic colleges, and as a visiting professor at five chiropractic colleges. He is past president of the International Chiropractor's Association, a member of the Board of Directors and chairman of the Committee on Policy and Definitions.

As a clinician, Dr. Barge has brought 17 chiropractors into direct practice with him and he has tutored over 40 interns in his clinic in La Crosse, Wisconsin. As a regular lecturer to the student bodies of various chiropractic colleges, Dr. Barge extends his influence, teaching young D.C.'s in the philosophy, science, and art of chiropractic. He is recognized as chiropractic's leading authority on scoliosis and he lectures regularly worldwide on the subject.

Torticollis was the second book in Dr. Barge's Trilogy of Chiropractic Technic texts. The First Edition was printed in 1979, the Second Edition in 1984 and now in 1998 he has produced this new text on the subject entitled, "Wryneck." In total he has now written nine texts on chiropractic and his writing efforts continue on. A listing and brief description of his texts is found in the back of this book.

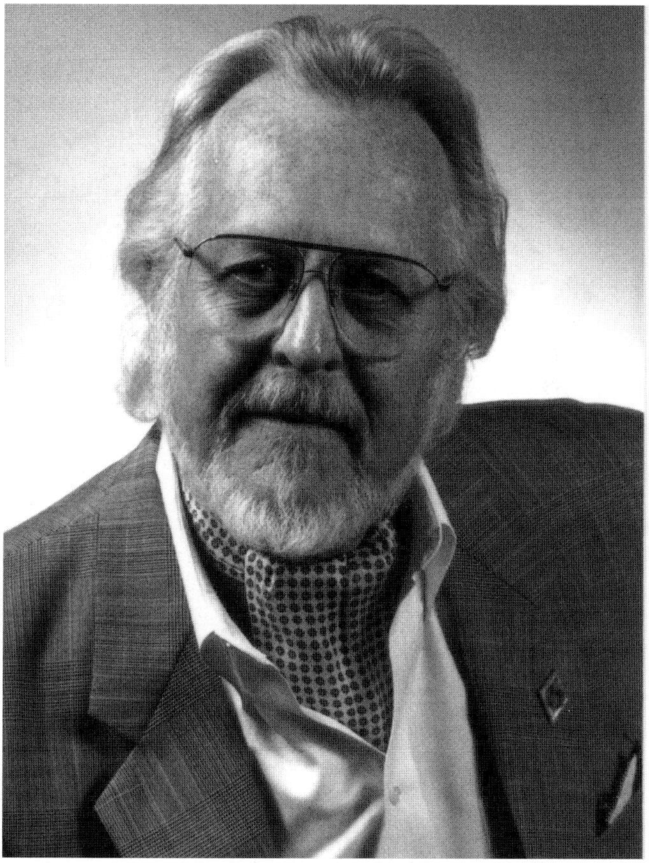

Fredrick H. E. Barge, D,C., Ph.C.
(Hon.) F.I.C.A., F.P.A.C., S.C.S.
Clinician, Author, Educator, Publisher
President Barge Chicropractic Publishing, Inc.

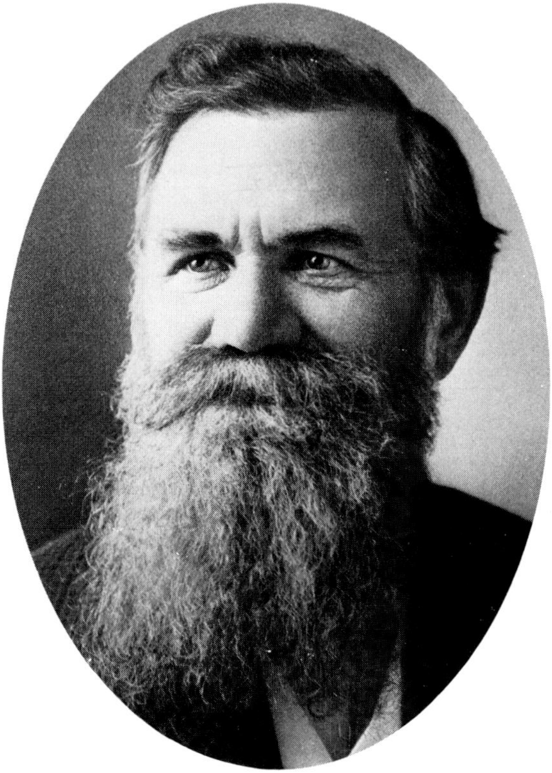

"As all conditions of wry-neck are caused by a displaced cervical vertebra, why not adjust, replace it?"[1]

D. D. Palmer

ACKNOWLEDGEMENT
Third Edition — 1998

I acknowledge the pioneer efforts of the chiropractors before me. Their results in the adjustment of this distinct and singular subluxation provided footsteps for me to follow in my investigation into the specificity of its correction. I wish to thank my early teachers in chiropractic, at both Palmer and Logan Colleges. Their instruction and counsel provided me with my basic understanding of the subject.

Acknowledgement must be paid to the technics developed by Dr. Clarence Gonstead, Dr. Hugh B. Logan, Dr. Otto Reinert, and Dr. W. Frederic Keck. A note of appreciation is in order to my good friend Dr. E. L. "Bud" Crowder for contributing a chapter and illustrations for this text and above all for his sage advice that has been a guiding hand in my professional life since my graduation from the Palmer School of Chiropractic in 1954.

A special note of 'thank you' goes to my good friend in chiropractic, Dr. LeRoy Otto. As a young man he was my protege, then my associate, today he serves the profession well and he has contributed a case study to this edition along with illustrations of the adjustment of infants. To Drs. Joan Fallon, Peter Fysh and Douglas Cox, I extend gratitude for their permission to quote in entirety their papers published in the I.C.A. Review and J.C.C.P. To the I.C.A., my professional organization, a thank you for permission to republish these papers and the paper by Dr. Gutmann from Germany. The writings of these fine doctors have greatly enhanced the contents of this text and the purpose for which it was written. Dr. Maxine McMullen's gracious help and permission to quote and reproduce illustrations from the Journal of Clinical Chiropractic Pediatrics is certainly appreciated and her leadership of the I.C.A.'s Pediatric council has been significant contribution to the entire chiropractic profession. The care of children goes well beyond the orthopedic problems so many adults seek chiropractic for. The far-reaching effects of chiropractic care in the organic, systemic and infectious problems of children provide concrete proof of the efficacy of the chiropractic principle.

I must not fail to thank the authors and publishers of the texts I have quoted from in this text. Their writings and research have enhanced my ability to explain the complexities of this condition and have lent supportive evidence to my theories on the disc block subluxation. For their names and text books I refer you to the bibliography. And may I also acknowledge the support of the chiropractic colleges; their curricular acceptance and sale of my texts through their bookstores, has been particularly gratifying to me and has made my continued writing efforts possible.

And a final note of thank you to my father H.A. Barge D.C., though handicapped in that he could only adjust with his right hand, his concept of "pulling" the spinous process of the involved vertebra lead me in the right direction in the adjustic correction of this subluxation.

In the final analysis an author's success in any scientific literary effort is based upon its acceptance by those for whom it was written. And thus to you my peers, my colleagues and friends, the students in the chiropractic colleges, the many readers of my texts in the chiropractic profession, a special and heartfelt thank you!

Fred H. Barge, D.C., Ph.C.

TABLE OF CONTENTS

PREFACE 1998

I graduated from the Palmer School of Chiropractic in 1954. In 1955 I traveled to St. Louis and pursued a nine-month post graduate course at the Logan Basic College of Chiropractic. Upon returning to my home town of LaCrosse, Wisconsin, my father Henry A. Barge, D.C. insisted that I spend some time with his classmate and seat partner in college, Dr. Clarence Gonstead of Mt. Horeb, Wisconsin. My father and Dr. Gonstead graduated from the Palmer School of Chiropractic in 1923. Their class was appropriately named the 'Crusader' class as I was told by my father that within six months of graduation 50 percent of his class were in jail or under litigation for practicing medicine without a license. There were over 500 graduates in the "Crusader Class."

For the next two months I visited Mt. Horeb every weekend to follow Dr. Gonstead around and observe his procedures. Dr. Gonstead carried on a full schedule of practice even on Sundays. By this time in my life as a young D.C., I had observed numerous chiropractors adjust patients with torticollis, but the explanation as to the WHY of the tortuous position of the patients cervical spine and the x-ray analysis of this cervical subluxation was still not clear to me. The teachings I had received offered no explanation in regards to the vertebral locking so evident in this acute subluxation.

In viewing torticollis as a young practitioner, I had one thought in mind — find the subluxation and correct it with an adjustment. How, was the question! Most certainly it should be done in a way which would give the patient the least discomfort and yet do the necessary job. . . move the vertebra into an improved position. In most cases of lateral torticollis you could have the patient lay their head in your hand. That is to say, if the patient's head was tipped to the left shoulder, you could stand on the right side of the patient, reach around with your right hand and have the patient lay his/her head in your hand. Therefore the common master cervical rotary adjustment could be used but this move lacked specificity. Palpation of the cervical spine and x-ray analysis revealed a spinous process deviation of a singular vertebra to the convexity of the patients head tilt. Wrapping my hand around the posterior aspect of the patient's neck and pulling the spinous process became a more specific and very effective adjustment. I became aware that a transverse contact with P to A line of drive into the concavity of the torticollis curve was also effective. This indicated to me that if the spinous was right, the body left, and head tipped to the left . . . a disc wedge must be open, on the right side and the x-ray analysis of acute torticollis victims verified my determinations. But why was the spine held so rigidly in this position? This same tortuous positioning was evident in low back disc conditions and thus my investigations and research into tortipelvis and torticollis. My first book, "Tortipelvis" was published in 1976 and I followed that book with its companion text "Torticollis" in 1979. A second edition of "Torticollis" was published in 1984, and in 1995, I began developing this new text on the subject of torticollis, its analysis and adjustic correction; VOL. IX WRYNECK.

Throughout the past two decades my viewpoints in respect to the cause and correction of this singular subluxation remain essentially the same. Recent medical viewpoints support my conclusions and empirical evidence continues to support the specific adjustic correction of this disc lesion subluxation. With two new chapters on history, pediatric adjusting and a chapter on the upper cervical specific approach to torticollis; along with the viewpoints and technics of the other noted chiropractic clinicians this text is now completed. It is my wish that it will provide for the practitioner a practical guide to the cause, the specific radiographic analysis and correction of the torticollis subluxation. Yes, torticollis **is** a subluxation.

"Enuf" Said,

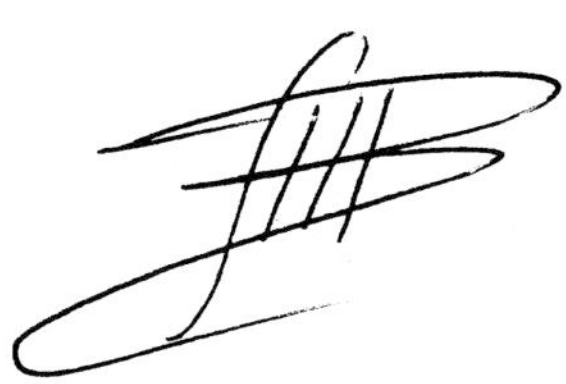

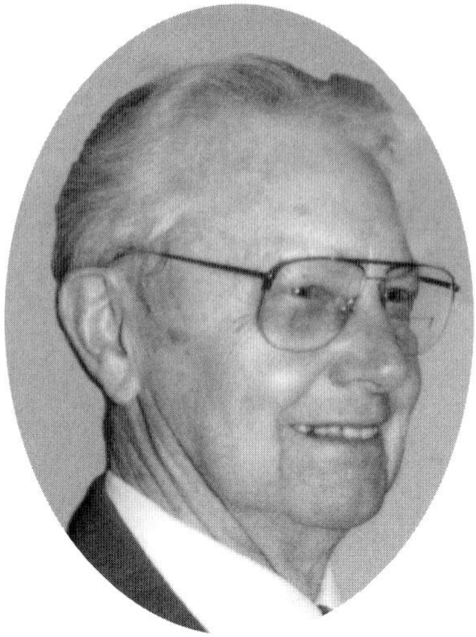

Drs. E. L. (Bud) and Juanita Crowder. My friends throughout my life in chiropractic. To my knowledge, Dr. Bud Crowder has trained more student interns than any other chiropractor. Mentor to many, respected by all, he has contributed the Foreword and a chapter on toggle recoil adjusting to this text.

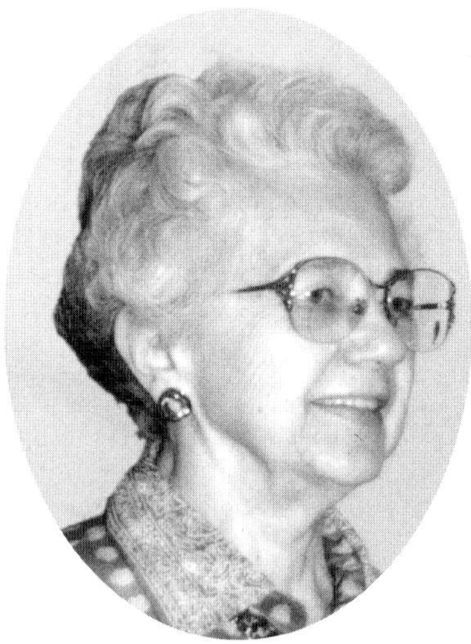

Dr. Juanita Crowder's father, also a D.C.. invented the "Nicholas" side posture table, in my opinion, the very finest toggle table; it is still produced by The Lloyd Table Company.

FOREWORD

Great leaders have much in common, all have intrinsic wealth derived from personal achievement and commitment to a worthy cause.

The drive and devotion Fred Barge has for chiropractic inspires countless others to reach for greater professional achievement. He proudly continues the heritage of the Barge family as true pioneers, teaching others, not only through words but with actions.

Brought together in this volume are fundamental principles and professional wisdom born from a commitment and dedication to chiropractic excellence.

Torticollis deserves the attention given by Dr. Barge. So long a mystery —not life threatening— but always an impediment and a pain in the neck.

The Barge text, **"WRYNECK,"** suggests a protocol for specific assessment and specific correction of the torticollis malady. It is refreshing to encounter precision from a health care giver.

Thanks to Dr. Fred Barge for his leadership and his passion for excellence.

E. L. Crowder, D.C., Ph.C.

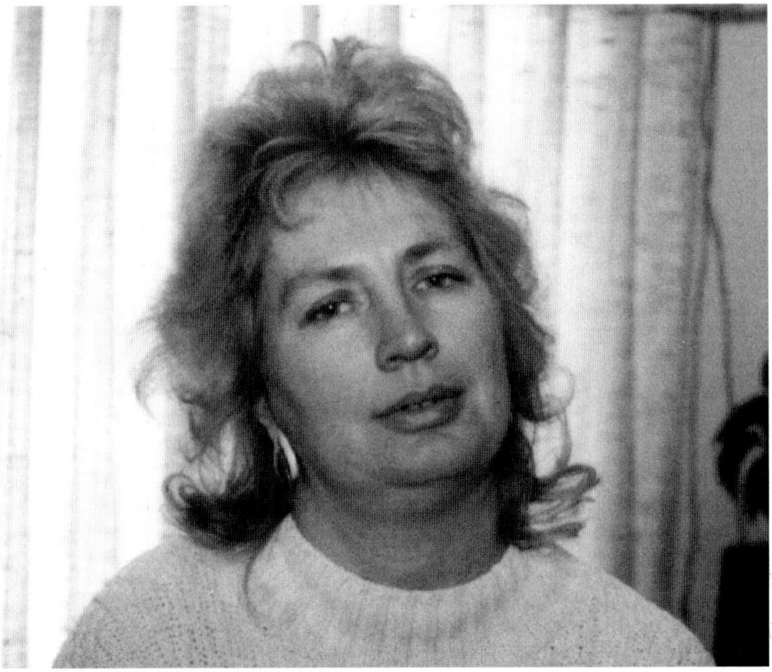

(Ill. Intro-1)

The classic positioning of the patients head and neck in torticollis.* The head is tipped to one side and the face is rotated away from the side of lateral tipping. Torticollis commonly affects the right side.

* Printed with patient permission, Judith Ibarra

INTRODUCTION

TORTICOLLIS — (as defined by Dorland's Medical Dictionary) - "A contracted state of the cervical muscles, producing twisting of the neck, and an unnatural position of the head."

If this definition is correct and torticollis is caused by muscle spasm then how could proper chiropractic adjustic procedures correct torticollis, sometimes instantaneously and commonly within a few hours after the adjustment? Only difficult and neglected cases require a series of spinal adjustments. This definition has some truth in the description of the symptomatic picture, but not causation; TORTICOLLIS IS A SUBLUXATION!

"Wryneck" they used to call it ... the neck has gone awry. Now most certainly it has, and it is extremely painful if not impossible for the patient to move it out of its anatomically locked position. No, the spine is not assuming an antalgic position, it is in a state of anatomical malposition and lock. We have here a rotatory disrelationship and disc wedge subluxation, wherein the nucleus pulposus of the disc has shifted to one side creating vertebral rotation, facet separation and the resultant state of anatomical lock. Given rest and time, torticollis is commonly self-limiting. During rest as the discs expand when the weight is released from them, they spread the vertebrae apart; nuclear and vertebral repositioning is facilitated and often accomplished. Therefore, rest has its way of producing self repair. In infants the tortuous position of head and neck can become chronic with resultant disfigurement of the hapless child. In adults, if the subluxation is below the third cervical and the body does not achieve subluxation correction, it produces a rotatory scoliosis in adaptation, and thus the victim at least has an objectively straight neck. But then the chronic subluxation can, and often does, cause neurological involvement and degenerative articular deterioration.

Being commonly self limiting in its symptomatic syndrome, torticollis will **seemingly** respond to aspirin, muscle relaxers, neck braces, and physical therapy. This response takes time, many days, weeks, and in some cases, even months. Chiropractically, the results are gratifying and often instantaneous.

For many years this condition, medically speaking, was thought to be caused by muscle spasm. So convinced were they of the muscular cause of this problem that surgical incision of the sternocleidomastoideus muscle was a frequent mode of treatment. In my early years of practice I saw a goodly number of post surgical scars on cases that had been thusly treated for "wryneck."

From the many sources I have on hand in my extensive library of early chiropractic writings I can truly say that our teachers of the past agreed that torticollis was a subluxation. For instance, Dr. James N. Firth, D.C., professor of Symptomatology at the Palmer School of Chiropractic, co-founder of The Lincoln School of Chiropractic and author of the text "Chiropractic Symptomatology"[2] (later editions, "Chiropractic Diagnosis") stated this under torticollis:

"This is caused by a local subluxation in the cervical region, which impinges the motor nerves leading to the muscles affected, and especially affecting the spinal portion of the spinal accessory nerve which is distributed to these two muscles."

It is the author's opinion that when, in rare instances, true muscle spasm exists in this malady, it is the result of the nerve root impingement caused by the subluxation. As I have stated in earlier writings, chiropractic has lost much to the grindstone of time. May the future see us correct this error. Today the veracity of our early analysis as to the cause of torticollis being a subluxation is being continually validated and medical texts do mention the subluxation cause. Later in this text I will quote from some of the more noted medical authors and their description of this subluxation.

In this text, "WRYNECK", VOL. IX, I endeavor to explain the mechanics of this subluxation, the cause of the vertebral locking and its adjustic correction. The mechanical fixation results in the tortuous twist of the cervical spine so classically seen on (Ill. Intro. 2) from D. D. Palmer's 1910 text.

No, torticollis is not caused by muscle spasm! That painful reflex muscular tensions follow certainly cannot be denied . . . but they are a result of the malposition, fixation, and the neuroforaminal insult of this disc block subluxation. The words of chiropractic's founder are as true today as when he uttered them in 1910.

"As all the conditions of wry-neck are caused by a displaced cervical vertebra, why not adjust, replace it?"[1]

D. D. Palmer

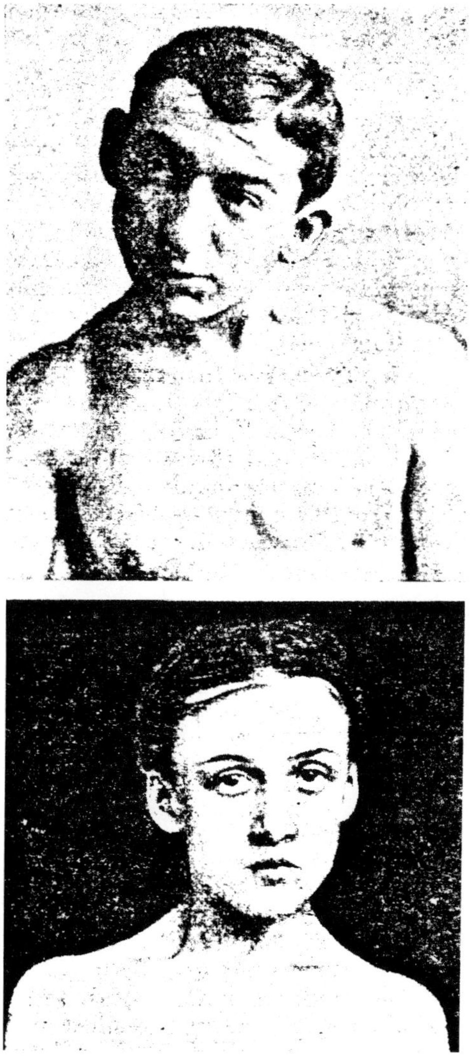

(Ill. Intro-2)

From D. D. Palmer 1910 text[1], The Science, Art and Philosophy of Chiropractic, The Chiropractor's Adjuster*. With credits to: "Taken from Whitman's Orthopedic Surgery, Published by Lea and Febiger, Philadelphia."

*Courtesy of Palmer College of Chiropractic.

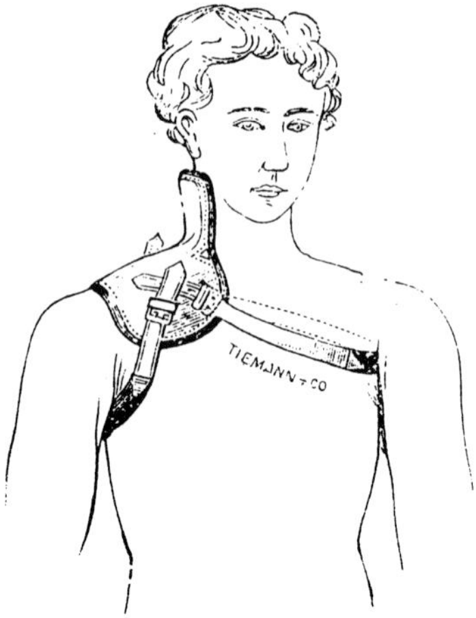

Splint for Wry Neck.

(Ill. I-1) The apparatus recommended by Dr. Holt, to “relieve incurable cases.”

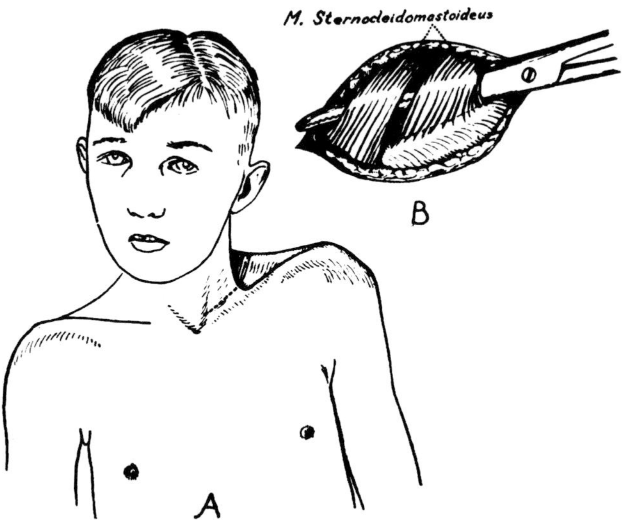

Operation for torticollis. A, Line of skin incision. B, Clavicular end sternal attachments of sternocleidomastoid muscle withdrawn from wound and divided. (From Speed, J.S., and Knight, R. A.: Campbell's Operative Orthopaedics, 1956, The C. V. Mosby Co.)[3]

(Ill. I-2) A method of surgery.

CHAPTER I
HISTORICAL OBSERVATIONS

Torticollis, I am certain, has always been a malady of fully erect man and a literature search into my own personal library reveals that the condition was well described in the medical texts of the late eighteen hundreds.

In the classical medical text book by William Osler, M.D., "The Principles and Practice of Medicine"[4], the noted medical physician ascribes the condition of "Torticollis; Wry neck" as being "chiefly though not solely" due to spasm of the muscles supplied by the accessory nerve. Now, I have in my collection both the first and third edition of this text and the wordage is the same in both. On pages 1064 the good doctor states;

"Congenital Torticollis — This condition, also known as fixed torticollis, depends upon the shortening and atrophy of the sterno-mastoid on one side. It occurs in children and may not be noticed for several years on account of the shortness of the neck, the parents often alleging that it has only recently come on. It affects the ***right side*** *almost exclusively. A remarkable circumstance in connection with it is the existence of facial asymmetry noted by Wilks, which appears to be an essential part of this congenital form. It occurred in 6 cases reported by Golding-Bird. In congenital wryneck the sterno-mastoid is shortened, hard and firm, and in a condition of more or less advanced atrophy. This must be distinguished from the local thickening in the sterno-mastoid due to rupture, which may occur at the time of birth and produce an induration or muscle callus."* (emphasis added)

Note that in this quote Dr. Osler mentions that most commonly torticollis is on the right side and facial asymmetry commonly accompanies the problem.

In 1896 J. H. Kellog, M.D. in his book, "The Home Hand-Book of DOMESTIC HYGIENE AND RATIONAL MEDICINE"[5], The noted Obstetrician and Gynecologist had this to say in respect to treatment;

"Treatment, — Wry neck sometimes resists the most energetic treatment. The majority of cases, however, can be relieved, and in time cured. Experience shows the best remedies to be the application of electricity, massage of the neck, hot and cold to the upper spine, rest, and warm baths. Incurable cases may be relieved by an apparatus (Fig. 321)." (Ill. I-1)

"THE PRACTITIONERS MANUAL"[6], A Condensed System of Medical Diagnosis And Treatment", by Charles Warrenne Allen, M.D., was written in 1898. In this text Dr. Allen makes the observation that is common throughout all early literature on torticollis, that is; the patient's head is tipped to one side and rotated away from the side of lateral tipping. (Ill. Intro. 1 & 2) I will now quote from page 781 of this text.

"Wryneck may be congenital, in which case the shortened sterno-mastoid undergoes atrophy and a hardening process. Facial asymmetry usually accompanies it. Partial rupture of the fibres of the sterno-cleido-mastoid during delivery, with intra-muscular hemorrhage and hematoma, is frequently followed by permanent muscular contraction. In tonic torticollis ***the head is drawn over with the occiput toward the shoulder of the affected side and the chin is thrown up in the opposite direction****."* (emphasis added)

In regards to prognosis Dr. Allen states;

"PROGNOSIS in the acute form is good. Recovery takes place often without special medication. In the chronic form the condition may persist or return even after the most active measures.

"TREATMENT — drugs and palliative measures rarely succeed in the chronic form. In recent cases massage does well, and hypnotism has had reported cures to its credit. Resection of nerves appears to offer the only radical course, and this, unfortunately, gives at times but temporary relief. The spinal accessory is the nerve usually resected.

In 1901 L. Emmett Holt A.M., M.D. wrote a book entitled, THE DISEASES OF INFANCY AND CHILDHOOD.[7] In it he makes some extensive and astute observations in regards to the so called tumor, or hematoma, associated with torticollis.

"Hematoma of the Sterno-Mastoid. — Hematoma, or, as it is sometimes called, induration of the sterno-mastoid muscle, leads to the formation of a tumor in the belly of the muscle. It is a rare condition, usually noticed in the second or third week of life, and it disappears spontaneously, without causing any permanent deformity. The tumor varies from three quarters of an inch to one inch and a half in length, being about the size and shape of a pigeon's egg. It is movable, almost cartilaginous to the touch, and sometimes slightly tender. The situation of the tumor is usually about the centre of the muscle. There is no discoloration of the skin.

In about two thirds of the cases it occurs after breech presentations. It is much more frequent ***upon the right*** *than upon the* *left side. In twenty-seven cases collected by Henoch the right side was involved in twenty-one and the left in only six cases.* ***The explanation of this difference is to be found in the obstetrical position.*** *Rarely, both sides may be involved.* ***The head is usually inclined towards the shoulder of the affected side and rotated towards the opposite side.*** *The tumor is frequently discovered by accident. Often it is the slight rotation of the head which is first noticed. Hematoma of the sterno-mastoid is frequently mistaken for an enlarged lymphatic gland; its position, however, is diagnostic. The swelling slowly diminishes in size, and in most cases by the end of the third month has entirely disappeared. Occasionally a slight torticollis remains for a longer time, but in the majority of cases the recovery is perfect.* ***Hematoma of the sterno-mastoid is due to the twisting of the head during parturition.*** *It is not an evidence of the employment of any improper violence in delivery. The twisting of the head produces laceration of some of the blood-vessels of the muscle, and in some cases there is doubtless rupture of some of the fibres of the muscle itself. Following this there occurs a certain amount of inflammation of the muscle and its sheath. The tumor is due partly to blood-extravasation and partly to inflammatory products. In one or two recent cases in which the sheath of the muscle has been opened it has been found filled with blood. Usually the inner border of the muscle is the part most affected.*

The prognosis for complete recovery is good. The condition requires no treatment. ***Operative interference is positively contra-indicated****."* (emphasis added)

Now you see that this medical physician is quite positive indeed that "operative interference is positively not indicated." Yet up into this past decade I have personally seen this procedure advocated medically (Ill. I-2 page xx), (and I might add solved chiropractically.)

Dr. Holt emphasizes his opinion that the condition occurs before birth by saying;

"While it is possible that the deformity is sometimes the consequence of injury received during delivery, the cause of most of the congenital cases goes back to conditions existing before birth. It may be compared to club-foot, and may be due to a faulty position of the child in utero."

Sir William Osler also made the observation that — *"Golding-Bird concludes that the facial asymmetry and the torticollis are integral parts of one affection which has a central origin and is the counter part in the head and neck of infantile paralysis with talipes in the foot."*[4]

Both these doctors felt that the position in utero that created (in their opinion) torticollis was similar to the cause of "club-foot."

In Dr. Holts book clearly describes his opinion on torticollis and through an illustration he depicts the directional malposition of the neck caused by the vertebral locking of this subluxation. He, of course, as the majority of medical doctors hold today, attributes the cause to muscle spasm.

"Torticollis — Wry-Neck . . . In simple sterno-mastoid spasm the head is inclined to the affected side and rotated toward the opposite side; the chin is raised, and the ear approaches the clavicle."[7]

In respect to treatment this text states;

"The first indication is to remove or treat the cause where one can be found. Malarial cases require quinine; rheumatic cases are benefited by rest in bed, hot applications, counter-irritation, friction, and sometimes by anti-rheumatic remedies. Cases which have lasted a month usually require some orthopaedic head-support, and those which have lasted six months or more are rarely cured without a surgical operation. This may be either a subcutaneous tenotomy or myotomy of the sterno-mastoid, or an open incision. Whitman gives the result of thirty-two cases admitted for treatment to the hospital mentioned, as follows: In 17 in which the deformity had lasted less than six months, 10 were cured, the average duration of treatment being three months; 4 were improved, and 3 not improved, the average duration of treatment in these cases being ***eleven months****. Of 15 cases in which the deformity had lasted over six months, none were cured and only 6 improved, after an average of about eight months' treatment. In the foregoing series of cases the treatment consisted mainly in the use of orthopaedic apparatus; later results from incision have been considerably more favorable. But these figures show how serious a matter is an old case of torticollis, and emphasize the importance of resorting to efficient measures early in the disease."*[7] (emphasis added)

It is appalling to think of any child going through eleven months of questionable treatments for that which can easily be handled by two to three chiropractic adjustments. It indeed was a fortunate child whose parents took him/her to one of the early practitioners of chiropractic rather than an M.D. and so too today. I will agree, however, that an "old" case of torticollis is serious indeed and in my opinion, may well lead to the serious condition of clonic or spasmodic torticollis; and this persistent subluxation is most commonly unyielding to chiropractic care. But let us carry on with more historical observations.

Dr. Glentworth Reeve Butler, A.M.,M.D. in his book, "THE DIAGNOSTICS OF INTERNAL MEDICINE"[8], 1902 gave the usual graphic description of torticollis:

"The head is inclined toward the affected side, the chin raised, and the head rotated to the opposite side."

As it is often said, a picture speaks more clearly than words and in "DIFFERENTIAL DIAGNOSIS AND TREATMENT OF DISEASE"[9], by Augustus Caille, M.D., 1907, I copy with credits the photograph and treatment found in this text. (Ill. I-3)

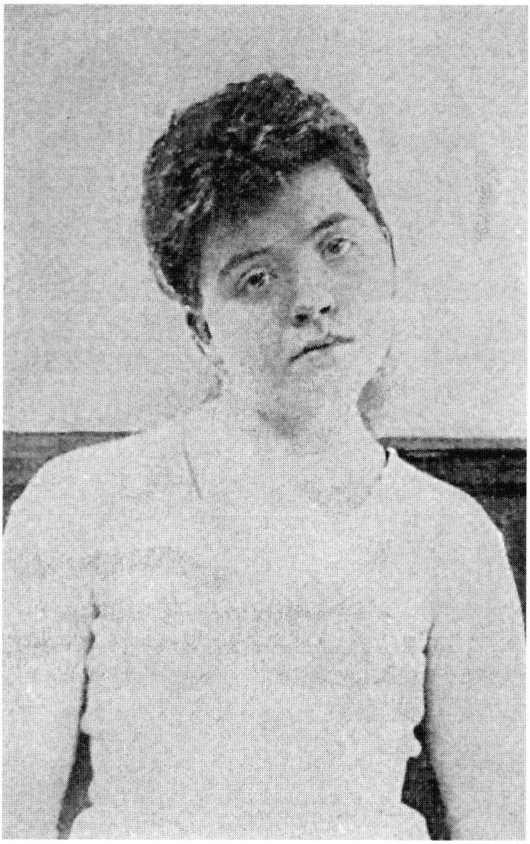

(Ill. I-3) Fig. 186.–Torticollis showing Facial Asymmetry.[9] See also *(Ill. I-4)* page 6.

"TREATMENT — (1) Medicinal, (2) mechanical, (3) operative, all of which is described in the chapter on Orthopaedics. Where it appears as an acute condition, rheumatic, or from some other infection, commonly described as a stiff neck, ***a forcible bending in the opposite direction, a painful procedure, will often give immediate and permanent relief.*** *When the underlying cause is unknown, we may begin treatment by giving first a laxative and subsequently quinine or salicylate of sodium, to be followed by manual or vibratory massage."*[9] (emphasis added)

Illustrations I-3 and I-4 are clear indications of the consequences that evolve from the uncorrected torticollis subluxation. The brutal treatment described in the last paragraph was most certainly a crude adjustment.

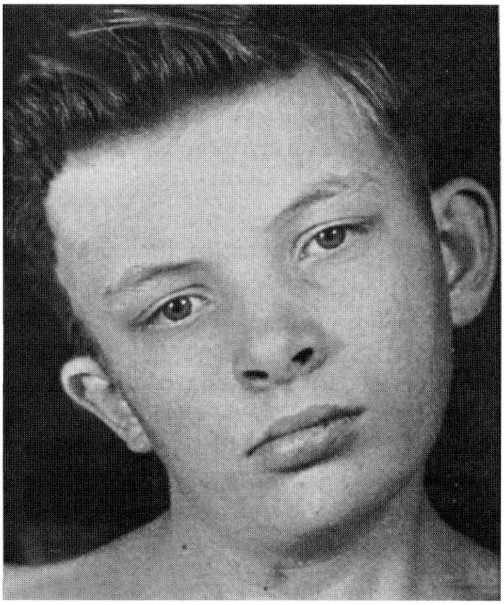

(Ill. I-4) Fig. 419 "TEXT BOOK OF PEDIATRICS",*[10] Nelson eighth edition, 1964, W.B. Saunders Company. "Congenital torticollis, untreated until age 12 years. Note wry neck and deformity of face." Facial asymmetry.

I could go on through the years in my collection of texts but from the foregoing, one can see that this malady was well recognized and treated in a variety of ineffective ways and the surgical procedures persist virtually the same today in medicine.

In his 1910 text D. D. quoted 20 medical authorities on

* I acknowledge the kind permission of the publisher to reproduce this illustration.

torticollis, seven of the 20 implicated birth injury. After summarizing their treatments he said:

"I have quoted twenty authors on wry-neck so that the reader may become acquainted with its symptoms and know the different opinions which various orthopedists and medical men entertain concerning its cause and the different methods of treatment they recommend. In summing up their different methods of treating wry-neck, I am led to say of them as did Moore of medicines: the very fact that so many methods of relief have been recommended, is evidence that they are all disappointing."[10]

He then went on to say;

"The pathological conditions existing in torticollis were, ofttimes, demonstrated by autopsy. The contracted muscles were examined macroscopically and microscopically, but the cause continued to be speculative and unknown. Even the discovery, made known by post mortem examinations, that cervical bones were distorted and dislocated, was of no value because it was not used. No one thought of replacing vertebrae or would have dared to try to replace them had the thought been conceived. Neither, previous to my discovery, had the idea that, by replacing them, they would grow back to their normal shape, ever entered the mind of man. Thousands of orthopedists, anatomists and pathologists were anxious to relieve these unfortunates, but their knowledge of anatomy and orthopedy did not enable them to do so."[1]

Before I close this chapter on historical observation, I feel compelled to quote again from D. D. Palmer's text page 187 as he quotes a most horrible form of cure of torticollis referred to as "The Hanging Cure."[1]

"Hanging from the neck by a rope has become a recognized form of treatment for certain nervous diseases at the National Hospital for the paralyzed and epileptic in Bloomsbury. In wry-neck in particular, this hanging is said to have given results, certain cases totally unrelieved by other more conservative methods of treatment responding well to this strenuous cure. The apparatus used consists of a metal tripod eight feet in height, with a pulley at the top. Over this pulley is passed a rope attached to two large metal stirrups, well padded with leather, one of which fits beneath the patient's chin and the other beneath the protruding part of the head. The principle of the treatment is that the weight of the patient's body is used to stretch the contracted neck and muscles, which cause the head to be held on one side.*

*See Author's Note next page.

"'We begin the treatment,' said one of the hospital staff in explaining it, 'by gently pulling the free end of the rope until the patient is raised up on his toes. After being kept in this position for a few seconds he is given a few moments rest. The second time he is raised a little higher, so that more strain falls on the neck's muscles. The process is continued every morning for a fortnight, the dose being gradually increased until toward the end of the treatment the patient can stand being suspended clear of the ground for twenty or thirty seconds.

"Immediately after each morning's treatment the patient is at once put back to bed, where he stays until the next morning's treatment. While this hanging cure has given good results in certain cases, it must not be understood that we treat all wry-necks in this way.'"

Then D. D. said;[1]

"Suspension by the neck is orthopedical. It has been practiced many years; it is given in orthopedic books. Thomas H. Story, D.C., of Los Angeles, CA, has been using that form of treatment for eight years.

As all the conditions of wry-neck are caused by a displaced cervical vertebra, why not adjust, replace it?" (emphasis added)

Thus I end this chapter on historical observations.

Author's Note

It is interesting to note that the "clinic" mentioned on page 7 was designated as a treatment center for the "epileptic." My very first patient was an epileptic boy who gained excellent results under chiropractic care. In my 43 years of practice I have cared for many cases of epilepsy with gratifying results. It will be proven someday that the upper cervical subluxation is a major cause of epilepsy.

It has been the author's contention, that swollen synovial membranes surrounding the odontoid process, press against the transverse ligament and the medulla oblongata causing epileptic seizures. The swelling is caused by the Atlanto/Axial subluxations articular disrelationship which causes stretch stress to the synovial membranes that surround the odontoid process.

CHAPTER II
MODERN MEDICAL HISTORY

Chiropractic history records the adjustic correction of this subluxation. Palmer, Firth, Forrestor the M.D., D.C. of National College, all early chiropractic authorities advised adjustment. All spoke to the subluxation and if they spoke of muscle spasm or contraction it was in relationship to the nerve irritation caused by the subluxation.

Dr. Forrestor of the National College of Chiropractic said this in his 1915 text, "PRINCIPLES AND PRACTICE OF SPINAL ADJUSTMENT"[11];

"Treatment — Adjust the cervical vertebrae. Massage and electricity are useful adjunct measures in these cases."

Yes, chiropractors in the liberal and conservative chiropractic schools and colleges agreed that subluxation was the cause and the correction was the adjustment.

But now let us take a leap in time to 1944 and the highly respected medical text entitled FUNDAMENTALS OF INTERNAL MEDICINE[12] by Wallace Mason Yater. Here we see that the author admits to the futility of medical therapeutical intervention.

"Torticollis, or cervical spasm, belongs in this group of dyskinesias. It consists of constant or transient spasms of the sternocleidomastoid muscle with rotation of the head to one side. In such cases the muscle on one side is often found to be considerably hypertrophied. Torticollis is sometimes seen in diseases of the vertebrae as in rheumatic myositis, but the etiology is usually obscure. It usually persists throughout a lifetime, often becoming more severe and spreading to other groups of cervical muscles. Practically no form of treatment is curative. Very often the spinal accessory nerve is cut with temporary relief, although with paralysis of the muscles affected. However, it has been noted that after a period of time the torticollis has spread to adjacent muscles of the neck. Orthopedic measures are equally ineffective."

And in respect to the muscular excession so commonly used medically since the turn of the century, Bernard S. Epstein, M.D. in his book, "THE SPINE A Radiological Text and Atlas"[13], 1962, states;

"Congenital Torticollis — This condition was recently studied

by Hulbert (1950), who reviewed 100 cases of torticollis and 117 cases of sternomastoid tumors. These were subdivided into postural and muscular groups. Congenital postural torticollis is present at birth and is not associated with sternomastoid tumor. The condition is transient and does not require operation for relief. Congenital muscular torticollis may be preceded by a sternomastoid tumor which is evident in about 20 percent of cases on physical examination. Most of these respond spontaneously and leave no deformity. Excision in childhood is ***inadvisable.*** *There are no definite associated skeletal changes in the cervical spine with either condition."* (emphases added)

With this last sentence you can see that they certainly missed the vertebral misalignment of the subluxation. But now, as we approach the turn of the century some medical texts are attributing torticollis to a subluxation. For instance, in "MUSCULOSKELETAL DISORDERS"[14] by Robert D. D'Ambrosia M.D. 1977, it illustrates on page 195 a picture of a seven-year-old child in the typical positioning of torticollis. With the kind permission of the publisher, I have reproduced the photo and the author's comments.

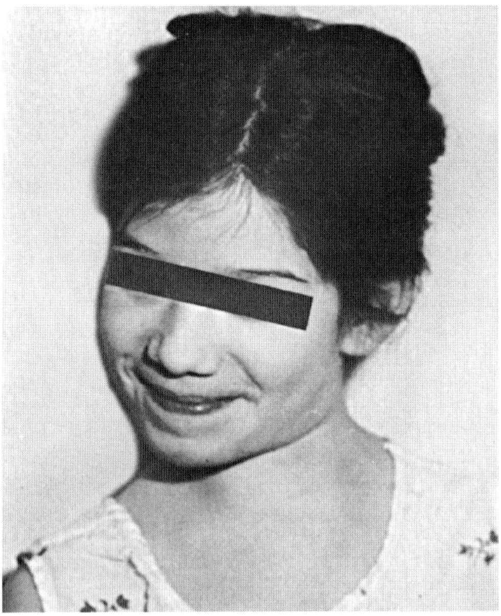

(Ill. II-1) "Seven-year-old child with torticollis for four months following a febrile illness of chicken pox. (A) The head is tilted to the left and the chin rotated to the right."*[14]

* Permission granted and credit to the J. B. Lippincott Company, Philadelphia, Pennsylvania.

And on page 201 the author relates to a subluxation;

"Acquired torticollis may occur in children as a result of mild trauma. The etiology is rotatory subluxation of the atlas on the axis, probably secondary to laxity of the capsular ligaments of those joints. The position of the head and neck is with the head tilted to the side of subluxation with the chin rotated in the opposite direction."[14]

Now we are starting to get somewhere in respect to medical understanding. They relate to a subluxation of Atlas on Axis. Their observation is correct in respect to the rotation of Atlas on Axis, but in my opinion, the subluxation is a **disc** lesion subluxation and there is no disc between C 1 and C 2. The subluxated vertebra is commonly the Axis. The Atlas rotation, the turning of the head away from the lateral bend, is an antalgic position in response to the painful articular strain caused by the open facet and articular lock of the Axis subluxation. I'll explain this later but allow me to go on with medical observations in respect to the subluxation cause of this malady.

In the first edition of "CLINICAL BIOMECHANICS OF THE SPINE,"[15] 1978, the authors make an observation similar to that of Yater. On page 206 authors White and Panjabi state;

"The right unilateral anterior rotary subluxation shown in Figure 5-17 would be expected to have a torticollis with the head "cocked like a robin, listening for a worm." There is lateral bending of the head and neck to the right and rotation of the head to the left. Rotating the head away from the direction that it faces, toward the subluxed side (in this case rotation of the head to the right), is difficult, if not impossible. However, rotating it further in the direction that it faces, to the left, is not particularly difficult. The head is tilted toward the side of the subluxation or dislocation and rotated away from it. The muscles may or may not be in spasm."

On page 207 of the aforementioned text, they show x-rays of the distortion and one can quite clearly see the rotation of the Axis spinous and even ascertain the disc wedge between Axis and C 3. The text goes into detail on traumatic subluxation of the Atlanto-Axial articulations and the drawings are beautifully done. I pass no judgements pro or con on their observation **except** that I contend the torticollis subluxation has a disc lesion origin and therefore is not an Atlas subluxation, it is most commonly found at Axis and third cervical and less commonly involves the lower cervical vertebra. It is encouraging however, to see medicine finally recognizing that subluxation does exist and to openly admit today that adjustic procedures do have merit. Of course, they use the term manipulative therapy, to essentially place such procedures under the auspices of common domain therapeutics. The adjustment is chiropractic's own terminology and is appropriately applied to a joint that is misaligned. You can manipulate any joint subluxated or not. **But**, you can only adjust something that is not in alignment, thus adjustment **is** the appropriate term when applied to the correction of a joint malposition. And as I have afore stated, torticollis **is** a subluxation.

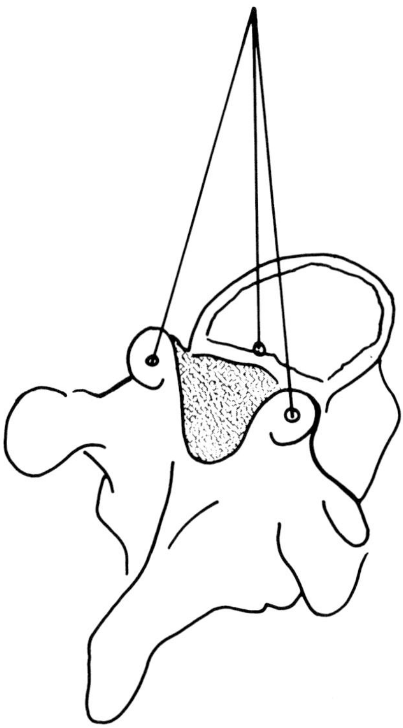

(Ill. III-1) The authors' "Tripod Theory" of weight bearing in the lordotic regions of the spine, places the weight bearing factor upon the facets and the posterior aspect of the vertebral bodies. The facets in the lumbar and cervical spine are meant to bear weight, they function in a closed state one to the other. In the final analysis, in the upright stance of the human body, the facet joints bear the shear force of the lordotic curves of the cervical and lumbar spine.

During periods of growth, weight borne to a greater degree on the posterior aspect of the vertebral bodies than on the anterior creates vertebral wedging. This results in vertebral body growth that produces the typical wedge shaped bodies of lumbar and cervical vertebrae, higher in dimension on the anterior than they are on the posterior. Hueter-Volkmann rule.

CHAPTER III
SPINAL ANTHROPOLOGY

Quoting from the first volume in my trilogy of technic texts, TORTIPELVIS VOL. I[16]: *"Anthropology, the science of the origin of, the development of man. Anthropoid, resembling man, the anthropoid apes are the tailless apes which include the chimpanzee, the gorilla, the gibbons, and the orangutan. Man believes that it is his mind that truly sets him apart from the other anthropoids. Certainly they have a physical make up very similar to ours; their arms, legs, shoulders and pelvic girdle, the opposing thumb, all make them able to function in a manlike way. Mentally, however, they cannot compete with man and thus they are placed in a lower evolutionary level in the order of life forms on this planet. Placed there, of course, by we who perceive ourselves as the ultimate of the creator's creations. But man's mind alone is not the only superiority that he has developed over the anthropoids. Man alone can walk in the full upright posture, man is truly biped."* (Ill. III-3 page 15)

Quoting from the excellent text 'BACKACHE ITS EVOLUTION AND CONSERVATIVE TREATMENT'[17], *"The spinal changes in modern man have allowed the centre of gravity of the trunk to be brought back to lie above the acetabulae. This has resulted in a lengthening of the lumbar spine and a lumbar lordosis which is peculiarly human and only associated with the final few degrees of uprightness of the trunk."*

Herein lies the key to the superiority of man's spinal development. Man alone has developed the secondary A to P curves of the human spine. (Ill. III-6 page 17)

The secondary curves of the human spine (the cervical and lumbar lordoses) remove the weight bearing burden from the vertebral bodies and discs in these regions. The weight bearing burden is then focused upon the facets and the posterior aspect of the vertebral bodies, see (Ill. III-1) on the opposite page. This weight bearing factor is responsible for the boney density of the cervical and lumbar facets (Wolf's Law) and the wedging of the vertebral bodies which are greater in height on the anterior and less high on the posterior (Hueter-Volkmann rule).

The discs in the lordotic regions of the spine are not meant to bear weight, they give shape and flexibility to these freely movable portions of the human spine. Only in the thoracic spine are the bodies of the vertebrae and the discs subjected to the weight bearing load. The thoracic spine has little movement in comparison to the cervical and lumbars and the discs in comparison are thin and appear rudimentary in development.

When normal lordotic curves exist in the cervical and lumbar regions little disc pathology occurs, even in later life. However, when kyphotic change occurs in these regions, disc pathology also becomes evident. Thus present concepts of the role of the intervertebral disc must change. I have written more comprehensively on this subject in TORTIPELVIS VOL. I[16], 4th edition, but for the sake of this text, that deals with the cervical spine, I will now refer you to (Ill. III-2) below.

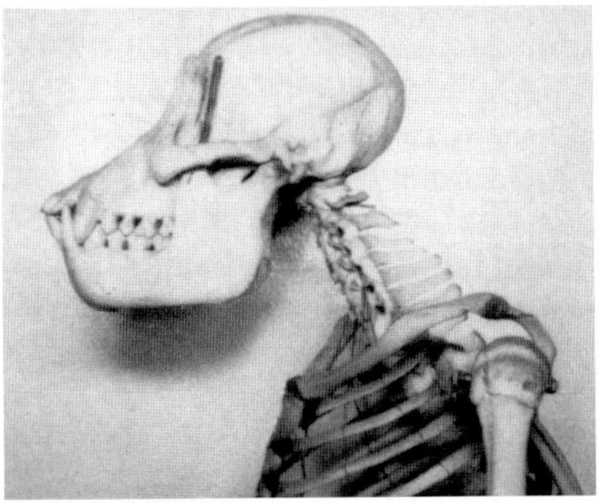

(Ill. III-2) The cervical spine of the orangutan.* Notice the long spinous process' for ligamentous and muscular attachment necessary to support the head in an erect position.

The foramin magnum is not centrally located in the skull and the massive jaw structure indicates the weight bearing factor is borne forward of the occipital condyles. The cervical spine is not lordotic, it retains the simple primary curve that is exhibited throughout the entire length of the spine. (Ill. III-5 page 16)

Only in man do we see a reorientation of the condyles and the enlargement of the occipital region of the skull. Man's head is poised, balanced so to speak, upon the leaf spring configuration of the human cervical spine. (Ill. III-4) The anterior curve of the cervical spine absorbs the shock of upright stance, it is the shock absorber not the discs. The secondary curves of the human spine must be developed and nurtured for man's spine to function properly as a biped. The reciprocal curves of cervical lordosis, thoracic kyphosis and lumbar lordosis are the true

*Courtesy of Palmer College of Chiropractic, osteological collection.

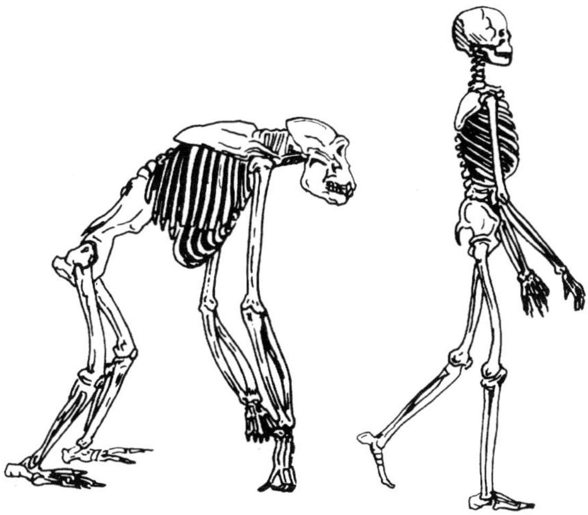

(Ill. III-3) The spine and posture of the gorilla as compared to man.

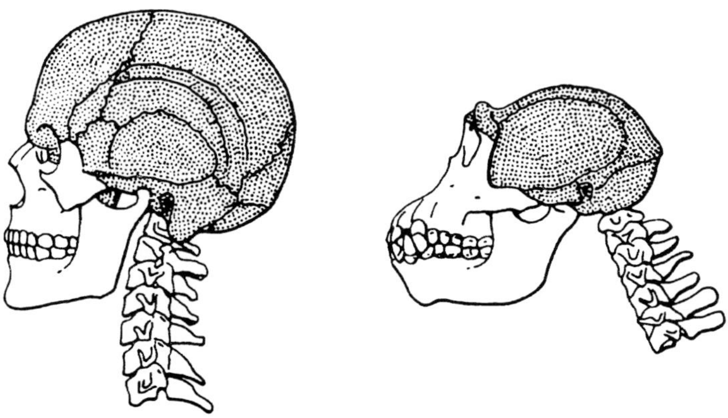

(Ill. III-4) Side view of the cervical spines of modern man and the chimpanzee. (After Boule)

shock absorbers of the erect human spine. I ask you to reflect upon the so-called Williams exercises used for so many years by the medical profession and some chiropractors. It is this author's contention that such flexion exercises should be eliminated from the normal regime of physical education. They are contra-indicated in most spinal conditions, being destructive to the secondary curves and abusive to the intervertebral discs. With this final comment I will return to the intended purpose of this text, a definitive study on the subluxation of torticollis.

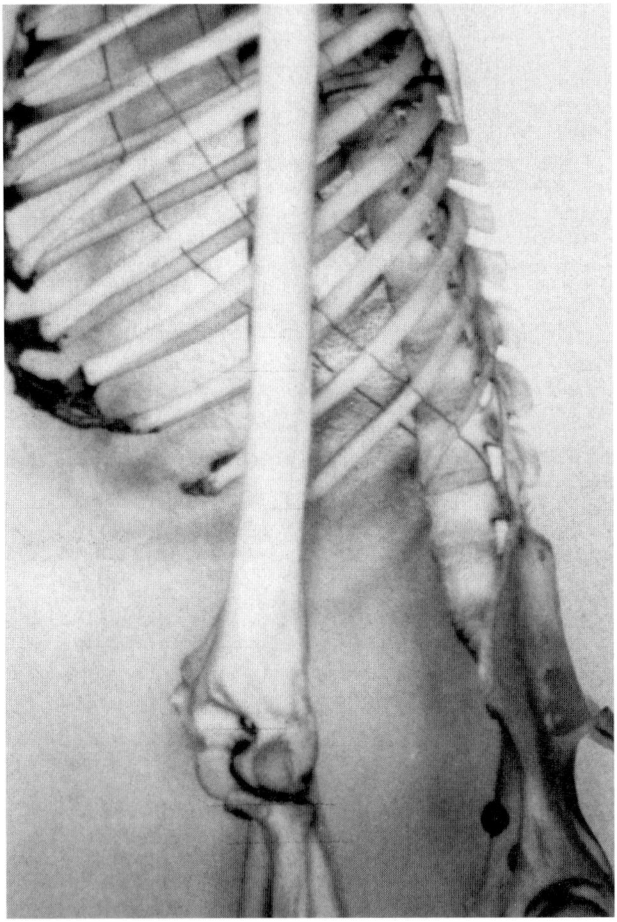

(Ill. III-5) The lumbar and thoracic spine of the orangutan*. The entire spine of this anthropoid ape (as is true of all anthropoidea other than man) is a simple C shaped uniform curve. Only man has developed the secondary cervical and lumbar lordotic curves.

*Courtesy of Palmer College of Chiropractic, osteological collection.

NORMAL SPINAL CONTOURS

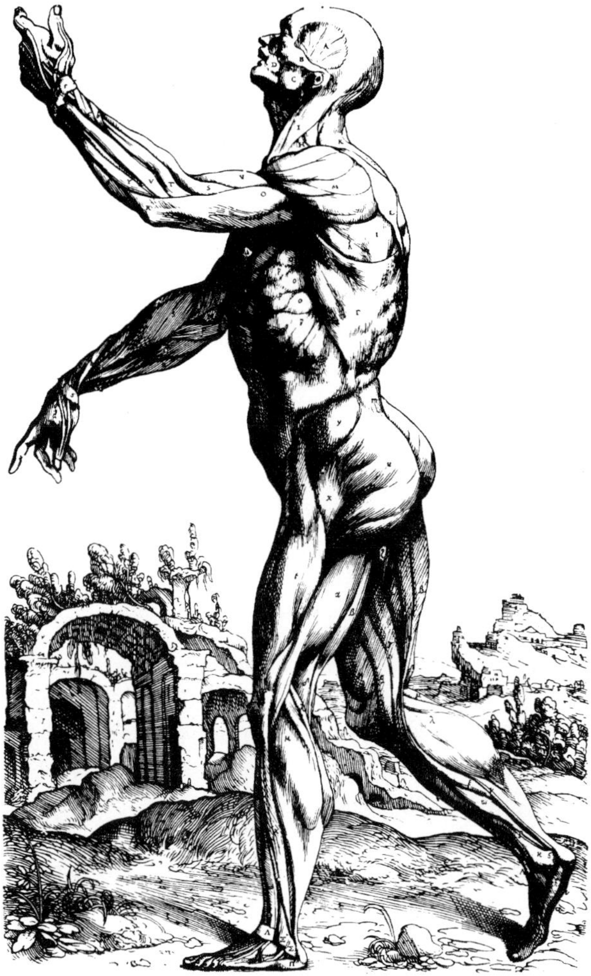

(Ill. III-6) From the anatomical drawings of the famed sixteenth-century physician Andreas Vesalius*. Notice the pronounced curves of the entire spine of this illustration; prounced in comparison to drawings seen today. Could it be that man through the ages has reduced these normal contours through sedentary occupations and improper exercises? I believe this is to be true. In the third text of this chiropractic technic trilogy, SCOLIOSIS VOL. III, I discuss the relationship of the normal lateral contours of the human spine (sigmoid curve) and the so-called "idiopathic" scoliosis.

*The Anatomical Drawings of Andreas Vesalius, Bonanza Books, New York.

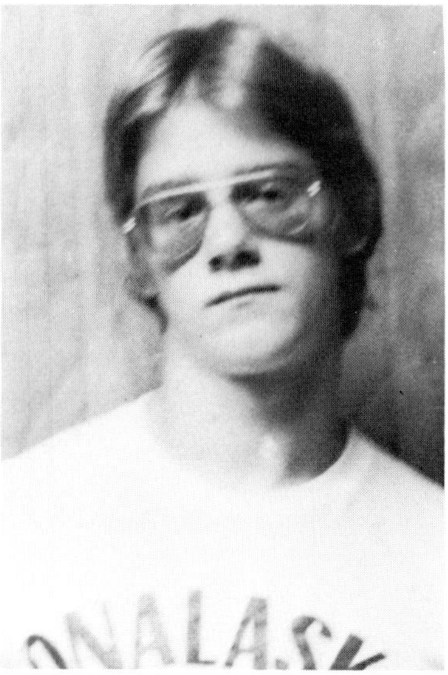

(Ill. IV-1) Lateral Torticollis*

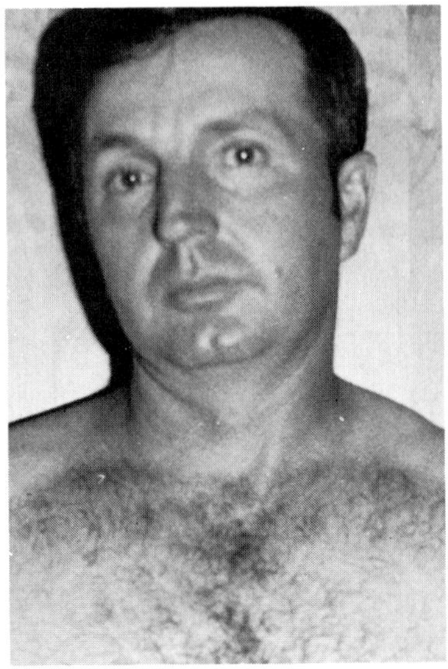

(Ill. IV-2) Lateral Torticollis*

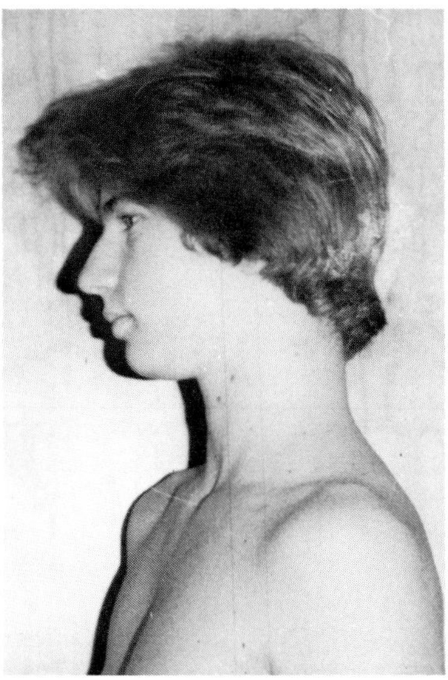

(Ill. IV-3) Anterior Torticollis*

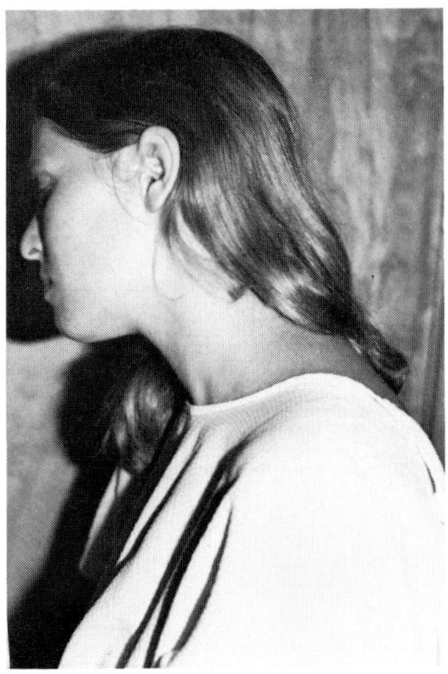

(Ill. IV-4) Anterior Lateral Torticollis*

* All photos printed with the permission of the patients.

CHAPTER IV
CAUSATION

TYPES OF TORTICOLLIS

On the opposite page are pictures of actual cases of torticollis[18], the description follows below:

I Lateral Torticollis *(Ill. IV-1, and IV-2)*

Objectively this condition is difficult to mistake. The cervical spine is bent tortuously to one side with the face commonly turned away from the lateral bend. Children often endeavor to support their head by raising the shoulder on the same side. In all cases the patient is unable to move his/her head and neck out of its peculiar position. The rotation and disc wedge mechanics of the subluxation are explained in Chapter V.

II Anterior Torticollis *(Ill. IV-3)*

Anterior torticollis can be very severe, the head and neck will be bent anteriorly, in flexion; extension of the neck will be greatly restricted if not impossible. There is also some restriction to rotation and lateral bending of the cervical spine. In mild cases anterior torticollis can be termed the 'occult' or hidden torticollis, the patient only complains of minor discomfort and simply relates to having a "stiff neck." Such is the case on this illustration, the patient's cervical spine is only slightly bent forward.

III Anterior Lateral Torticollis *(Ill. IV-4)*

In this condition the patient's neck is held in flexion and bent to one side. It is simply a combination of anterior and lateral torticollis and there can be more than one vertebral subluxation involved in this condition. Anterior lateral torticollis is, at times, slower to respond to chiropractic adjustment.

IV Spasmodic Torticollis

"Colonic Torticollis," was the name first placed upon this nasty persistent muscle spasm of the cervical spine. The unfortunate victims of this mysterious malady suffer from muscle spasms that twist the neck into torticollis-like positions. I personally have seen cases wherein the cervical spines spastic contractions pull the neck backwards into full extension. The contractions, however, are spasmodic and the position is not that of the articular lock subluxation of true torticollis, the subject of this book. It is possible that this condition is the result of an unresolved torticollis subluxation and the author has seen some indication that this may well be true. I have personally had a number of cases of suspicious neck "tics" that have resolved completely upon vertebral adjustment. However, in the full blown case of spasmodic torticollis, I have seen no clear cut evidence of chiropractic correction. Surgical intervention is fruitless, recent experimental injections of botulism toxins have shown some results but the true causative factors remain unknown at this writing. It is my opinion that this problem is either the result of a chronic subluxation or an unknown intercranial lesion.

Author's Note
This text is not intended to discuss "Spasmodic Torticollis." This subject may be addressed chiropractically as research advances in the care of the unfortunate victims afflicted with this unusual malady.

Etiology

Definition: - the study or theory of the origin of any disease; the knowledge of origins.

In my text VOL. I, TORTIPELVIS[16], I went to great lengths to prove that the kyphosis lays the ground work for the disc lesion subluxation. In this way tortipelvis and torticollis are one and the same. They are disc lesion subluxations made eminently more probable by a lack of a normal anterior curve in the cervical and lumbar spines. According to the A.C.A.'s "Council on Chiropractic Orthopedics," *"A vertical line drawn from the apex of the Odontoid process should cross the anterior corner of C7."* Dropping a plumb line down through a normal cervical lordotic curve the axial line of weight bearing does not fall upon the discs. (Ill. IV-5) Look at line (A), this is the plane line of the facet. This plane line indicates the role that it plays in cervical support. The plane of the facets prevent anterior displacement of the vertebra. As you look at the curve of the cervical spine and the weight carried forward upon it, it becomes apparent that the facets *are* the really important weight bearing structures of the cervical spine.

The body plane line (B). It is actually slanted downward, it is not at a plane intended to bear the weight of the head - the discs are not intended to be weight bearing structures in the lordotic curves of the normal spine nor do they act like shock absorbers as was previously assumed. The shock absorber of the cervical spine is the **leaf spring** configuration of its lordotic curve. Only when flattening of the normal anterior curve exists do the discs bear the weight of the head.

Note also that the size of the facet mass (C), compared to the body of the vertebra. Upon examination the combined size of the two sets of facets, equals the size of the vertebral body itself. The point I am trying to make is that they have reorientated themselves in man to bear the shear force of upright posture in the lordotic regions of the spine.

THE NORMAL CERVICAL LORDOTIC CURVE

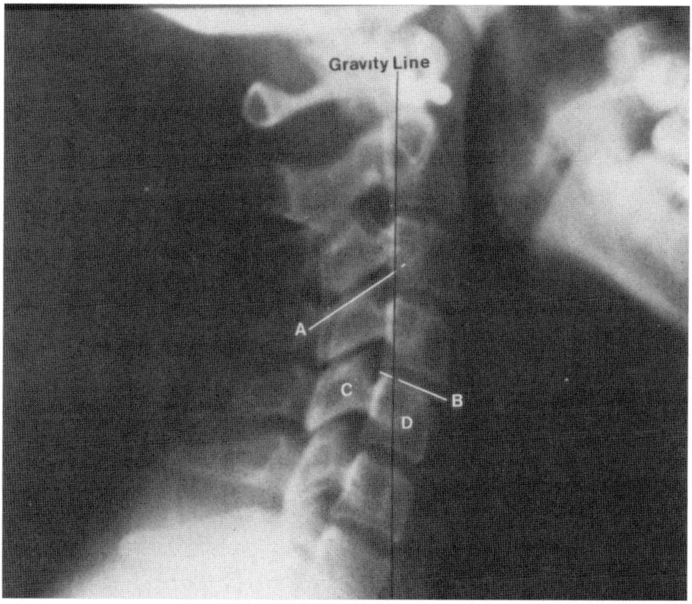

(Ill. IV-5) In the normal cervical lordotic curve, notice how the weight of the head is borne by the cervical spine.

In the excellent text CLINICAL BIOMECHANICS[19], Chapter 7, pages 320, 321, The Cervical Region; author R. C. Schafer D.C. explains the weight bearing factors of the cervical spine this way.

"APPLIED ANATOMY"[19]

"In the healthy cervical (or lumbar) spine that presents a moderate degree of lordosis, a good share of weight bearing is upon the zygapophyses because the line of cumulative loading of compressive forces is quite posterior to the center of the vertebral bodies. This produces a considerable degree of normal articular jamming as the result of loading that tends to restrict excessive rotation. That is, the rotary motion that occurs at the zygapophyses does so upon relatively compressed facets.

There is structural adaptation for this. For the normal adult spine, the cervical discs average 3 mm in thickness, there is a 2:5 disc / body ratio, a 4:7 nucleus / anulus ratio, and the nucleus sits in a position that is slightly posterior to the center of the disc. ***In addition, the surface area of the cervical facets is larger in proportion to the surface area of the vertebral body than at any other region of the spine.*** *This contributes greatly to the overall segmental base of support in the neck. In fact, the weight-bearing surfaces of the two facets equal more than half (67%) that of the centrum.* ***In addition, the superior facets below the axis face posterosuperior and medial to compensate for the normal anteroinferior tilt of the vertebral bodies.***

The more the cervical curve becomes flattened, the more superimposed weight is shifted to the discs. With the shifting of the normal compressive forces at the posterior toward the anterior of the motion unit, the discs are forced to carry more weight and a greater responsibility in cervical stability. In time, this unusual compressive force on the nucleus can produce degenerative anular thinning, spurs, ebernation, and Schmorl's nodes. The posterior joints become relatively lax and predispose retropositioning and posterior subluxations." (emphasis added)

Author Schafer's observations concur with mine. My first edition to torticollis was published in 1977, Dr. Schafer's book was published in 1983. For further information and corroboration of the viewpoints I have brought forth on this subject I would heartily recommend that the reader pursue reading his text. It is more complete and comprehensive in its biomechanical explanations of cervical movement that go beyond the purposes of this text.

In the kyphotic cervical spine, the plumb line falls upon the discs. The kyphosis necessitates that the discs too become weight bearing structures, a burden they were not intended to bear. We contend that the cervical zygapophyseal articulations (facets) are meant to function in a closed state one to the other. The shear force they bear make them the actual weight bearing articulations of the cervical spine. This produces a high inter-facet force that prevents retrolisthesis and undue rotation of the individual vertebral segments.

When the normal anterior (lordotic) curve of the cervical spine flattens it creates the following:

1. The weight of the head is borne directly by the discs.
2. Without the anterior curve, shear force against the facet joints is reduced producing articular laxity. This laxity creates a tendency for rotational subluxations, posterior subluxations, posterior/lateral disc wedging, and torticollis.

THE KYPHOTIC CERVICAL CURVE

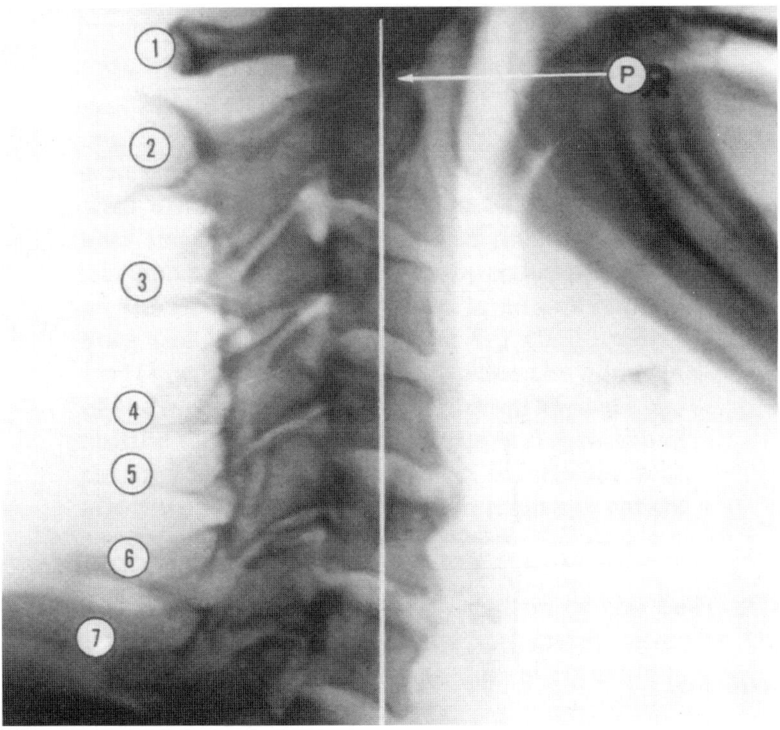

(Ill. IV-6) Above the 6th cervical vertebra we have a complete flattening of the normal anterior curve. In the kyphosis, the discs bear the weight of the skull, the facets become articularily loose the nucleus of the disc becomes the fulcrum of support to the vertebra above.

THE DISC BLOCK SUBLUXATION

A.P. VIEW

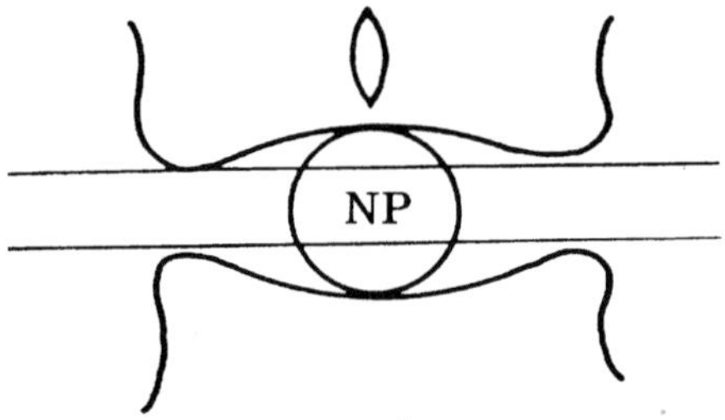

A
NORMAL DISC

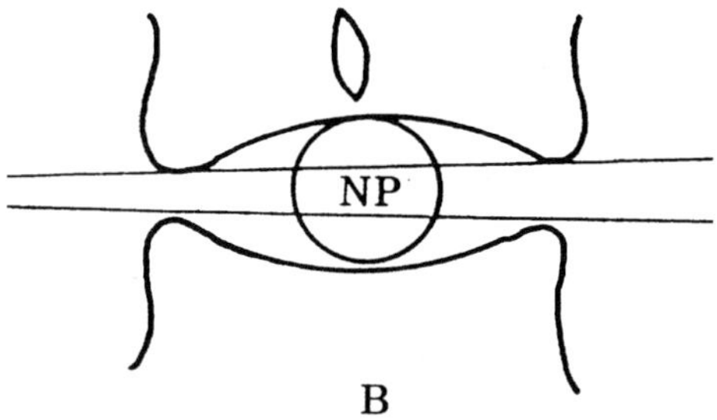

B
LATERAL TIPPING
(disc wedge)

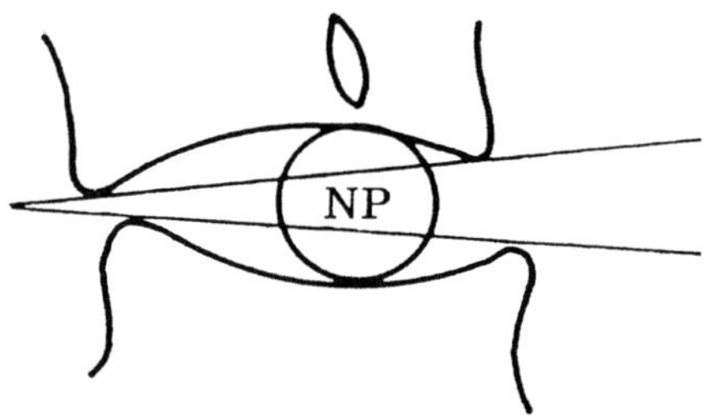

C
NUCLEAR SHIFT
(increased disc wedge and rotation)

(Ill. IV-7) The weight upon the discs allows the nucleus to act as the fulcrum of support to the vertebra immediately above. The nucleus, in its central position in the disc substance, bears weight like the fulcrum of a teeter-totter, and it is subject to lateral and posterior shifting.

Rotation and Disc Involvement on the A.P. X-ray

Allow me to again illustrate and quote from my first text VOL. I, TORTIPELVIS:[16]

"Normally, the anterior to posterior view of the disc space would give a picture similar to two concave plates with concavities opposing each other, (Ill. IV-7A); with a lateral tipping (Ill. IV-7B); with a disc block subluxation (Ill. IV-7C). Notice the disc compression and shifting of the nucleus pulposus toward its open border. As the nucleus pulposus shifts to one side so does the fulcrum of support for the superior vertebra. Look again at (Ill.IV-7C). Notice the position of the nucleus. See how the fulcrum of support has shifted to the right allowing the vertebra above to tip to the left creating an inferiority and allowing for the body of this vertebra to rotate towards its inferior border."

The last sentence relates to the gravational rotation of the body of a vertebra to its inferior border. This statement refers to Dr. Hugh B. Logan's rule of lumbar vertebral rotation.[20]

"The body of the lowest freely movable vertebra always rotates toward the low side of the sacrum or the foundation upon which it rests."

In other words the vertebra rotates towards its low side, the narrow side of the disc wedge.

I contend Dr. Logan's rotational rule also holds true in the cervical spine. The cervical and lumbar curves of the human spine have a great deal in common but this book is not meant to belabor detail and we will assume that the reader's knowledge is complete along these lines. Following Logan's rule, let's look at some x-rays of the normal rotatory scoliosis in the cervical spine to show you how the rule applies to the cervicals (Ill. IV-8 and IV-9).

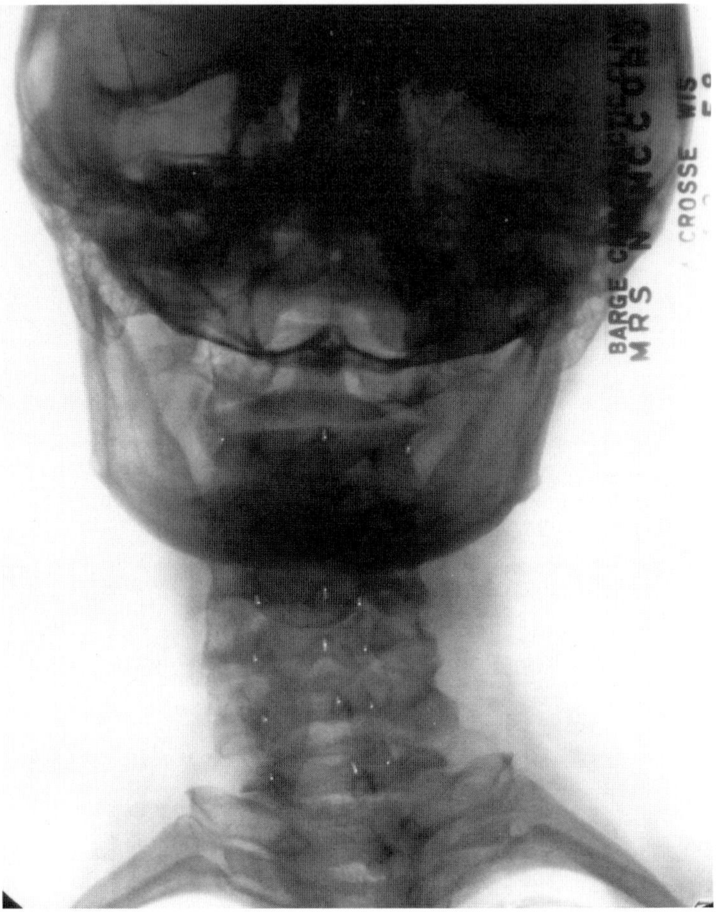

(Ill. IV-8) Measuring from the junction of lamina to like points on the lateral borders of the vertebral bodies dimensional measurements are ascertained. The wide side of the vertebral body is the side of vertebral body rotation. Disc wedges are also drawn with the use of a ruler or gliding parallel ruler. *(See Chapter VII, X-ray Analysis.)* In the common rotatory scoliosis all vertebral bodies are rotated to the convex side of the lateral curve and all disc wedges are open to this side. On the x-ray above, it is easily seen that the vertebral bodies are wider on the left than the right. Millimeter measurement will ascertain the degree of the rotations and also point out significant rotational disrelationships and contrarotations.

COMMON ROTATORY SCOLIOSIS

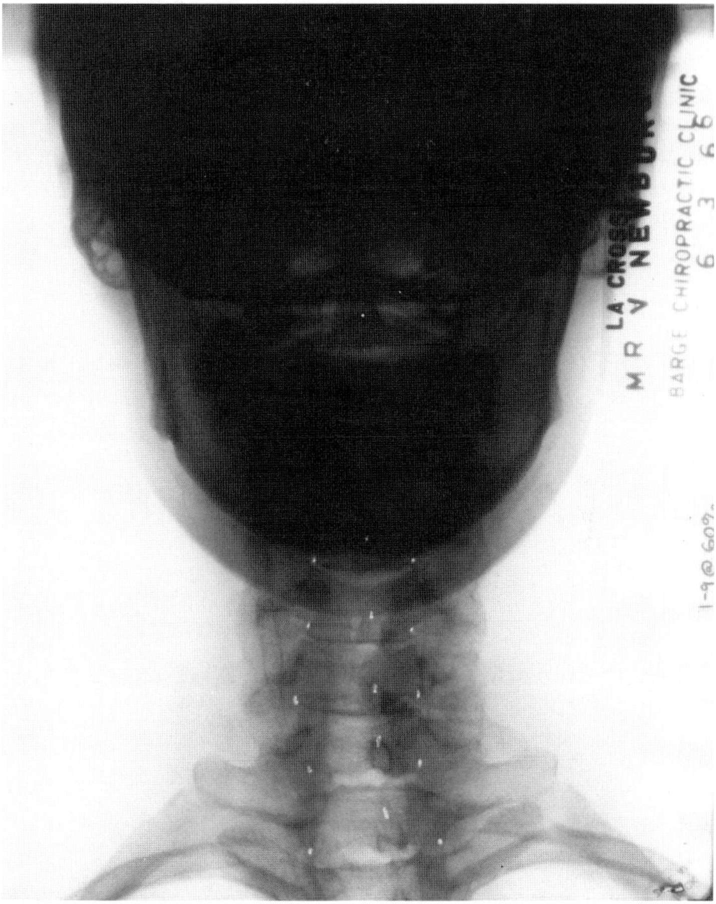

(Ill. IV-9) Rotatory scolioses as pictured on these two facing pages are usually adaptations to lower vertebral rotational distortions. A full spine x-ray study is often necessary to determine the underlying cause of the rotatory scoliosis. The complete study of this condition is found in my third text, SCOLIOSIS VOL. III. Because of vertebral rotations and disc wedges, cervical rotatory scoliosis (especially combined with a degree of kyphosis) is very prone to attacks of torticollis; in children, torticollis is commonly an early sign of curvature.

On the x-ray above, it is easy to see that the body dimensions are wider on the left. The beginning of a thoracic curvature is also evident.

It should be apparent to the reader that the author holds that the kyphotic change in the cervical spine sets the stage for the torticollis subluxation. This then posses the question, WHY the kyphosis? There are two major factors in the lack of the development of the normal sigmoid curve in the human spine. One is the way we handle our children as babies and in youth. The other factor is faulty behavior of the young childs balance mechanisms. In the next chapter we discuss the development of the normal sigmoid curve from infant to adult. Chapter XI discusses spinal balance and the "Righting Reflex."

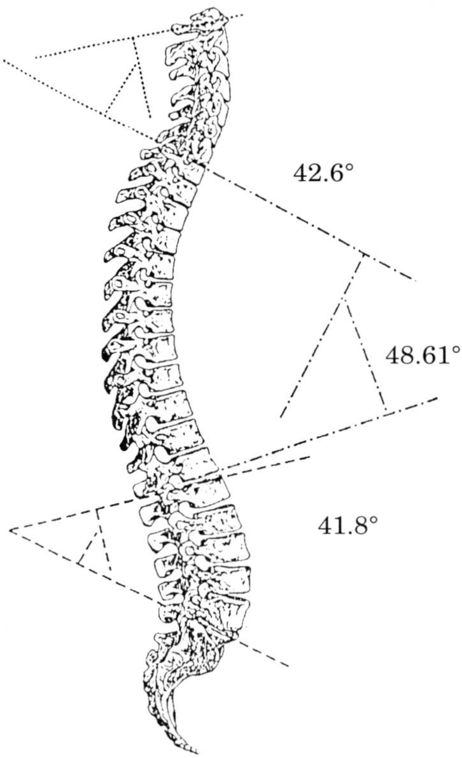

(Ill. IV-10) In 1983 the research completed by the author, and staff members of The Barge Chiropractic Clinic, was delivered in a paper at the "Biomechanical Conference on The Spine" in Boulder, Colorado. The methods and results of this study are written in the author's VOL. III SCOLIOSIS[21], 2nd Edition 1986 and 2nd Expanded Edition 1996; see also page 47 of this text.

CHAPTER V
THE DEVELOPMENT OF THE SIGMOID CURVE

Kyphosis in the Lumbar and Cervical Spines

Why is the population of this country so prone to kyphosis? To answer this question, I quote from my first text, "The Development of the Kyphosis", VOL. I, TORTIPELVIS.[16] "*When a child is in the womb and when first born, its spine configuration is that of a figure C (Ill.V-1). The secondary curves of the spine have not yet been formed. The early days and months of a child's life are of utmost importance in the development of the sigmoid curve of the human spine. Most mothers realize a new born baby cannot support the weight of its own head. Its little neck wobbles and strains to hold its head upright. These motions and exercises by the baby develop the muscles of the cervical region and begin promoting the development of the first secondary curve of the spine, the cervical lordotic curve.*

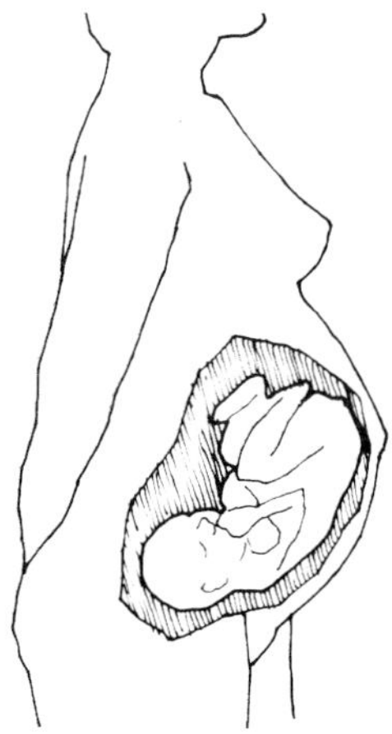

(Ill. V-1) In utero the spine held in its primary curve.

"One of the best possible positions for a baby when it's awake and amusing itself is on its stomach. This position allows complete freedom for the baby to lift its head and develop the arch in its neck, (Ill. V-2). It also lays ground for the second secondary curve, the anterior lordotic curve of the lumbar spine, (Ill. V-3). Just watch an infant lying on its tummy, hands in the air, feet in the air, head up, smiling, wiggling, kicking, and chortling as it

exercises its little body. It is developing the spinal muscles and contours in preparation for the upright posture of man. The next movement to develop the lumbar arch is ***creeping and babies today simply are not allowed to creep enough.*** *(Ill. V-4)*

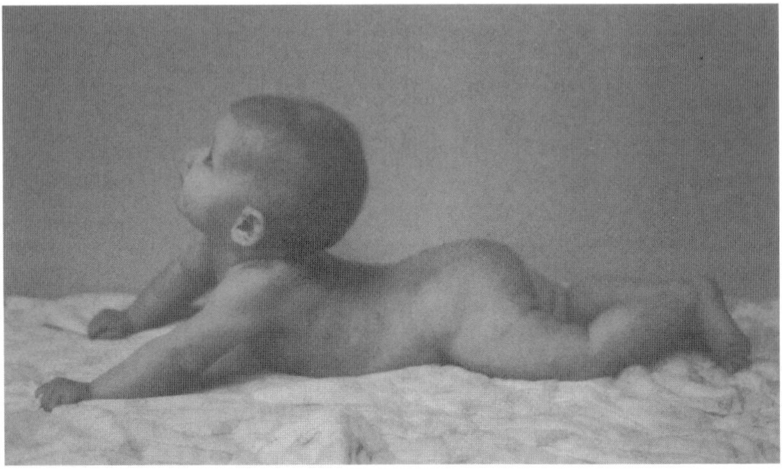

(Ill. V-2) Baby* lying on floor exercising and creating the cervical lordotic curve.

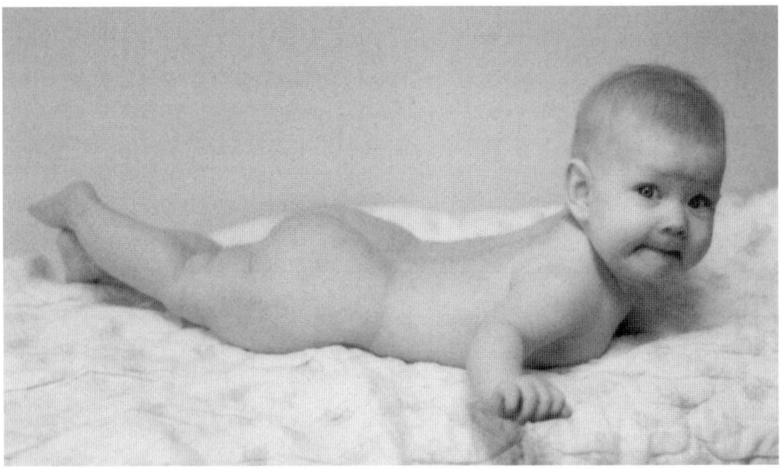

(Ill. V-3) When the baby* raises its legs it encourages the development of the lumbar lordosis.

*Baby Amanda, daughter of Drs. Patricia and Michael Berkley, the author's granddaughter.

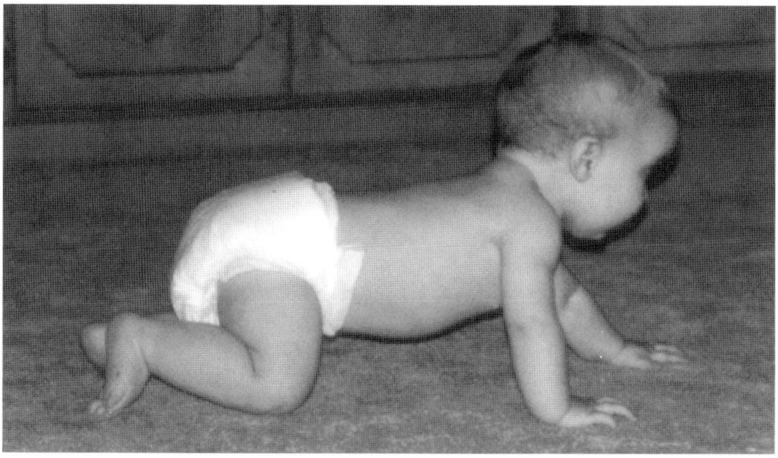

(Ill. V-4) As the baby* creeps, the sacrum tips to the posterior at its apex. The spine **hangs** between its support at the acetabulum and the shoulder girdle. The weight of the abdomen pulls the lumbar spine down and nurtures the development of the lumbar lordotic curve.

The Swingy Swings and Other Contraptions

"For the convenience of the busy mother many contraptions are made to pacify and occupy the baby. None is more dangerous for the baby's spine than the SWINGY SWING or the spider-legged walker (sometimes with wheels). The swing contraption lulls the child into oblivion and holds the spine in the old figure C posture. It hinders the development of the secondary curve of the lumbar spine. The walker introduces them to propelling themselves with their feet and to erect posture before their spine and pelvis are developed properly for the upright posture. Both train the baby's balancing mechanism (the labyrinth of the inner ear) to accept upright posture. This leads to early walking by the baby. Urge is created for the infant to be upright and standing erect. The crib and playpen too, are prone to force a baby to attempt standing up. As soon as the baby is able to grasp the bars of its confinement, the only way to go is up! Again the upright posture is assumed before the lumbar spine has begun to form its normal anterior curve. All this leads to a flat lower back which is called kyphosis.

"Combine this poor start for the infant's spine with the enforced sitting activities of youth; the ride to school in the

* Brittani, the daughter of Dr. and Mrs. David Ragland.

bus; the classroom sitting; studies at night; sit-ups and bending over to touch the floor in physical education class; then on to college and more sitting; riding in low cars which do nothing to encourage the lumbar arch, and for many, sitting jobs at work. All are adequate reasons for the development of the chronic kyphosis in today's adult population."[16]

Now, I have written here of the lumbar kyphosis. Just how does this relate to the cervical kyphosis? Although, the cervical lordotic curve is the first secondary curve to be developed in the spine, maintenance of this normal lordotic curve requires the proper development of the lumbar curve. In other words, without the proper development of the lumbar curve, the cervical lordotic curve often does not maintain itself. With a lumbar kyphosis the spine endeavoring to achieve erect posture flattens all normal curves and the ramrod spine is developed. (Ill. V-5)

The reciprocal curves of the human spine, cervical lordosis, thoracic kyphosis and lumbar lordosis are nature's bastion of defense against lateral deviation of the spine and vertebral subluxations. These curves should be nurtured in youth and not destroyed by improper exercises. The development of a normal lumbar lordosis maintains the thoracic and cervical sagittal curves. On the next two pages I have illustrated two x-rays of spines with diminished sagittal contours.

If one finds a true kyphosis in the cervicals in an otherwise normal spine, it is most likely due to vertebral subluxation, a whiplash injury, a congenital anomaly, occupational adaption, a fetal delivery trauma or an uncorrected anterior torticollis subluxation. We should be careful to avoid the development of the cervical, and especially the lumbar, kyphosis in children as it is the beginning of the most serious spinal problems … torticollis, tortipelvis, scoliosis, vertebral and disc degeneration.

LATERAL VIEW
OF THE SPINE

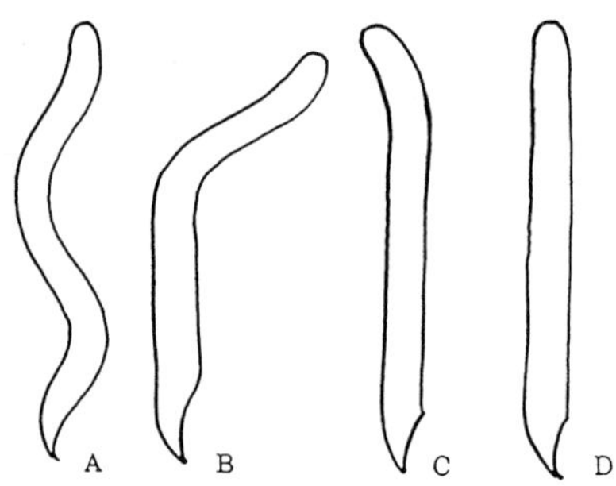

(Ill. V-5)

KYPHOTIC CHANGE Lumbar-Cervical

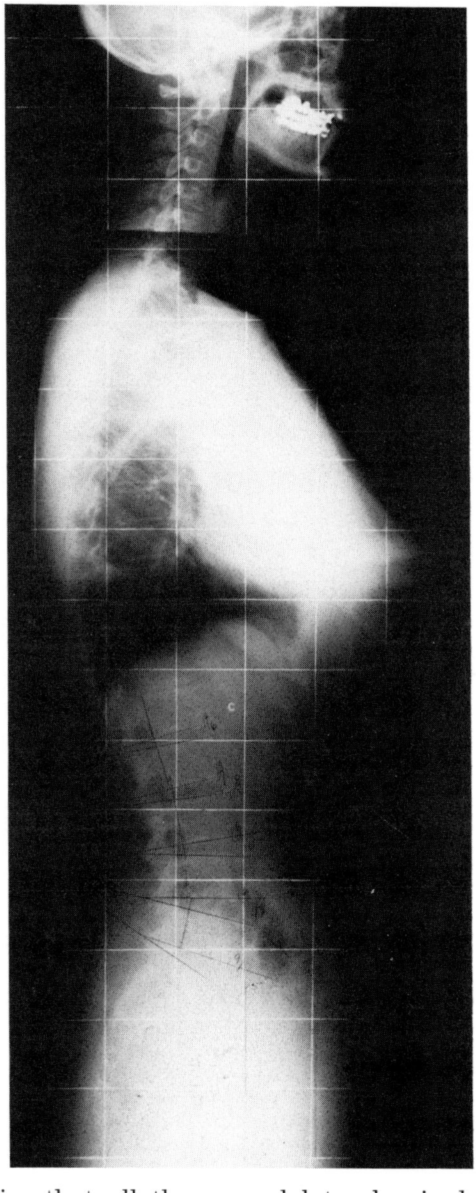

(Ill. V-6) Notice that all the normal lateral spinal curves are diminished. This is a typical example of the ramrod type lateral full spine x-ray found in spines associated with the disc block subluxations and curvature; the so-called military spine.

KYPHOTIC CHANGE Lumbar-Cervical

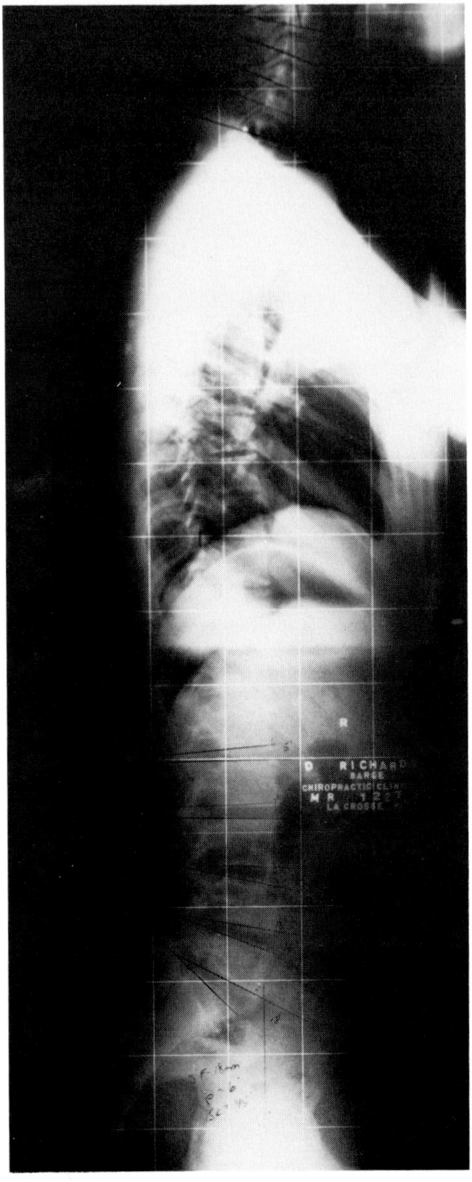

(Ill. V-7) There is some attempt on the part of this spine to maintain a semblance of the normal cervical curve. This case exhibits a double major rotatory scoliosis on the A.P. view. These lateral x-rays show some double imaging in the mid-film area as they are taken in two exposures.

CONCLUSION
Chapters I – V

To this point we have endeavored to establish and explain the predisposition for torticollis, the flattening of the normal cervical lordotic curve. The lack of the normal anterior curve places the weight-bearing burden of the head inordinately upon the discs. The inter-facet shear force is reduced and the vertebrae are then more easily involved in rotatory and retropositioning subluxations. Also, when the weight is borne by the discs the nucleus of the disc assumes a function much like the fulcrum of a teeter-totter. It, in effect becomes the fulcrum of support for the vertebra immediately superior to it. The kyphotic cervical spine is thus an articularly loose and poorly supported group of articulations. The disc bears weight in a way not intended by nature and thus the cervical spine is prone to the peculiar disc lesion subluxations of torticollis. Initially the chiropractor must recognize the subluxation, correct it, and eliminate the immediate problem. Secondly he/she should endeavor to improve normal spinal contours and thus reduce the distortion that allowed the acute subluxation to manifest itself. The past two pages illustrate x-rays showing kyphotic flattening of the normal lordotic curves of the human spine. In such cases the thoracic spine is actually hypo-kyphotic, and a thoracic hypo-kyphosis necessitates the development of a cervical kyphosis. (Ill. V-5 page 32)

I contend that drastic changes must be made in today's exercise programs taught to our youth in schools and colleges, and in the handling of our infants we must allow adequate time for natural development of the secondary curves of the spine. Encouraging a child to walk too soon can be ruinous to proper spinal development. It can produce a lack of normal lordotic spinal curves and lead to a lifetime of spinal problems.

It bears repeating that it is my opinion that the practitioner should consider juvenile torticollis to be a symptom and a sign of curvature and/or scoliosis.

LATERAL TORTICOLLIS*

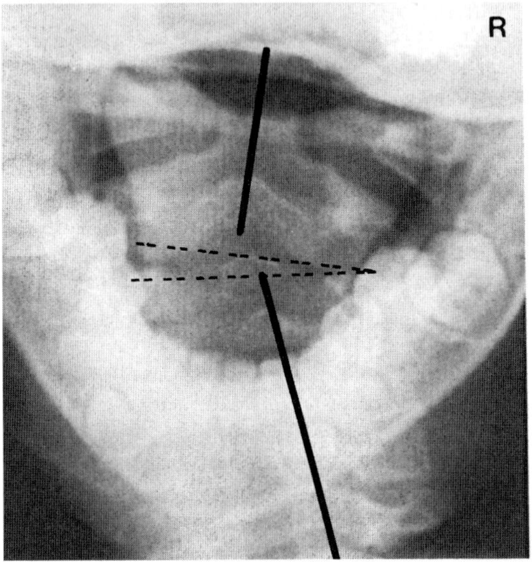

(Ill. VI-1) This A.P. x-ray[22], viewed from the posterior, (the usual chiropractic manner) exhibits a right lateral torticollis. Note the disc wedge between Axis and C 3. The body of the Axis is rotated away from the open side of the disc wedge in relation to C 3. The classic disk block subluxation of torticollis. The spinous of Axis moves towards the convexity of the curve in relation to its articular mate below. The Gonstead listing would be Axis P.L.S., this is the teeter-totter principle explained on the next few pages.

* X-ray courtesy, Journal of Clinical Chiropractic Pediatrics, Vol. 2 No. 2, Oct. 1997; International Chiropractors Assoc.

CHAPTER VI
THE MECHANICS OF TORTICOLLIS

As described on page 19 I have categorized torticollis thusly.

I Lateral Torticollis
II Anterior Torticollis
III Anterior Lateral Torticollis

In this chapter we will discuss the mechanics of each type separately starting with number I.

I Lateral Torticollis

Lateral torticollis follows the same nuclear-shift rule as in lateral tortipelvis of the lumbar spine. The nucleus pulposus shifts to one side, the vertebra tips to the other. The tipping of the vertebra superior to the disc wedge, creates an inferiority and the body of the vertebra rotates towards its low side. (Ill. V-1), the classic disc block subluxation.

The "Teeter-Totter Principle"

Let me expand on the nuclear shift principle and look at it in the light of the mechanical principle of the fulcrum. In the normal lordotic curve the nucleus of the disc has limited function in vertebral body balance, but in the kyphosis the weight bearing factor has shifted to the anterior, directly on the nucleus (Ill. IV-6 page 23) and the balance of the vertebra above is dependent upon the central position of the nucleus.

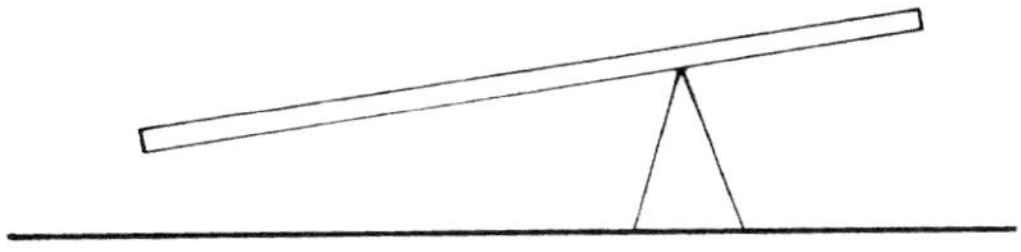

(Ill. VI-2)

Shift the fulcrum on a teeter-totter and the board drops to one side, so too in the spine, when the nucleus shifts from its central position the vertebra above tips to one side. The nucleus becomes the fulcrum of support for the vertebra immediately above. The articular laxity due to the kyphosis and the gravitational pull, causes the vertebral body to rotate towards its low side. Try to visualize this subluxation like the teeter-totter, toss in the "Logan"* principle of vertebral body rotation, and you

* The body of a freely moveable vertebra will rotate towards its low side, H. B. Logan[20]

will have the lateral torticollis subluxation clear in your mind.

The Nuclear Shift Rotational Principle

Referring to Dr. C. S. Gonstead's system of spinal analysis, the wedging of inter-vertebral discs is easily analysed. How then is one to ascertain evidence of nuclear shift other than the obvious wedging and/or narrowing of discs commonly seen on x-rays?

A great deal of interest in the disc lesion subluxation by the author led to a diligent study on our part to research thoroughly this type of vertebral subluxation. In a chronic rotatory scoliosis a peculiar disc wedge was often noted with the open side of the wedge on the concavity of the scoliotic bend. This was not typical, in that normally the open side of the disc wedges are on the convexity of a scoliosis and their apexes on the concavity of the curve. A contrarotation was also noted between the two vertebrae involved in this peculiar disc wedge subluxation. Other chiropractors active in research at this same time also noted this peculiar subluxation. Dr. Roy Hildebrandt and Dr. Otto Reinert were two with whom this author spoke.

Dr. Reinert made the following statement:[23]

"Any increase in the size of an inter-vertebral space on one side as compared with the other denotes a displacement of the nucleus pulposus to that side, provided there is also a relative rotation of the body of the superior vertebra to the side opposite increased intervertebral space."

In other words, if the vertebral BODY immediately above a disc wedge is rotated away from the open side of the disc wedge in relation to the vertebra immediately below, then the nucleus has shifted toward the open side of the disc wedge.

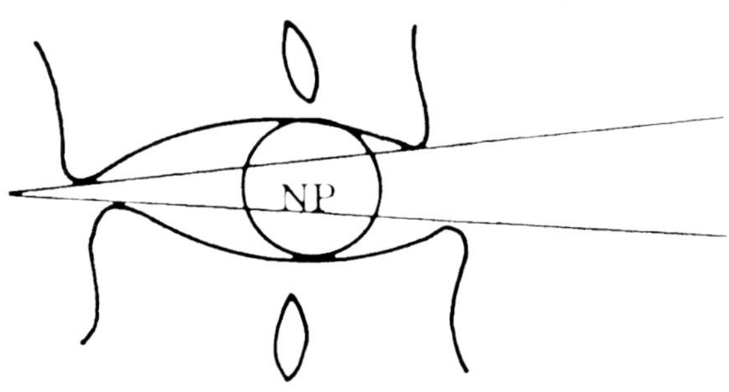

(Ill. VI-3) THE NUCLEAR SHIFT DISC BLOCK SUBLUXATION

A chronological summary:

1. Vertebral malposition (the kyphosis and/or lateral tipping).
2. Disc Wedge.
3. The nucleus of the disc shifts to the open side of the disc wedge producing an articular lock (disc block subluxation).
4. Rotation - the body of the vertebra, superior to the disc wedge rotates towards its low side in relationship to the body rotation of the vertebra below. (Ill. VI-3)

Try to visualize the explanation of this subluxation and you will then understand the mechanics of its adjustic correction. With the nucleus having lost its central position, the vertebra above tips to the side opposite the nuclear shift. The resulting inferiority causes the vertebral body to rotate towards its low side (narrow side of the disc wedge). The inordinate rotation "opens" the facet joint on this same side. In other words the facet separates *on the side of body rotation of the subluxated vertebra.*

The classic "disc block" subluxation. Now the complication of muscle fatigue, strain, pain, nerve root compression, etc. But muscle spasm? Most commonly no, only muscle splinting and strain as the body tries to support the upright posture of the head and neck. Adjusted properly this subluxation responds dramatically, without the use of any muscle technics or modalities.

It is the purpose of this text to explain this subluxation and describe its adjustic correction, but the principle of the nuclear shift subluxation must be clear in your mind before going beyond this point. I urge you to re-read the last two pages, (and Chapter IV for that matter) if there are any questions in your mind as to the mechanics of this subluxation it should be resolved now before you continue on.

On the next two pages we show sketches of the common rotatory scoliosis and the acute torticollis scoliosis. The cervical spine can be difficult to x-ray. The images on the A.P. film are often obscured by the mandible and the teeth. However, when one is aware of the mechanical principles of this subluxation it is easy to locate even though obscure. It is not necessary to ascertain the exact degree of contrarotation, but one must find the exact vertebra involved. Of course, I do not mean to infer that poor x-ray technic is excusable. The ideal should always be sought for, so that the exact degree of rotation and disc wedge can be ascertained. The objective symptoms indicate the side of disc wedge. The rotation of the vertebral body above the wedge will be away from the open side of the disc wedge in relation to the vertebra below. The mechanical principle of the subluxation determines the listing. In other words, if a patient comes in with his/her head tipped to the left (left torticollis) then a **significant** disc wedge will be seen converging on the left side. The vertebra above this disc wedge is the subluxated vertebra and its **body** will be rotated away from the open side of the disc wedge in relation to the vertebra below. (Ill. VI-5) The facet will be separated (open) on the **left**. The x-ray becomes most useful in determining the exact vertebra involved.

COMMON RIGHT ROTATORY SCOLIOSIS

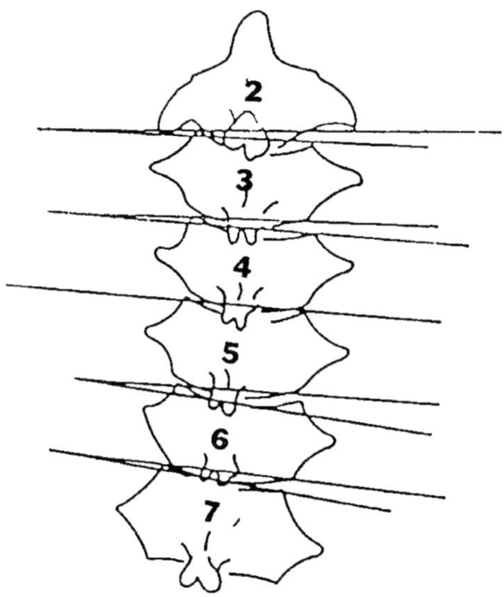

(Ill. VI-4) Lateral tipping of the cervical spine is accomplished by the rotation of the vertebral body's to the concavity of the curve. **In the common compensatory rotatory scoliosis the reverse is true, the vertebral body's rotate to the convexity of the curve (above).** The disc wedges are also open to the convexity of the curve to bring the spine back to plumb. Such cervical scolioses (which are most commonly compensations to curves lower down in the spine) are prone to torticollis. If the nucleus would shift from its central position in one of the disc wedges, a lateral torticollis subluxation would be the result. (Ill. VI-5).

ACUTE LEFT TORTICOLLIS SCOLIOSIS

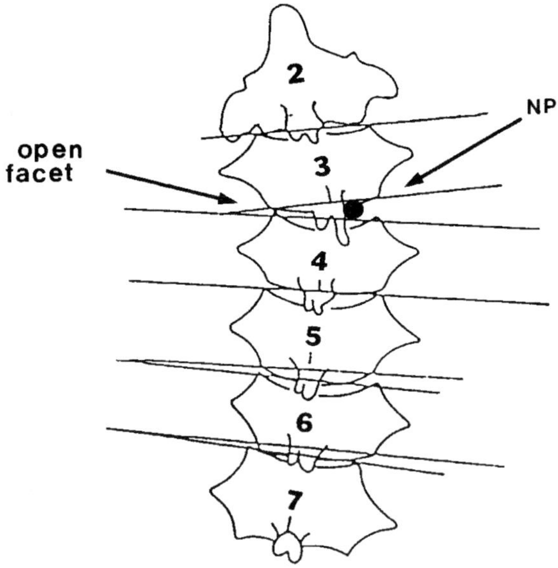

(Ill. VI-5) The acute subluxation is 3rd cervical. The nucleus pulposa (NP) has shifted from its central position in the disc space towards the wide side of the disc wedge. Notice the spinous process deviation of C 3 in comparison to C 4, it has moved toward the **convexity** of the curve. Measuring from the junction of the lamina of C 3 to like portions of its vertebral body the rotational disparity is clear analytically, the vertebral body is rotated towards the **concavity** of the curve. The facet will be **open** (separated) on this same side. The spine **tips** dramatically away from the wide side of the disc wedge.

The Atlas will rotate to the posterior on the side opposite the lateral bend. (Ill. VI-6) In the author's opinion this is an antalgic rotation. The turning of the head and face, away from the open facet of the torticollis subluxation, relieves the capsular strain of the facet separation (Ill. VI-7).

The mode of rotation of the skull being the rotation of Atlas on Axis, the Atlas simply rotates to relieve pain; the Atlas rotation should not be assumed to be a subluxation.

ACUTE LEFT LATERAL TORTICOLLIS
(From Above Down, Atlas Rotation)

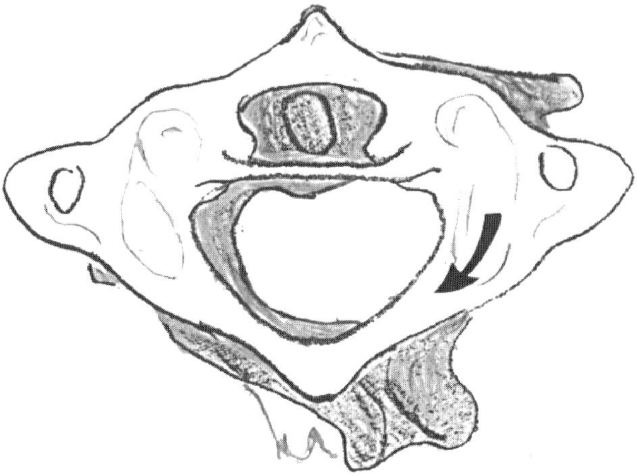

(Ill. VI-6) As explained on the preceding page, the author holds that the appearance of an Atlas subluxation is purely due to its antalgic rotation. On the illustration above, the Axis is the torticollis subluxation, its spinous is to the right of the C 3 spinous below. There is a disc wedge between Axis and 3rd on the AP x-ray (Ill. VI-7), the wedge converges to the left. The body of the Axis rotates to its low side separating the facet joint on the left. (Ill. VI-7, next page). Atlas rotates to the right and posterior endeavoring to ease the capsular strain between Axis and 3rd on the left.

The Atlas rotation is antalgic in nature, and it also allows the head to face forward. The Atlas is not "fixed" or "locked" on the Axis. This is evident as, when asked, the patient can turn their head further in the direction it is facing (in this case right) but not to the side of lateral bend, as this would aggravate the **open facet** between Axis and C 3 on the side of lateral bend (in this

ACUTE LEFT LATERAL TORTICOLLIS
(Posterior View)

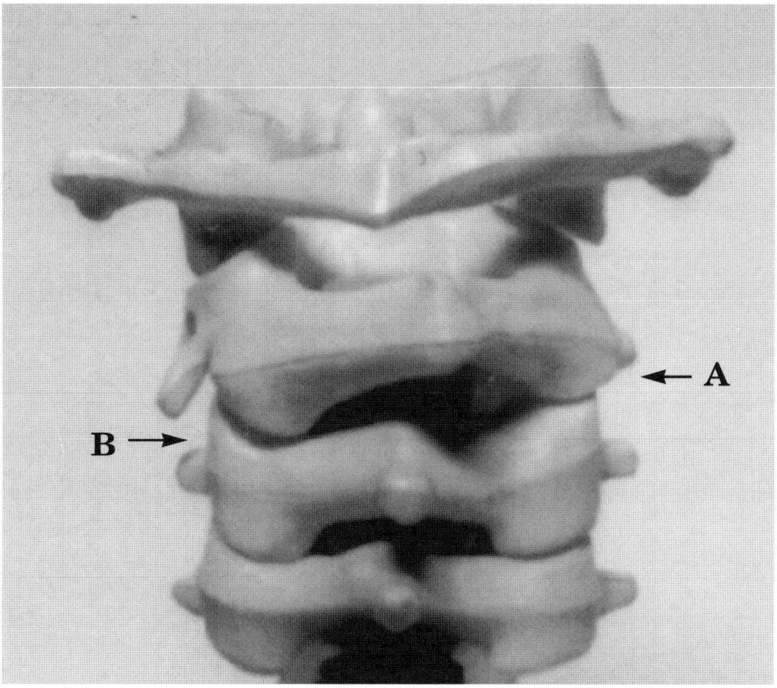

(Ill. VI-7) Here we have the torticollis subluxation of Axis explained on the opposite page. Note the facet of Axis on the right glides up on its articular mate below (A); this is the side of spinous process deviation. The contralateral facet (B) is distracted, **open** as I say, due to the vertebral body rotation towards the converged side of the disc wedge. The Atlas rotates to the posterior on the right attempting to ease the situation. **Due to the rotation of Axis, the Atlas transverse may palpate anterior but in its relationship to Axis, it is rotated posterior on the right. I contend that this rotation of Atlas is antalgic and not a subluxation.**

LATERAL TORTICOLLIS
(Before)

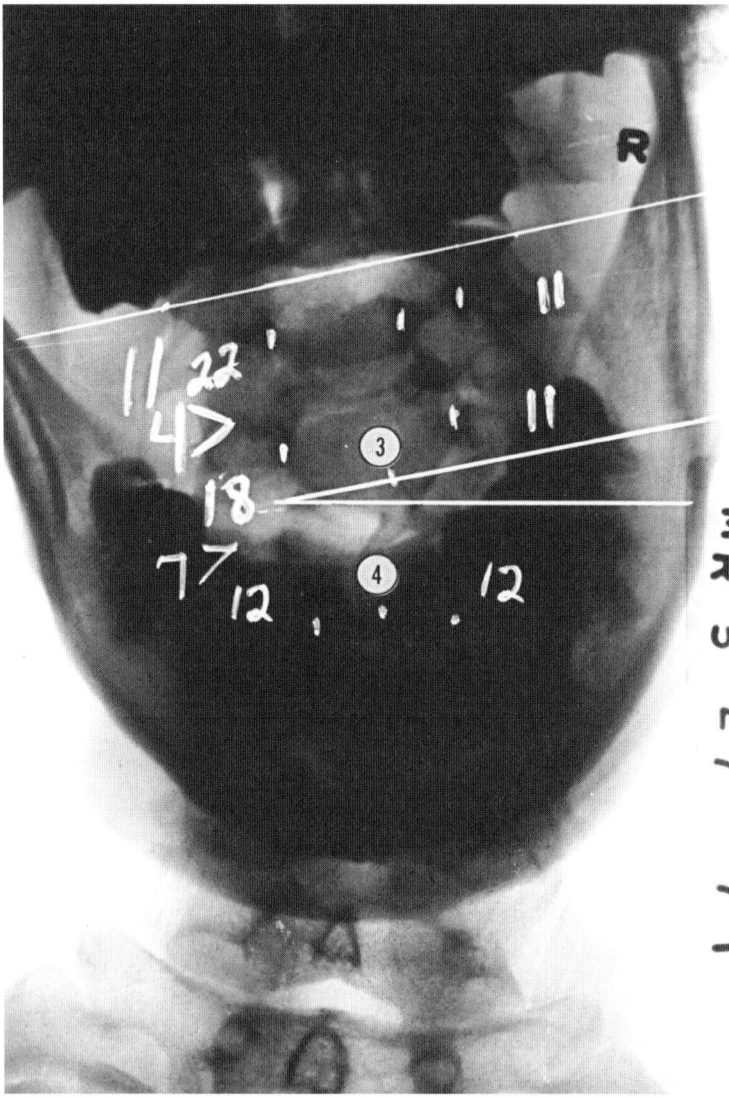

(Ill. VI-8) Third cervical subluxation, left lateral torticollis. Note the disc wedge and contrarotation. The 4th cervical is rotated 0mm, the 3rd cervical is rotated 7mm body left away from the wide side of the disc wedge in relation to the 4th cervical. There is also a 4mm rotational difference between Axis and 3rd, **but no disc wedge**.

LATERAL TORTICOLLIS
(After)

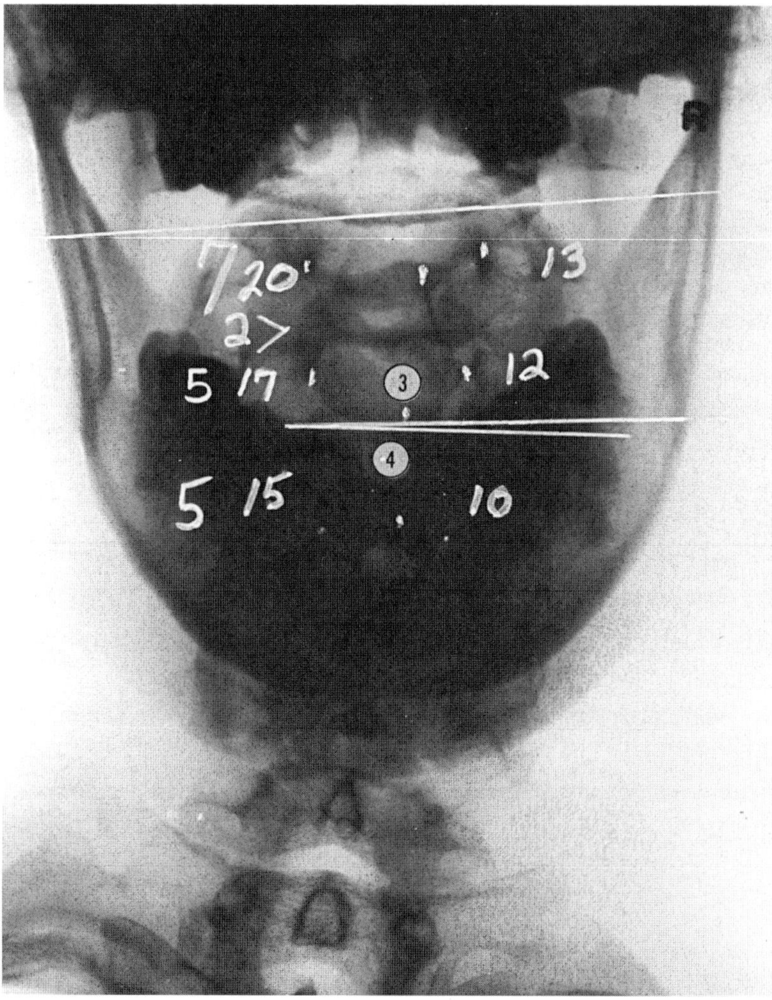

(Ill. VI-9) This dramatic set of before and after x-rays shows immediate reduction of the torticollis subluxation. An adjustment was given as described later in this text. The disc wedge has been dramatically reduced and the contrarotation eliminated.

Sitting cervical A.P. and lateral x-rays were taken, the x-rays were immediately developed and analyzed — an adjustment was given with the patient still sitting in the radiographic chair and the "after" x-ray was then taken.

II Anterior Torticollis

In this particular subluxation there is a posterior shifting of the nucleus pulposus. As in lateral torticollis a cervical kyphosis usually predisposes the spine to this problem. Normally there should be a nice rounded lordotic curve in the cervical spine.

I have held forth throughout this text my opinion that the sagittal curves of the human spine are reciprocal. Therefore the cervical lordotic curve is necessitated and nurtured by the existence of the thoracic kyphosis. In 1985 I presented my research paper on the normal degrees of the lumbar, thoracic, and cervical sagittal curves at The Biomechanical Conference on the Spine in Boulder, Colorado. I have also presented this research in the third text of this trilogy, VOL. III SCOLIOSIS, 2nd edition[16]. For the reader of this text I present below part of this research.

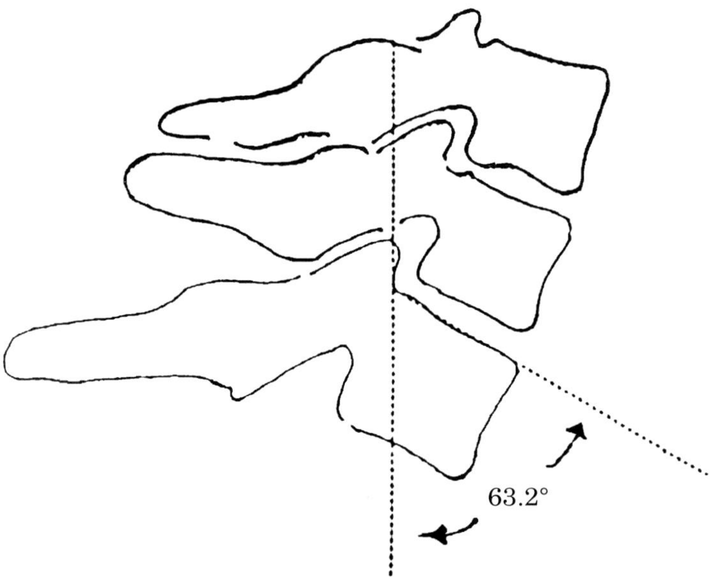

(Ill. VI-10) **The First Thoracic Angle**. I contend that the first thoracic vertebra is the base of the cervical lordotic curve and much like the sacrum in the lumbar spine its angle determines, to a great degree, the degree of the cervical lordotic curve.

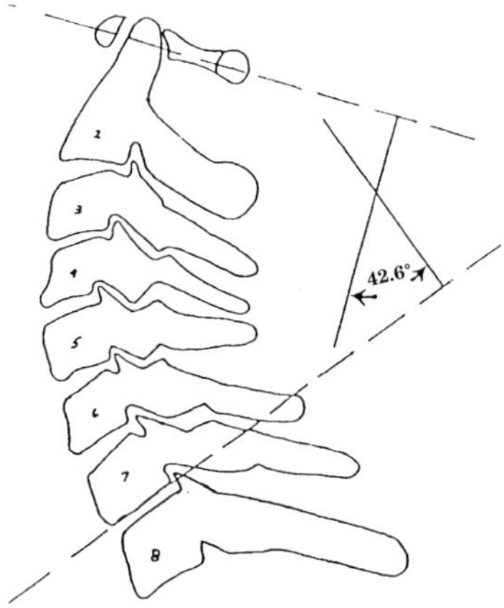

(Ill. VI-11) **The Normal Cervical Curve**

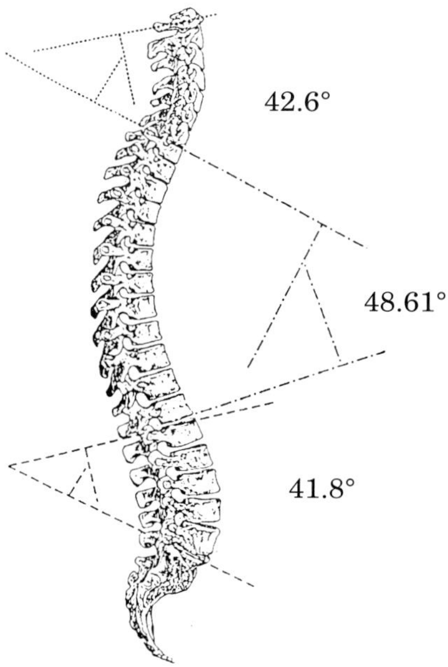

(Ill. VI-12) **The Normal Sigmoid Curve***

RANGES of Normal

CERVICAL	THORACIC	LUMBAR
Range 28°-60°	Range 39°-58°	Range 35°-54°
Average 42.6°	Average 48.61°	Average 41.8°

*For the complete study on The Normal Sigmoid Curve see author's VOL. III SCOLIOSIS, 2nd Edition.

ACUTE ANTERIOR TORTICOLLIS
(Before)

(after on page 49)

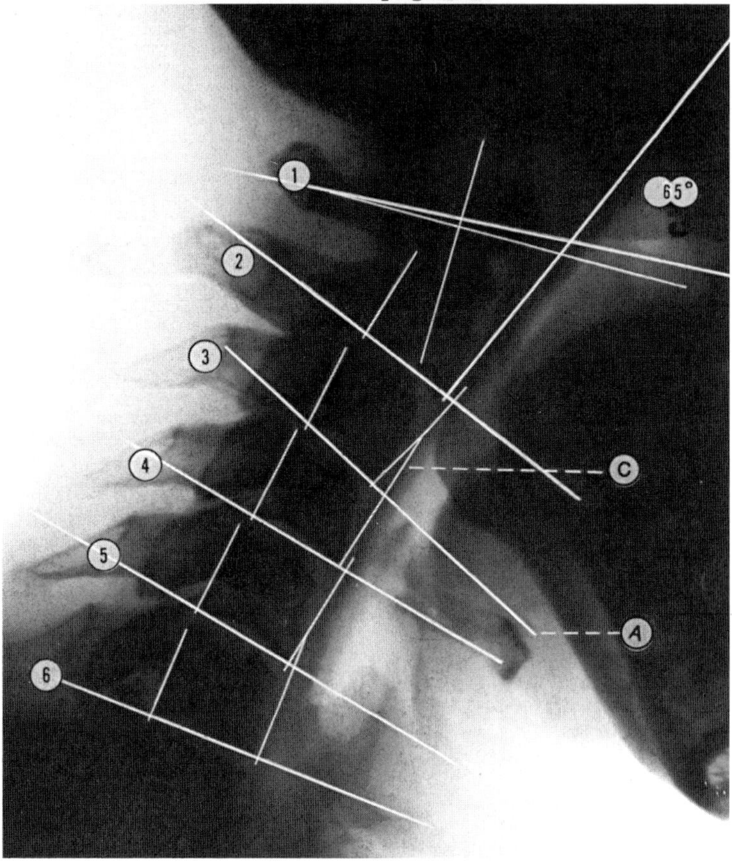

(Ill. VI-13) In the normal cervical spine, plane lines drawn across the inferior aspect of the vertebral bodies should be parallel or converge to the posterior. Notice the convergence of plane line A to the anterior. This indicates a shifting of the nucleus pulposus to the posterior between C 3 and C 4, a classic disc block subluxation. In the author's opinion the shifting of the N.P. causes the articular lock in torticollis, in this case 3rd cervical. In anterior torticollis, the patient's neck inclines forward due to the articular lock of the disc block subluxation. In most cases the patient cannot extend his/her neck without severe pain and great difficulty. This patient could not extend his neck at all. He was positively locked in this position.

ACUTE ANTERIOR TORTICOLLIS
(After)
(before on page 48)

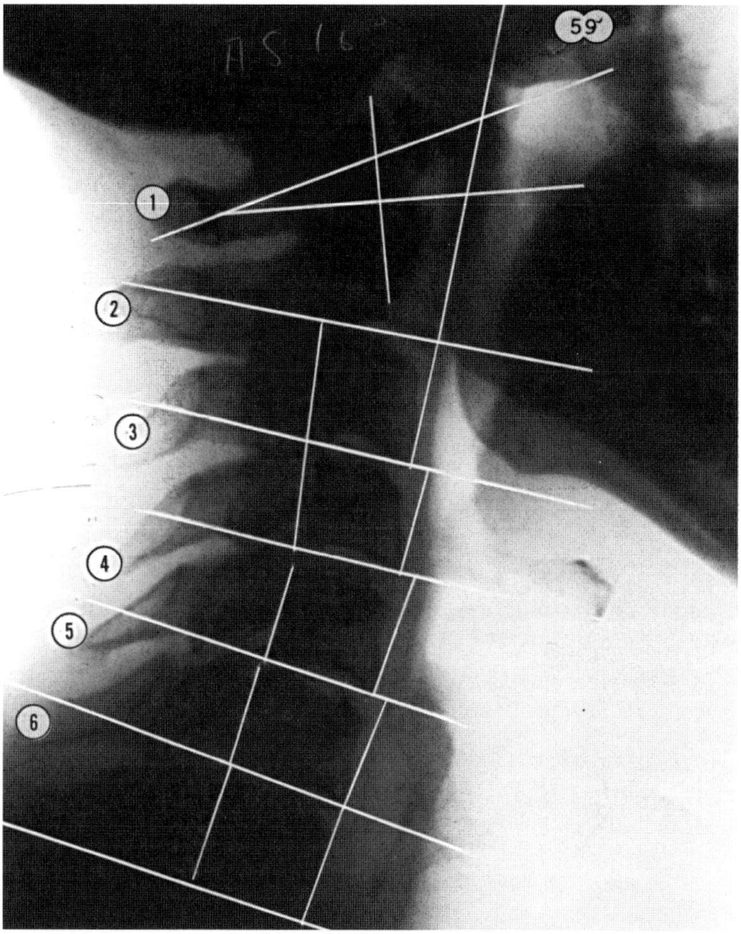

(Ill. VI-14) Dramatic change is evident on this x-ray. The adjustment used was the Keck move described in Chapter IX. The patient responded dramatically to the first adjustment and was fine after the third visit. He had suffered three weeks before coming under chiropractic care. Notice now that the body plane lines are parallel or converge to the posterior. The perpendicular lines (c-opposite page) now do not collide. This method of lateral film analysis has been developed by the author. It is described and explained on Chapter VII pages 63 - 67.

ACUTE ANTERIOR TORTICOLLIS
(Before)
(after on page 51)

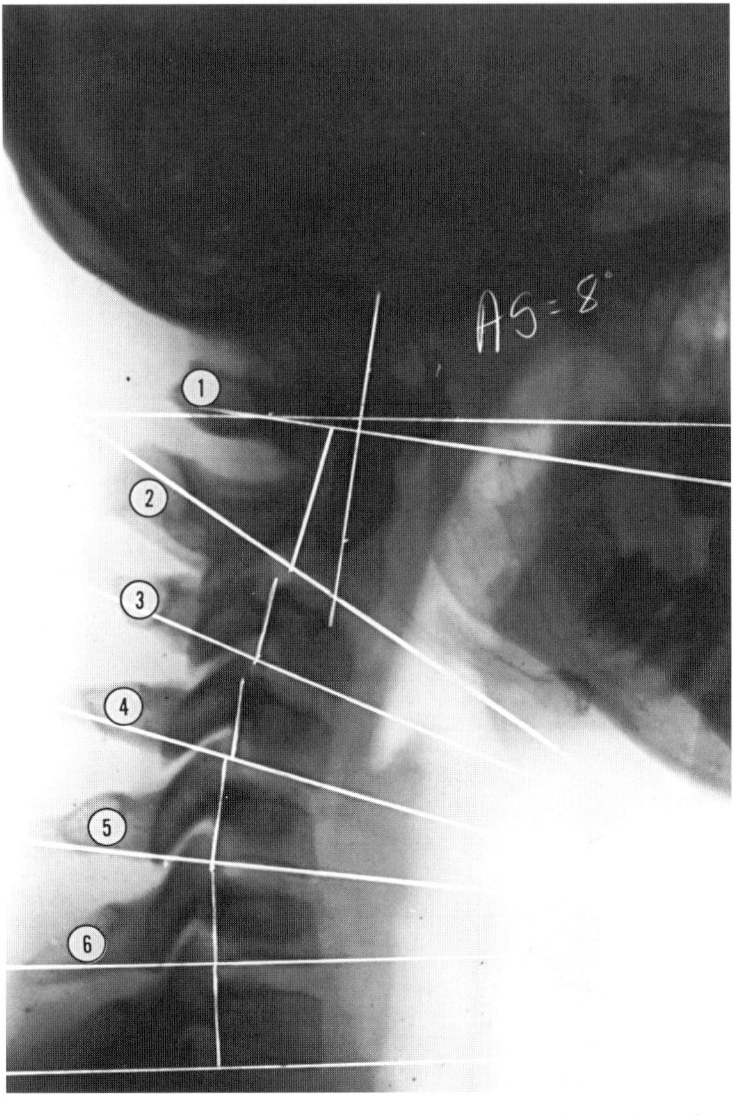

(Ill. VI-15) In my opinion the 4th cervical is the culprit here, although the Axis is also involved. The patient is a young female age eleven. She complained of a stiff neck since rough-housing with her brother the night before.

ACUTE ANTERIOR TORTICOLLIS
(After)
(before on page 50)

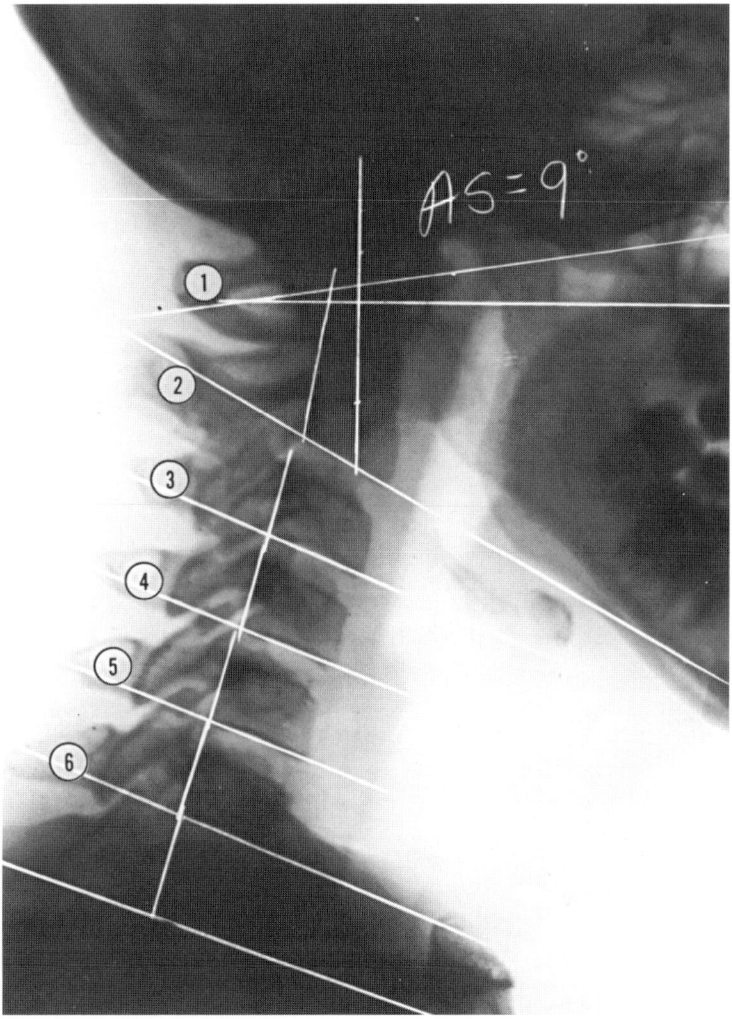

(Ill. VI-16) Four days between adjustments - We took the x-rays before adjusting the second time. Note the improvement. Axis is still involved somewhat, but the reverse curve is gone and the patient is much relieved. A total of three adjustments completely solved the problem. A.P. x-rays were taken, but were not significant in this case. 4th cervical was adjusted on the first visit, Axis was adjusted after this x-ray was taken.

III Anterior Lateral Torticollis

Anterior lateral torticollis is simply a combination of the two conditions. The patient's head will be bent to one side and forward. The nuclear shift will be posterior lateral. The A.P. and lateral x-rays will indicate posterior, lateral disc wedge. The nuclear shift rotational principle of lateral torticollis will be present on the A.P. film.

It is often found in anterior lateral torticollis that more than one vertebra (and disc) is involved in the analytical syndrome. For instance, the lateral torticollis subluxation exists at C 4 (Ill. VI-18) and the anterior torticollis subluxation at C 3. (Ill. VI-17) Thus a combination of adjustments is called for. The doctor may choose to use a sitting "spinous pull" move on the lateral torticollis subluxation and on the following day deliver a posterior cervical thrust on the keck pillow. The adjustment of this subluxation is described in Chapter VIII, but the reader must be aware at this time, that anterior lateral torticollis can involve more than one subluxation. If only one vertebra is involved, the disc then has a nuclear shift both lateral and posterior.

A. P. and lateral x-rays must be taken in torticollis. I cannot emphasize this point enough. Good x-ray evaluation is necessary in torticollis; especially in traumatic torticollis which, if instantaneous, can be a facet dislocation. (Ill. VI-19 page 54)

However, most often, especially in sports related trauma, torticollis appears a few hours after the injury. In these cases the argument could ensue as to the mechanics of the cause. However, such discussion would not contribute to the analytical conclusions arrived upon by the author. The disc block principle of the subluxation is apparent on x-ray. In most cases of torticollis you will find a combination of lateral and posterior nuclear shift. The anterior tipping of the patient's head is positive indication of the posterior shift. The lateral tipping of the head indicates lateral torticollis and the rotation of the chin is usually towards the side opposite that of the lateral bend. **In my opinion the turning of the head away from the open facet (side opposite the lateral bend) is an endeavor to ease the pain of the separated facet joint.** (See pages 42 and 43)

The objective symptoms of torticollis are interesting. The more proficient the chiropractor becomes in the objective and palpatory analysis of this disc lesion subluxation, the more prone he is to adjust without x-ray. Here I must say, again ... *x-rays are a must*. Often a patient will not properly relate the trauma involved in their problem. The patient may be reluctant to relate his/her injury; and the doctor may be dealing with more than a subluxation and in fact be faced with a facet dislocation. All palpation must be very gentle, heavy pressure against the capsular membranes of the "open" facet will elicit extreme pain and **produce** muscle spasm.

ANTERIOR LATERAL TORTICOLLIS

Lateral View

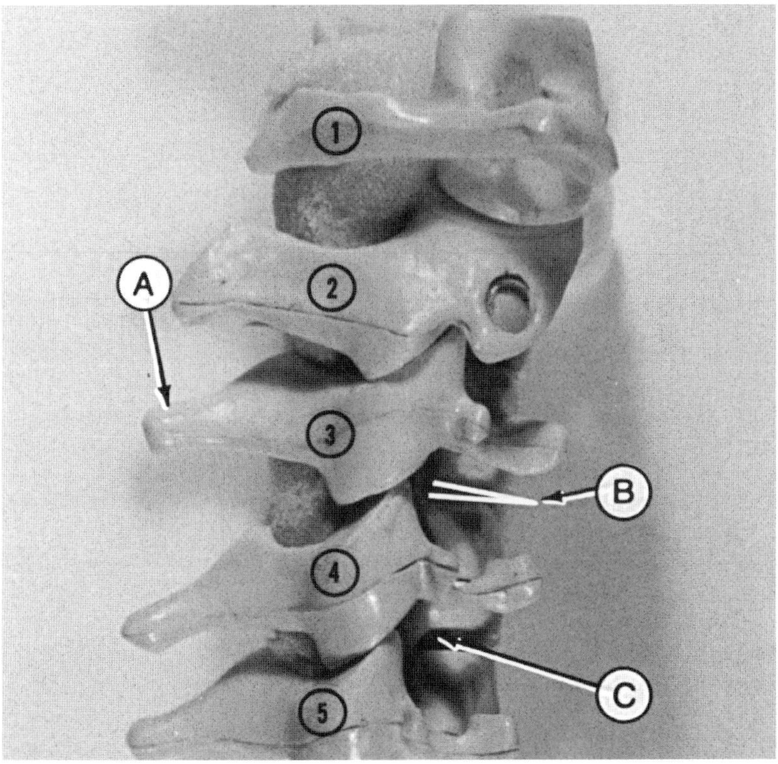

(Ill. VI-17) The 3rd cervical spinous is superior (A). A disc is wedged open to the posterior between 3rd and 4th cervical (B) this is the anterior torticollis involvement. Below this subluxation we have the lateral torticollis involvement of the 4th cervical, easily seen on (Ill. VI-18). Note here that on this lateral view you can see the facet of the 4th cervical riding up upon the facet of the 5th (C).

ANTERIOR LATERAL TORTICOLLIS

A.P. View

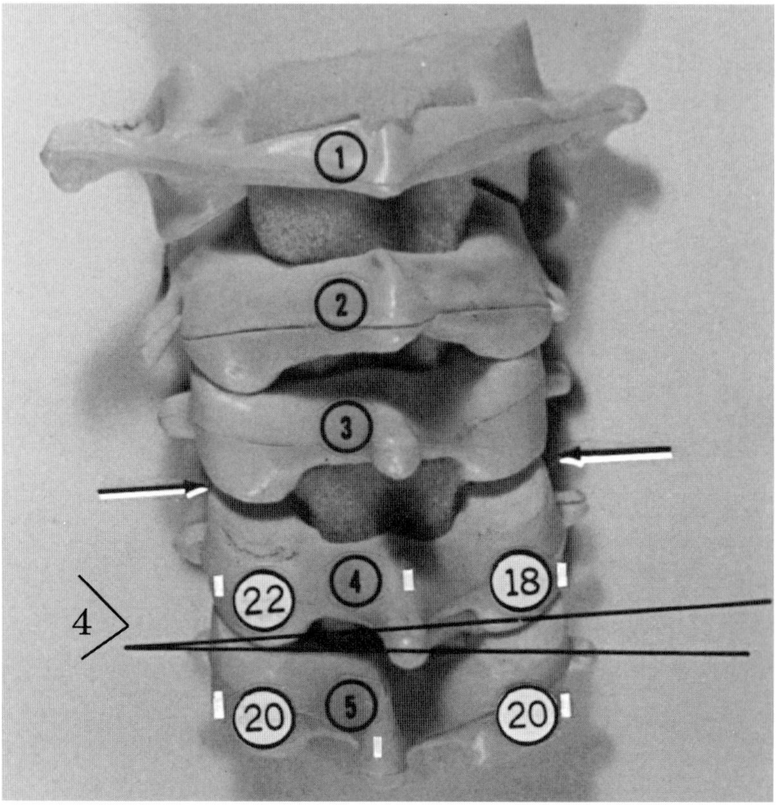

(Ill. VI-18) Notice the facets are open between the 3rd and 4th cervical vertebrae on both sides. The spinous of C 3 is superior in its relationship to C 4. Obviously the 3rd cervical is rocked forward and is the segment involved in anterior torticollis. (Ill. VI-17) Now notice the disc wedge between 4th and 5th cervical. The spine tips to the left above the level of the 5th cervical. The 4th cervical is rotated 4mm away from the open side of the disc wedge in relation to C 5, this is the lateral torticollis subluxation. The rotation of L 4 on L 5 "opens" the facet on the left.

FACET DISLOCATION

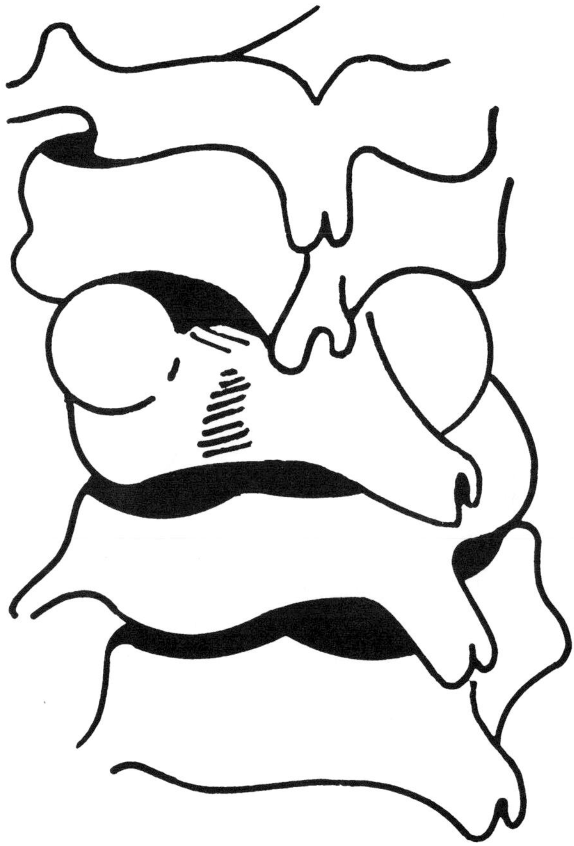

(Ill. VI-19) One can clearly see the superior articular surface of the vertebra immediately below the dislocated vertebra. The facet of the superior vertebra has slipped over the top of its articular mate.

The necessity of x-rays regardless of the degree of complaint is important. I personally believe that facet dislocation could be effectively reduced by proper chiropractic adjustment, but then too, I believe that many vertebral fractures and dislocations should be reduced by direct adjustment before surgical intervention. I look to the future for chiropractors to assert themselves into such areas, because I do not believe we shall be asked to provide our services!

SCOLIOSIS & TORTICOLLIS

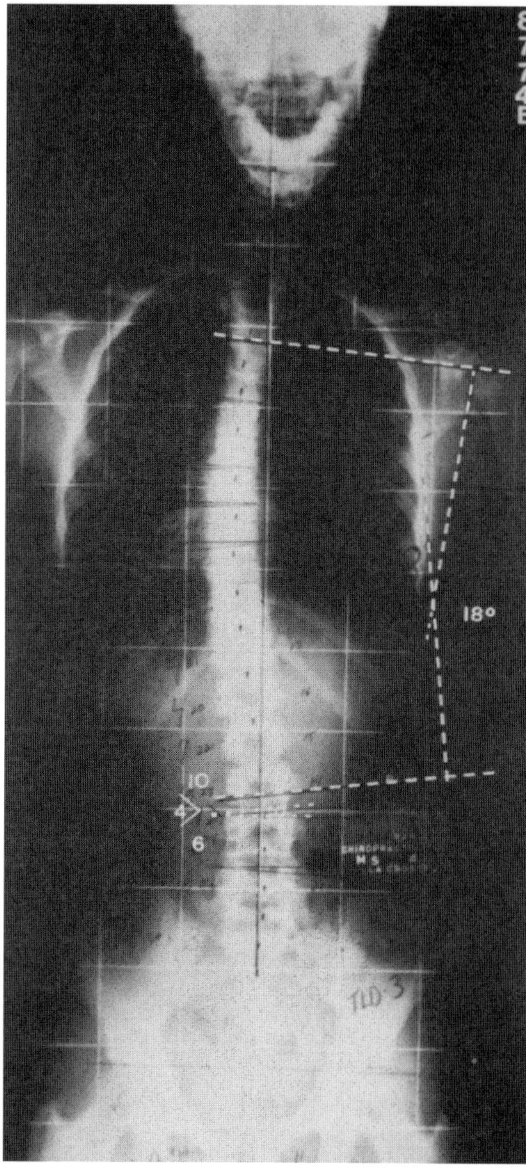

(Ill. VII-1) Mild scoliotic curves such as seen on the x-ray above led to frequent complaints of "stiff neck" and acute attacks of torticollis. This young female, age 14, was suffering from a mild attack of torticollis. Case #8774B, page 278 author's text VOL. III SCOLIOSIS.[21]

CHAPTER VII
X-RAY ANALYSIS

In my opinion, the cause of torticollis is a disc block subluxation. Therefore any cervical vertebra below the Atlas can be involved in this condition. A. P. and lateral x-rays should be taken for proper analysis. Regardless of the pain syndrome or the tortuous position of the neck take the x-rays ... either sitting or standing. If the cervical spine indicates a curve extending down into the dorsals, take a standing full spine x-ray, as often a dorsal or even a lumbar subluxation can be involved and should be adjusted.

Scoliosis predisposes a spine to both torticollis and tortipelvis subluxations. (Ill. VII-1) This factor will be discussed in Chapter XI, Initiating Factors. In youth reoccurring attacks of torticollis are often resolved when spinal balance is improved by the correction of the causes of an impending scoliosis. My text VOL. III SCOLIOSIS completely covers this subject but it should be sufficient to say here that we should look well to the configuration of the entire spine in all cases of torticollis, especially in young people and I repeat, torticollis is often a symptom of early scoliosis.

As I've said, take x-rays either sitting or standing as the position of the subluxation itself is not dependent upon posture. This is a true articular lock, and the subluxated vertebra's disrelationship with its articular mate is not changed by posture. If you asked me; do I have a preferred position for these x-rays? I would say, yes, standing ... The curve below the subluxation **does** change with posture and I consider the standing x-ray to produce a more accurate image as to what really happens to the entire spine during an attack of torticollis.

But remember both A. P. and lateral x-rays are a must as most often we are dealing with a posterior-lateral disc wedge. The nuclear shift is more commonly in both directions. The analytical interpretation of these two spinographic views gives a clear picture of the subluxation of torticollis.

I have separated this chapter into two parts.

1. **A.P. X-ray Analysis**
2. **Lateral X-ray Analysis**

1. A. P. X-ray Analysis

Using Dr. Clarence Gonstead's wedge line analysis one can easily determine disrelationships between the cervical vertebrae. Following what I've said in preceding chapters, you now realize that when a vertebral body immediately above a disc wedge rotates away from the wide side of the disc wedge in relation to the vertebra below ... this denotes a shifting of the nucleus to the wide side of the disc wedge. This contra-rotation is determined by measuring from the junction of lamina to like points on either side of the vertebral body. The wide side of the body dimension is the side of body rotation.

But remember, the rotational disrelationship between two vertebrae is a relative one. In other words, looking at the illustration (below) you will see that there is a disc wedge between C 4 and C 5 converging to the left. C 4 is rotated 1mm body left ... C 5 is rotated 3mm body right. So in relation to C 5 ... C 4 is body rotated 4 mm away from the wide side of the disc wedge. The facet is open on the left between C 4 and C 5.

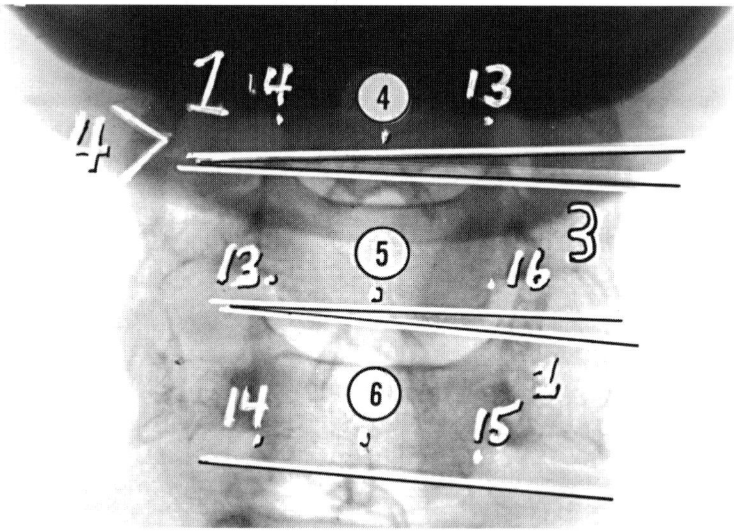

(Ill. VII-2) Relative Rotation

The very fact that this is a relative disrelationship (one vertebra to another) also makes it less important to consider the distortion factors of x-ray. So in regard to patient, bucky, tube alignment, (and the difficulties of placement in the tortuously bent spine of torticollis) remember you are only trying to determine the exact vertebra involved.

Draw your wedge lines between the vertebrae, then determine which vertebral body is rotated away from the wide side of the disc wedge (in relation to the vertebra below) and you have found the causative subluxation in lateral torticollis. On the following three pages you will find sketches and x-ray examples of A. P. film analysis.

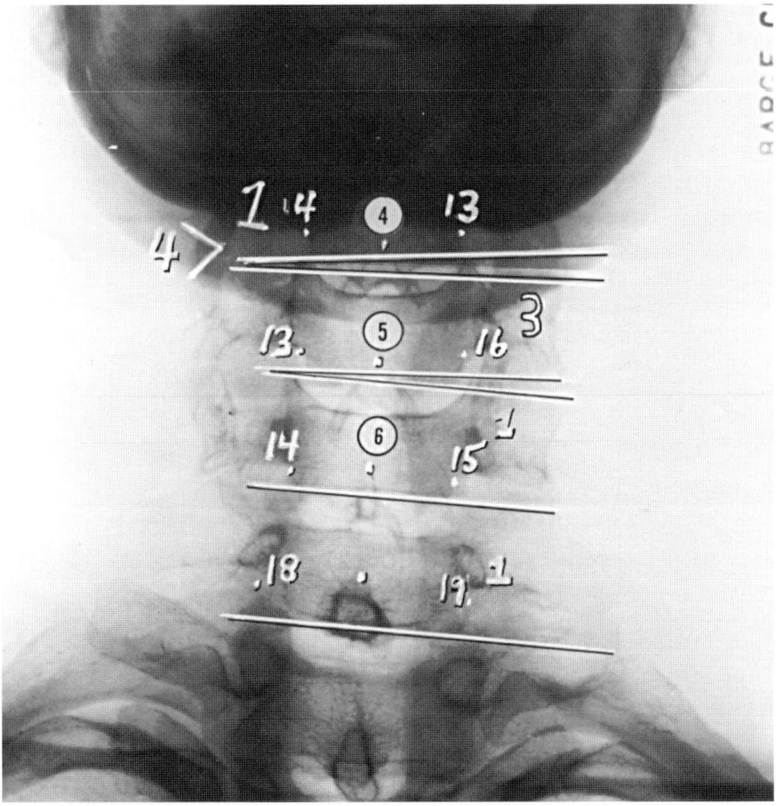

(Ill. VII-3) Using the Gonstead technic of drawing wedge lines between vertebrae, disc wedges are clearly seen. (Ill. VII-5 page 61) This is the complete x-ray of the cutaway view seen on the opposite page. This patient is in a mild state of torticollis, the body of the 4th cervical is rotated away from the open side of the disc wedge in comparison to the vertebral body of the C 5. The patient complained of a stiff neck with only mild restriction to a full range of rotation. In such cases a patient will experience a more limited ability to rotate their head toward the side of the

open facet (in this case left) as such rotation would tend to separate the facet further and create pain. **Pain upon rotating the head towards one side usually indicates that there is an "open facet" on that same side! Gentle** palpation must verify the open facet (this case on the left) in all such, analytically minor, vertebral misalignments.

Note the dots on the vertebrae indicating measuring points for rotation.

A.P. X-RAY ANALYSIS
Vertebral Rotations

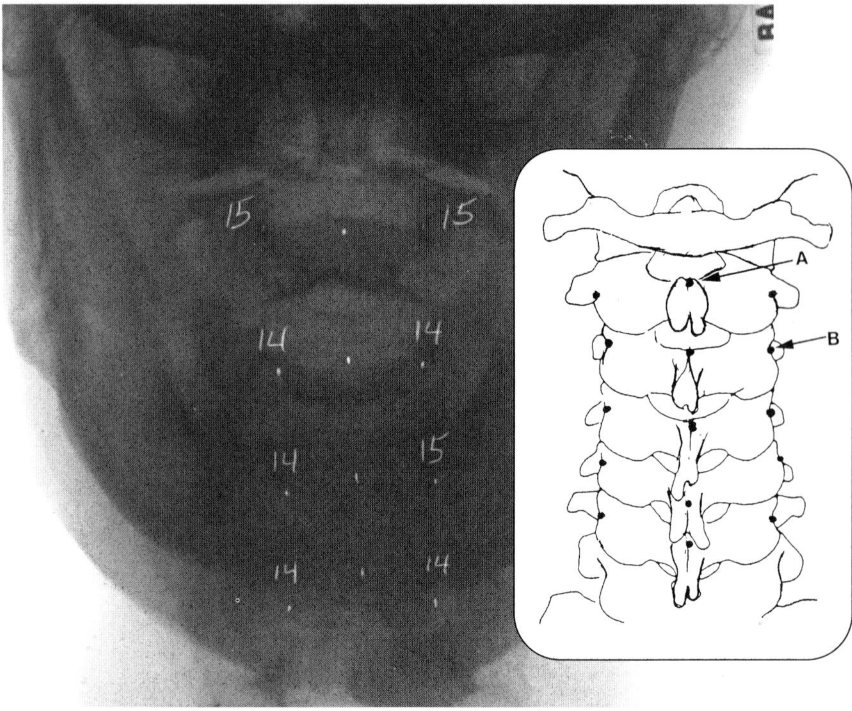

(Ill. VII-4) As mentioned on page 58, dot the junction of lamina (A) and like points on the lateral aspects of the vertebral bodies. (B) If the vertebral body is wider in dimension on one side than the other, this denotes that the body of the vertebra is rotated to that side.

This x-ray is interpreted for rotations only. The center line of the ruler is placed on the junction of lamina, its numerated edge on the body dots. The dimensions out to the body dots are then measured. Again, the wide side of the vertebral body is the side of **body** rotation.

WEDGE LINE ANALYSIS

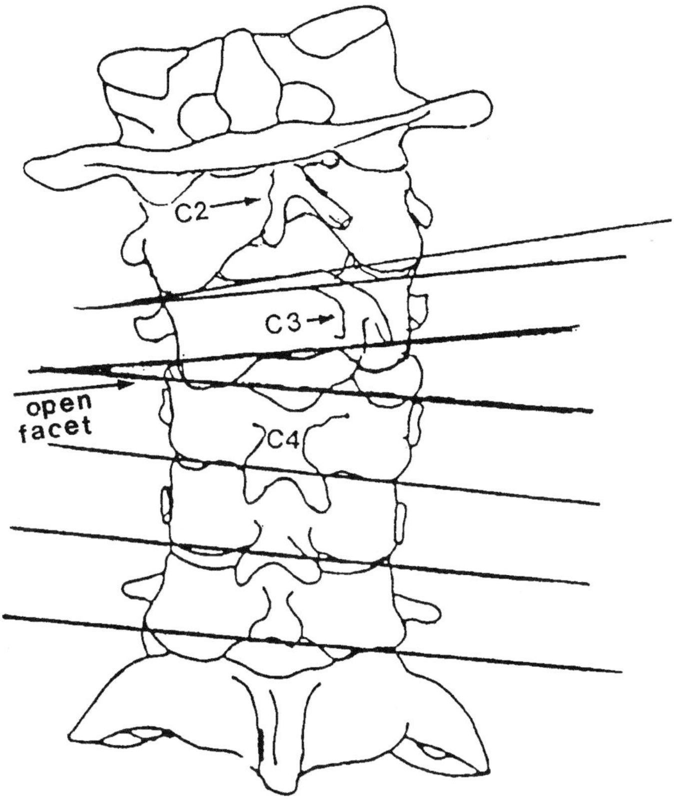

(Ill. VII-5) A credit to the chiropractic pioneer Dr. Clarence Gonstead is the wedge line analysis developed by him. Using a gliding parallel ruler he would compare the level of each vertebra, one to the other, in respect to later tipping. A disparity in the alignment indicated disc wedging between the vertebrae. It is important to check each vertebral body for wedging so that malformation does not interfere with proper disc wedge analysis. By gliding the parallel from the inferior to the superior surface of the vertebral body, body wedging can be easily determined and corrected for. If the top of the vertebral body is not parallel to its inferior border then the vertebral body is wedged and you must adjust the ruler accordingly.

On the schematic sketch above there is no evident disc wedging in the lower cervical spine. 3rd cervical, however, is dramatically tipped to the left. Using wedge line analysis the degree of disc wedging can be accurately determined. The body of 3rd cervical is rotated away from the wide side of the disc wedge in relation to C 4. Overriding of the facets and separation of their articular surfaces occurs on the narrow side of the disc wedge. **This is the open facet** found in the disc block subluxation of torticollis.

2. Lateral X-ray Analysis

Using a concept similar to that which we developed for the lumbar spine, an accurate method of lateral film analysis of vertebral subluxation can be achieved. (Ill. VII-6 opposite page).

1. First draw plane lines across the inferior aspect of each vertebra (A).
2. Next dot the inferior tip of the body of each vertebra (B) (When an exostotic spure develops here you must judge where the tip should be).
3. From the body dot, draw a perpendicular line up from the plane line, past the center of the vertebral body above (C).

Note on our illustration that lines (C) do not intersect. When there is a posterior nuclear shift (and thus a posterior disc bulge) these lines will intersect. In anterior or anterior lateral torticollis you will find these lines intersecting. This will be at one or two vertebral levels. Notice, also, that the body plane lines (A) converge to the posterior. In anterior and anterior lateral torticollis they often converge to the anterior.

The following sketches and x-rays graphically demonstrate our method of laterial cervical x-ray analysis in torticollis.

Our research thus far has indicated that a space of more than 3 mm between the perpendicular lines (D) indicates retropositioning.

Therefore, this lateral film analysis is not limited to torticollis, but is useful in general x-ray determination of cervical subluxations.

Remember, when a vertebra is retropositioned it intrudes on the dimensions of the intervertebral foramina on both sides, and augments the foraminal narrowing effect of vertebral rotations. Our points of reference for lateral film analysis in the *lumbar* spine are different than they are cervically. For readers interested in our system of lateral lumbar analysis I refer you to VOL. I TORTIPELVIS.

LATERAL X-RAY ANALYSIS

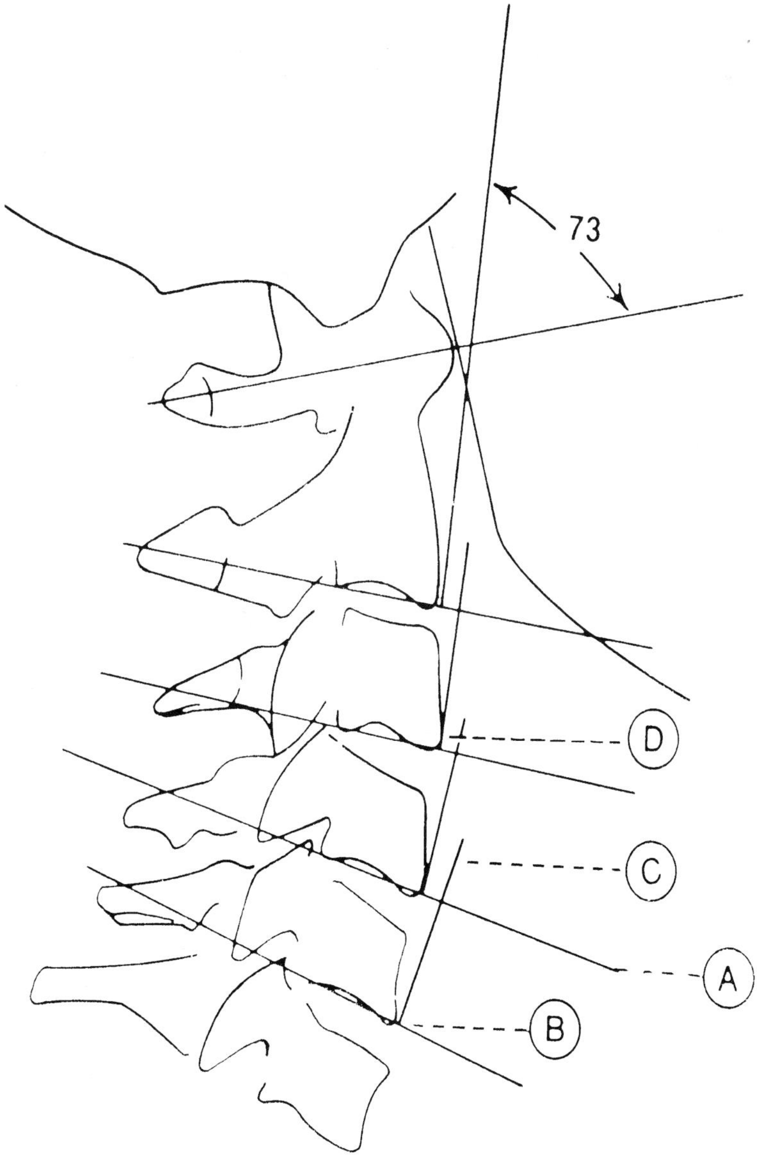

(Ill. VII-6) This sketch shows the analytical lines used by the author in lateral cervical x-ray analysis.

LATERAL X-RAY ANALYSIS

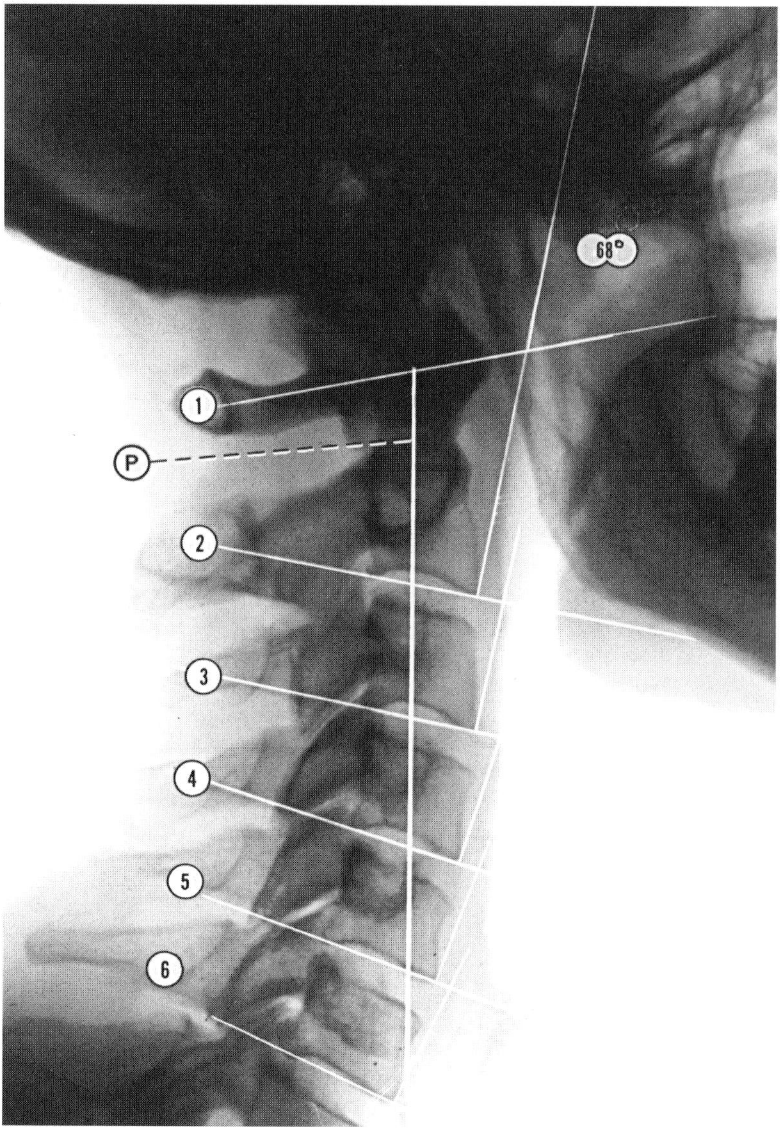

(Ill. VII-7) Here is how our film marking lines appear on a near-normal lateral 8x10 cervical x-ray. Notice the plane lines across the vertebral bodies are parallel or converge to the posterior and the vertical lines do not intersect. The plumb line indicates some flattening of the normal cervical curve on this x-ray (P).

LATERAL X-RAY ANALYSIS

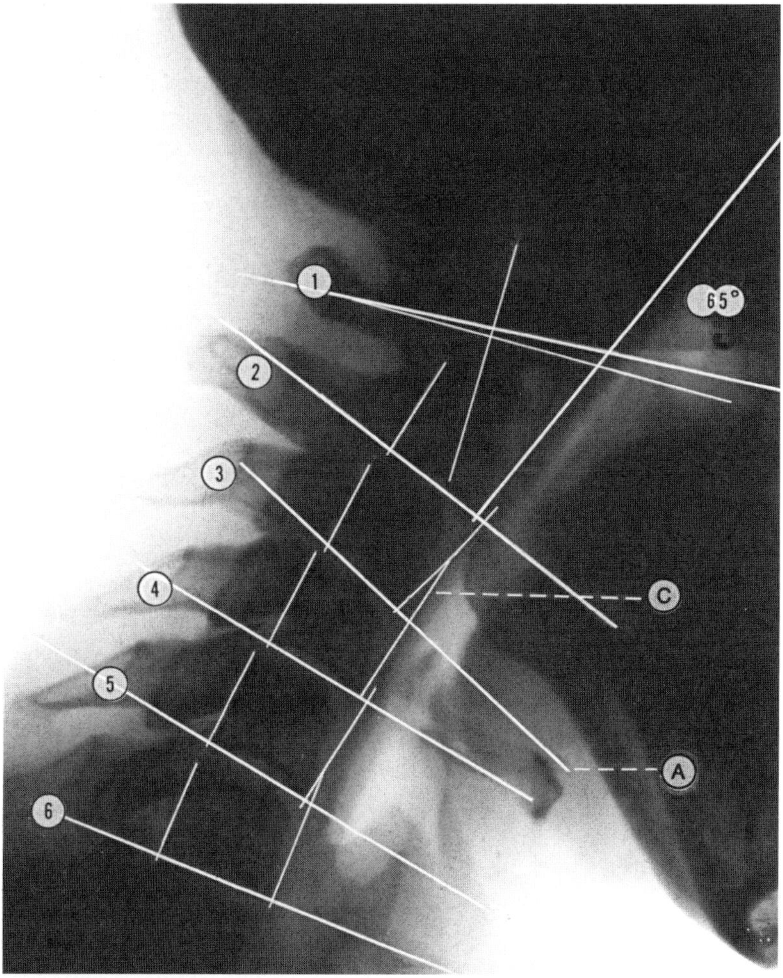

(Ill. VII-8) This is how anterior torticollis appears on x-ray using the x-ray analysis developed by the author. Notice how the body plane lines converge anteriorally between 3rd and 4th cervical (A).

The perpendicular lines (C) also intersect at this level indicating the 3rd cervical is the subluxation. These same guidelines show a secondary involvement of the 5th cervical. The disc between C 3 and C 4 is bulged posteriorally indicating a posterior shift of the nucleus pulposus. This is a classic example of the anterior torticollis subluxation.

ATLAS AXIS RELATIONSHIP
Lateral Film Analysis

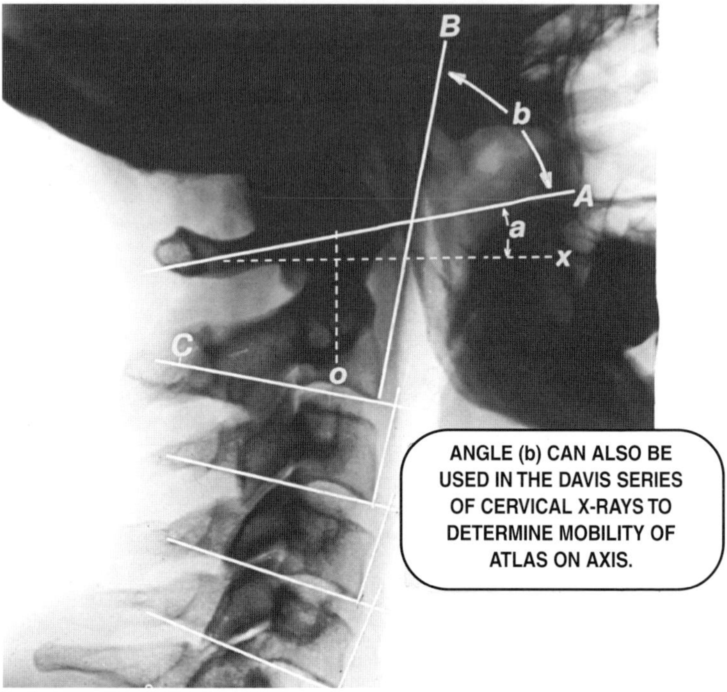

(Ill. VII-9) To determine the Atlas Axis relationship on the lateral cervical x-ray, the common angle used today is (a) above. In the determination of this angle a line is drawn through the odontoid process down into the body of Axis (o). Another line (x) is then drawn crossing the odontoid line at right angles (see broken lines above). An angle is formed by this line and its intersection with the Atlas plane line (A). This angle (a) is said to be normally four degrees superior to line (x).

Due to the obscurity of the odontoid and Axis body structures on some x-rays, the author has developed another angle (b). By continuing the vertical line (B) from Axis' body plane line (C) on up through the plane line of Atlas (A) an angle (b) is formed.

In our research with this angle we compiled 100 lateral cervicals. We carefully picked x-rays that showed normal lateral contours, without malformation and/or traumatic insult. The results of this research showed that in 68 percent of the x-rays this angle ranged between 55 and 65 degrees, while the average of all the films was 61.02 degrees.

ATLAS AXIS RELATIONSHIP
LATERAL FILM ANALYSIS
(Barge Method)

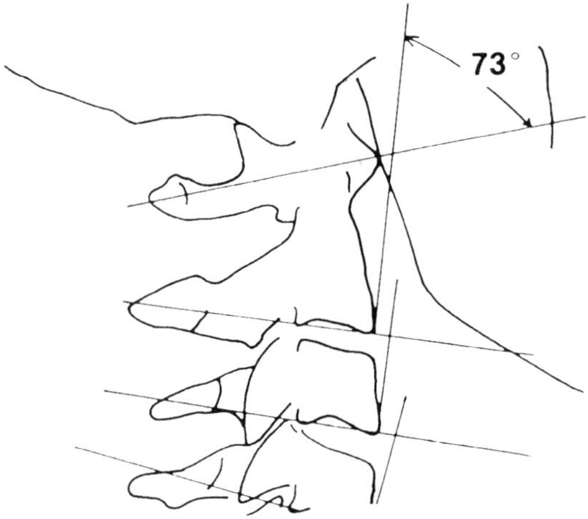

(Ill. VII-10) Draw a plane line across the base of Axis and erect a perpendicular up from its inferior tip. This line will intersect the Atlas plane line, the angle thus formed is a good indicator of normal Atlas Axis relationships.

This method of Axis Atlas analysis is very simplistically done and easy to accomplish even on poorly exposed films where the former odontoid line was impossible to ascertain.

RANGE 55-65 DEGREES
AVERAGE 61.02 DEGREES

Results of 100 patients' x-rays showing degrees of the Barge Atlas Angle

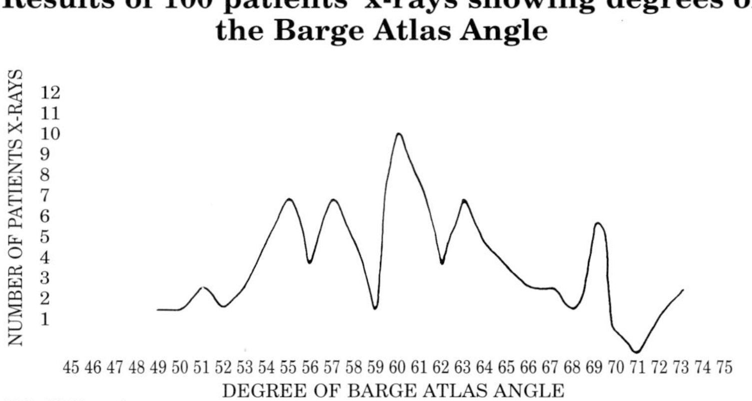

(Ill. VII-11)

X-RAY TECHNIC

As this book is not meant to be an x-ray technic manual we shall only briefly discuss the technic we use for x-raying these cases. Needless to say, in torticollis, the cervical spine is bent in a tortuous position, thus patient bucky placement can be difficult. An 8x10 cervical bucky is recommended for x-raying the severe cases. This bucky (used commonly by upper cervical specific chiropractors) can be tilted to better accommodate the tipped cervical spine found in severe torticollis. When the tortuous bend of the neck is not severe 14x36 A.P. and lateral views can be very revealing, as often lower spinal distortion has initiated the acute torticollis attack. Chapter XI illustrates such problems under "Predisposing Factors." Good bucky/patient central ray placement is, of course, to be sought for; but in this acute spinal condition the ideal is difficult to achieve. By using the 8x10 bucky we have found that even the most severe cases can be adequately x-rayed so that analysis will reveal the vertebra involved in this subluxation.

When taking the lateral x-ray, place the convexity of the cervical curve next to the bucky. In other words shoot into the concavity; to do otherwise will obscure the disc spaces. Take before and after x-rays to prove full recovery so that chronic malposition does not remain to create the need for adaptative curves. In all cases of reoccurring torticollis take full spine studies **standing.** Leg deficiencies and pelvic distortions grossly change when x-rays are taken lying down. 8x10 cervical x-rays can be taken sitting, standing, or lying down, as the level of the acute subluxation will not change.

To date the x-ray is our most useful tool to verify and identify the subluxation. My recommendation is to x-ray all cases.

Author's Note

For the reader interested in the typical and atypical disc block subluxations of the lumbar spine I refer you to VOL. I TORTIPELVIS[16], *the third and fourth editions.* VOL. III SCOLIOSIS[21] *discusses the role the disc block subluxation plays in the "idiopathic" rotatory scoliosis.*

CHAPTER VIII
THE PAIN OF TORTICOLLIS

The pain of the subluxation

To understand the pain of torticollis, we must understand the pain created by a subluxation. The pain of the subluxation results from the stress (or stretch) upon the ligamentous structures of the vertebral joints due to the malposition of the vertebra. Especially involved in this stretch reflex pain are the capsular ligaments of the facets, and the joints of Luschka, the latter are often called the unco-vertebral joints (see pages 70, 71, 72). In VOL. I, TORTIPELVIS, there is a thorough discussion of this pain reflex, including Dr. Skyrme Rees' and Dr. C. Norman Shealy's surgery for such pain syndromes. By denervating the capsular ligaments of the intervertebral joints these surgeons eliminate the pain of the subluxation without changing vertebral position. Dr. Rees surgically cuts these nerves; Dr. Shealy first burned them off, but now uses an injection of phenol. For reference on this surgery, I refer you to VOL. I, TORTIPELVIS, Chapter I, Second, Third and Fourth Editions.[16]

The capsular ligaments of the intervertebral facets (Zygapophyses) and the joints of Luschka are the major synovial membranes of the cervical intervertebral articulations.*

Synovial membranes are capable of eliciting much pain upon stretch stress. This happens to the capsular ligament when a vertebra rotates excessively and thus separates a facet joint. The ligamentum flava also comes into stress upon vertebral tipping, but it is a highly elastic ligament capable of withstanding stretch stress.

The causes of pain:

1. **The capsular ligament of the facet.**
2. **The capsular ligament of the joint of Luschka.**
3. **Strain to the annular fibers of the disc.**
4. **Nerve root compression.**
5. **Muscle fatigue and tension.**

Analyzing the vertebral subluxation's malposition can indicate to the doctor which tissues are receiving the most stress. Directing the line of drive of the adjustic thrust to relieve this stress corrects the subluxation and brings prompt pain relief. In torticollis one must also consider the nuclear shift and disc block peculiarity of this subluxation. With adjustic concern for

* Gray's Anatomy states that odontoid articulations have synovial membranes.

the nuclear malposition, dramatic correction is achieved (Chapter IX, The Adjustment).

JOINTS OF LUSCHKA

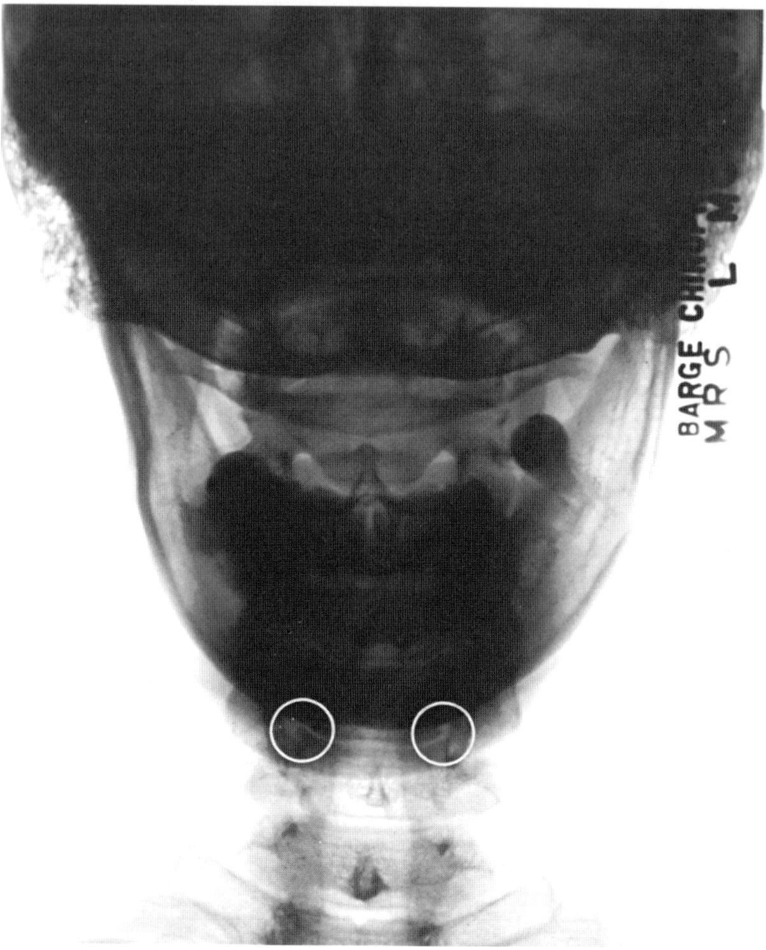

(Ill. VIII-1) Look at this x-ray and the x-ray on the opposite page. Notice the superior aspect of the vertebral bodies. On this x-ray they show only a slight "dishing" on their lateral edges, indicating very deficient joints of Luschka. All extremes and various degrees in between are found. The author's research indicates that individuals with large and steep joints of Luschka are difficult to adjust. The spinous pull move and the posterior cervical thrust (Chapter IX) are more easily accomplished.

JOINTS OF LUSCHKA

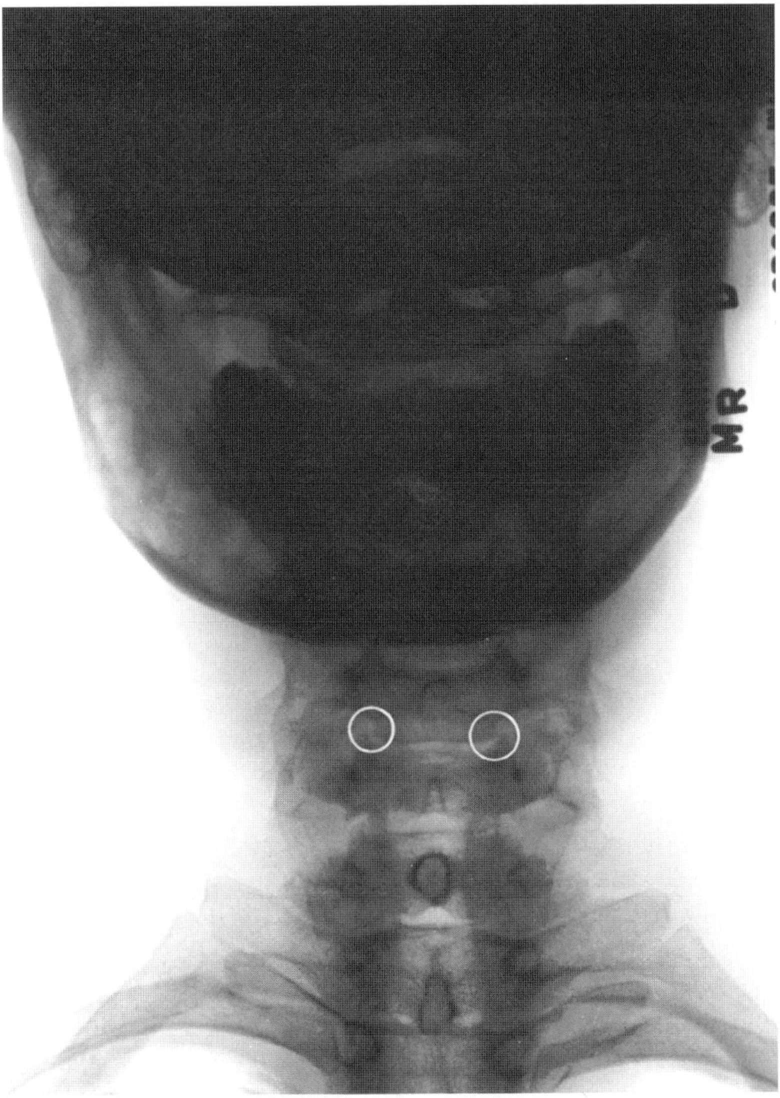

(Ill. VIII-2) The fully developed, steeply inclined joints of Luschka exhibited on this x-ray contribute to lateral vertebral stability. Notice your x-ray when you have a case that is difficult to adjust cervically. You will usually find such joint development. In the author's opinion, cervical spines thus equipped would be less prone to traumatic subluxation.

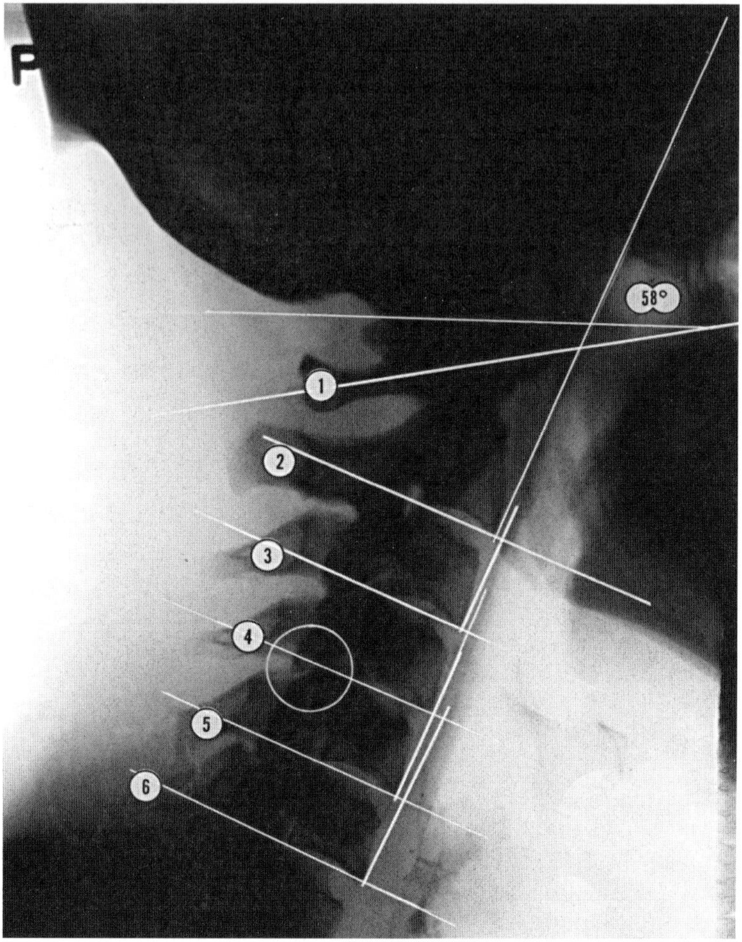

(ILL. VIII-3) The facet joints are surrounded by a capsular ligament. This ligament has some laxity and its fibers are optimally orientated to provide for a specific range of motion, but it will not withstand the stretch stress caused by the constant malposition of the torticollis subluxation without considerable inflammation and pain. As explained before, the facets are synovial joints and the capsular ligaments are synovial membranes capable of illiciting much pain upon stress. The author contends that capsulitis (caused by the malposition of the subluxated vertebra's separating the facets) plus the concomitant nerve root compression is the major cause of pain in all vertebral subluxations. (See page 255)

Stress Factors

The illustrations on the last three pages show the areas of synovial membranes in the cervical spine; namely the facets and the joints of Luschka. The inordinate rotation and lateral tipping of a torticollis (disc block) subluxation causes stretch stress to these membranes.

ROTATION - As the body of the vertebra rotates to the side opposite the nuclear shift, (narrow side of the disc wedge) it separates the facets on the same side. It also stresses the capsule of the joint of Luschka in a rotatory fashion. Now remember, the facets are meant to function in a closed state. The capsular ligaments have some laxity to allow for tipping and rotatory movement, but the constant stress of the torticollis subluxation's *facet separation and fixation* is intolerable, and thus the inflammation and pain. The undue vertebral rotation also compromises the size and shape of the intervertebral foramen on the side of the separated, "open" facet. (narrow side of the disc wedge, the side of convergence).

LATERAL TIPPING - The lateral tipping (caused by the nuclear shift and resultant disc wedge) may also stress the capsular ligament of the facet joint and the joint of Luschka on the wide side of the disc wedge, but this joint is not distracted (open) and the orientation of the capsular fibers allows for motion in this direction (one facet gliding up upon the other) so it is unlikely that this facet's capsular ligament is involved in the pain syndrome. However, the lateral tipping lowers the height of the foramen on the narrow side of the disc wedge and compromises its normal dimension, this in turn may cause nerve root compression.

NERVE ROOT COMPRESSION - On the closed side of the disc wedge, the narrowing and lowering of the height of the foramen, the separation of the facet joint and resultant inflammation results in nerve root compression and pain. Biochemical products of inflammation, turgidity within the foramen, demyelination and malnutrition of the nerve root, may also be implicated in nerve root irritation and pain.*

* See pages 255-273 for more information on nerve root irritation.

LEFT LATERAL TORTICOLLIS
(Posterior View)

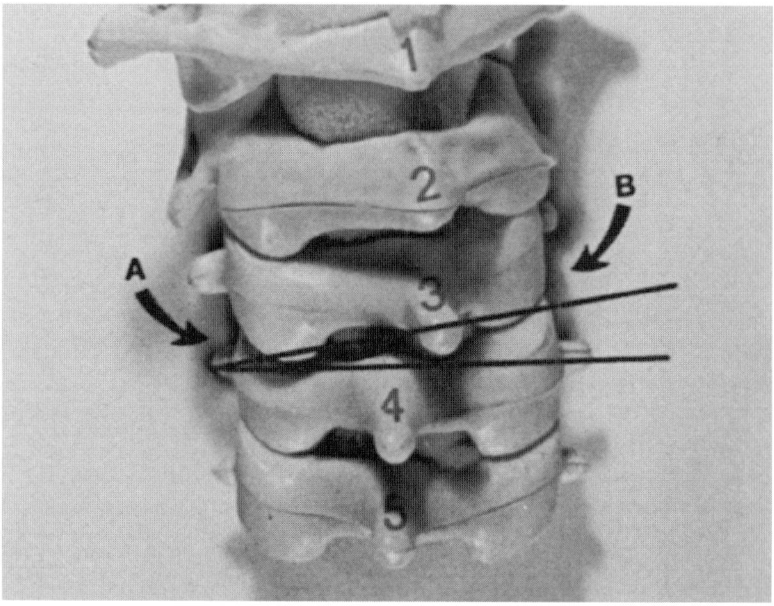

(Ill. VIII-4) Left lateral torticollis subluxation of the 3rd cervical vertebra. The listing of the 3rd cervical is spinous right, body left. (PRS Gonstead) The body rotation is away from the wide side of the disc wedge in relation to the 4th cervical. The facet of C 3 is "open" on the left. (A)

The nuclear shift, resultant tipping and rotation of the involved vertebra does not separate the facet on the open side of the disc wedge. It allows this facet to glide up upon its inferior partner. (B) The rotation of the vertebra away from the wide side of the disc wedge separates the facet on the opposite side, (open facet) (A). With the nucleus of the disc shifted to the right, the vertebra above has lost its fulcrum of support producing the vertebral locking I describe as the disc block subluxation. Feature the constant stress - also the muscle fatigue going on in the cervical spine. Rigidity sets in to safeguard against ligamentous damage and disc herniation. Only one type of movement will be allowed ... a movement which would close the facet and improve the lateral tipping. A chiropractic vertebral adjustment in this direction brings prompt relief and improved vertebral positioning.

It is important to notice that the facet on the wide (right) side of the disc wedge does not open, but glides up on its inferior partner. (Ill. VIII-4 B) This is the physiological movement that the fibers of the capsular ligament are optimally orientated to tolerate; although at the extreme range of their physiologically permitted limits they too could be involved in the pain syndrome of torticollis. However, palpation of this joint indicates it is less involved than the "open" facet on the side of the narrow disc wedge. It is wise not to pursue palpation of the facets too vigorously, as the aggravation of the pain is not worth the information gained. Palpation of the rotated spinous, along with x-ray, will determine vertebra involved.

LEFT LATERAL TORTICOLLIS
(Anterior View)

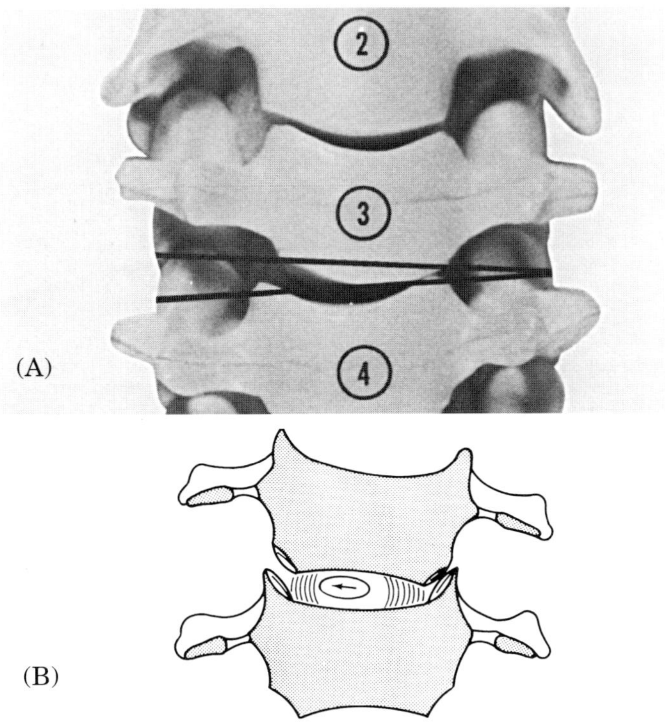

(Ill. VIII-5) An **anterior** view of the same left lateral torticollis shown on page 74 illustrates how the disc wedge is open to the would-be patient's right (A). It can also be noted on illustration (B), that the capsular ligament of the joint of Luschka would be stressed as the joint is separated on the right.

ANTERIOR TORTICOLLIS
(lateral view)

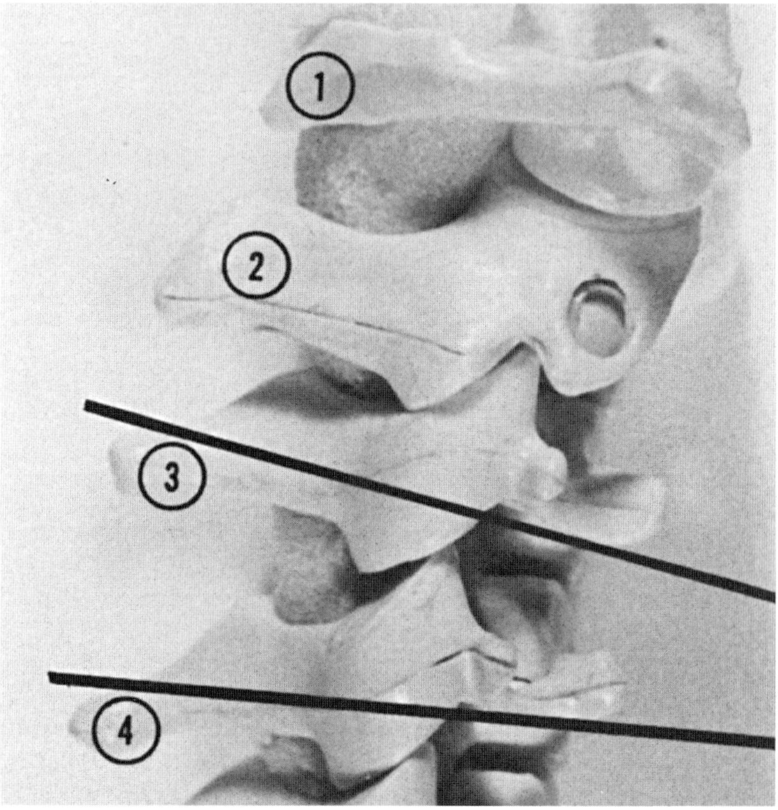

(Ill. VIII-6) This illustration is an example of an anterior torticollis subluxation of the 3rd cervical. Note how the body plane lines converge to the anterior between 3rd and 4th cervical. (see Chapter VII X-ray Analysis). It is clearly seen how the facets are separated between 3rd and 4th cervical. Notice that the 3rd cervical vertebra has also moved anterior. This plastic specimen exaggerates this involvement BUT anterior displacement is commonly true. The vertebra rocks anterior on its posteriorly shifted fulcrum (the nucleus). So, along with facet separation on both sides, we **have** a degree of anteriorlisthesis. **When using the posterior cervical thrust adjustment the line of drive must be superior to inferior (S to I) so as not to increase the anterior disrelationship!**

ANTERIOR TORTICOLLIS
(posterior view)

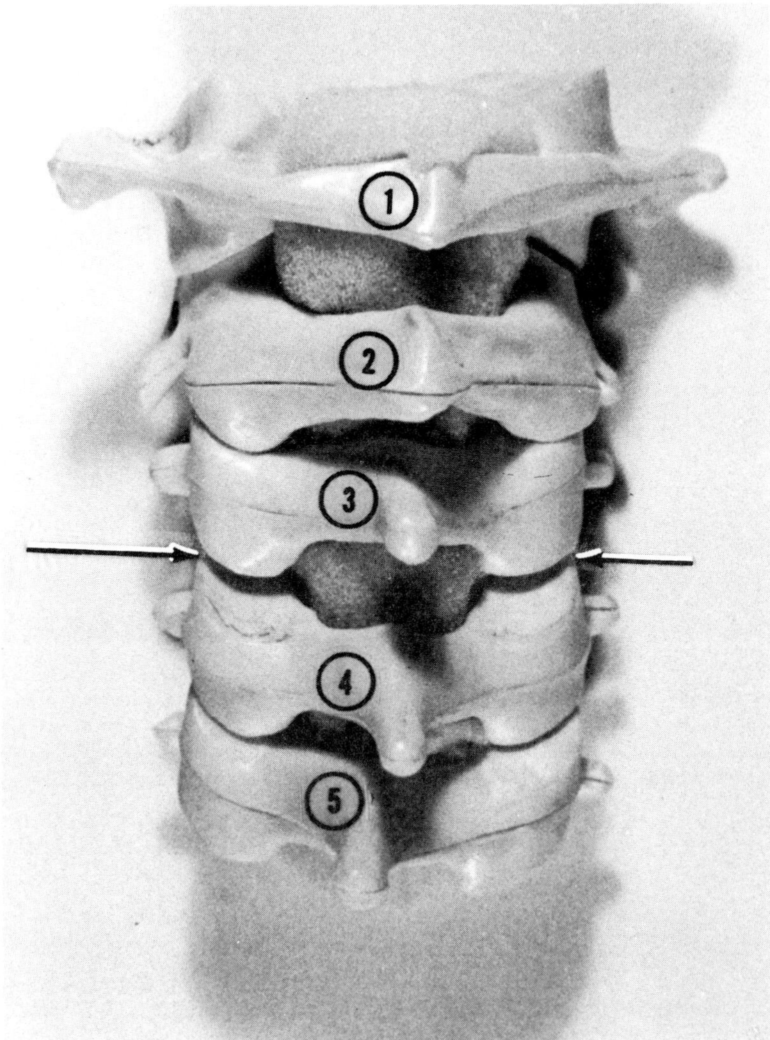

(Ill. VIII-7) This is the posterior view of the same subluxation as on illustration VIII-6. The spinous of the C 3 is superior and the facets between C 3 and C 4 are visibly open on both sides. See (Ill. V-18) page 54 for this same picture with wedge lines and rotational analysis.

ACUTE LEFT LATERAL TORTICOLLIS
Axis Subluxation

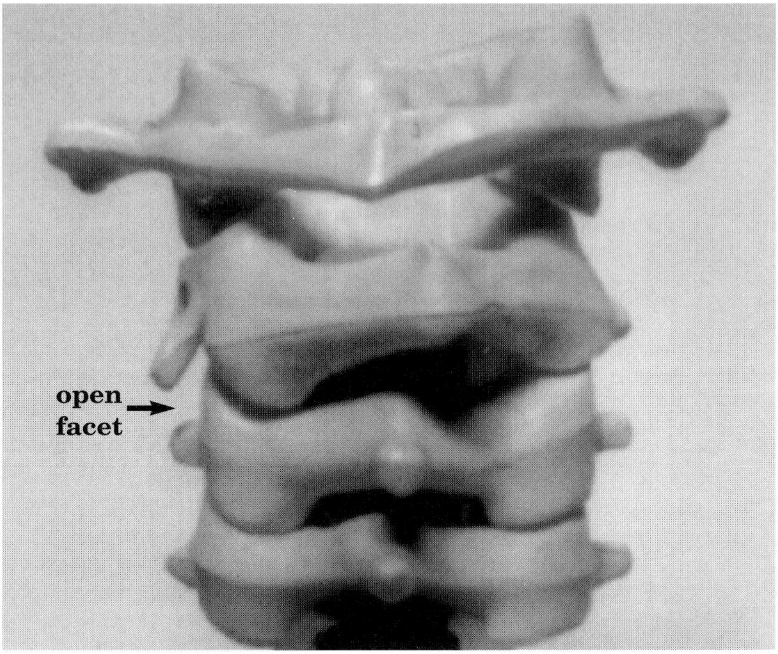

(Ill. VIII-8) I have illustrated above how the Atlas rotates towards the side **opposite** the open facet of Axis, which is involved in a torticollis subluxation. The Atlas listing would be posterior on the right. The Axis would be spinous right. The body of Axis rotates left towards its inferior side and the facet separates between Axis and C 3 on this same side (left). The head (chin and face) **rotate to the right** to ease the stress of the open facet. Atlas rotates posterior on the right in **relationship** to Axis. In my opinion, this is a compensatory rotation and not a subluxation. If you ask the patient to rotate their head further to the right they can usually do this without pain. They cannot, however, rotate their head left, towards the lateral bend, without severe pain as such movement would tend to separate the open facet between Axis and C 3 even more. I contend that the rotation of the face and chin away from the lateral bend is the only part of the torticollis positioning that could properly be termed antalgic. This antalgic rotation produces the Atlas rotation that can be misconstrued as a subluxation!

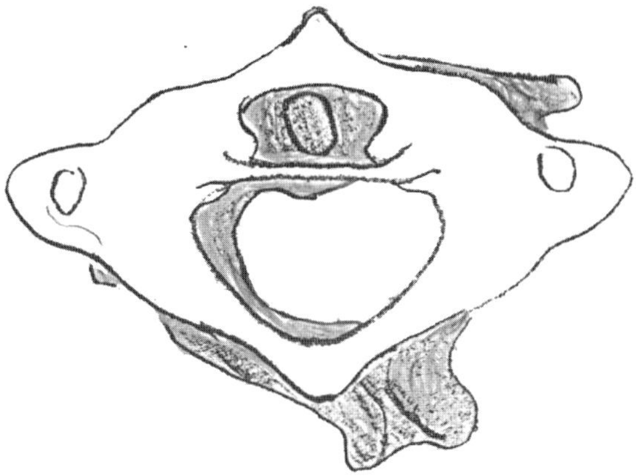

(Ill. VIII-9) With Axis spinous deviated to the right, Atlas rotates right to ease the stress on the open facet between L 3 and Axis on the left. (Ill. VIII-8, opposite page).

The pain of torticollis, in my opinion, is in the swollen articular membranes of the separated (open) facet joint of this subluxation. (Ill. VIII-8) Painful reflex muscular tensions follow as observed by Schmorl and Junghans. These muscular tensions attempt to hold the head erect and they are responsible for the head and face being turned **away from** the lateral head. This is an attempt to ease the strain on the capsular ligament of the open facet. This turning of the head (face and chin) away from the lateral bend is accomplished by the rotation of the Atlas on Axis. So the Atlas is rotated posterior on the side opposite the lateral bend.* In my opinion it **is not subluxated** but rotated to ease the pain of the open facet between Axis and C 3 on the concavity of the curve. This rotation could be termed antalgic. It is, however, the only antalgic part of the tortuous positioning of torticollis. Nerve root encroachment may in rare instances cause true muscle spasm in torticollis and this can be brought on by excessive palpation of the swollen capsular ligament. Pressure on this ligament can extend its turgid mass forward into the foramina thus irritating the nerve and causing the spasm. As I have said before and it bears repeating, the muscle tension and contracturing is not the cause of the problem, **it is the result**. The result of the mechanical malposition and nerve root encroachment of the subluxation. The opinions of other authors to the contrary have not altered my opinion, the cause of torticollis is a subluxation.

* in its relationship to Axis

The Disc Block Subluxation

The author contends that the disc block subluxation and its resultant articular lock is the cause of torticollis as it is the cause of tortipelvis in the lumbar spine. In these two acute spinal conditions *we **are not** dealing with an antalgic position* ... a position for relieving pain. The patient is not assuming this posture because it is more comfortable; the patient is locked in this position due to the nuclear shift involved in the subluxation. The nucleus has shifted to one side preventing the return of proper vertebral alignment: a disc block subluxation. In torticollis the rotation of the head away from the side of the lateral bend of the neck is the only part of the patient's position that can reasonably be assumed to be antalgic, as this rotation would tend to ease the stress of the capsular ligament on the narrow side of the disc wedge. It is opposite the body rotation of the subluxated vertebra and thus would ease the capsular stress.

In my opinion the tortuous tipping of the head and neck could not be the result of a disrelationship between Atlas and Axis alone. The extent of the lateral tipping of the head is commonly quite extreme and either the entire neck would be involved or a distinct disc wedge below the Axis would be necessary to create the acute lateral bend. My research to date indicates the latter to be true. So, I contend that the cause of the "acute list" (listing to one side) of torticollis is a subluxation between two vertebrae that share a disc. The subluxation of torticollis is most often found at Axis with C 3 and C 4 not infrequently involved. The segment involved tips due to a shifting of the nucleus of the disc to one side. The **body** of the vertebra above the disc wedge rotates towards its low side (H. B. Logan rule) and separates the facet (open facet) on this same side putting stretch stress on its capsular ligament. To ease the strain on the capsular ligament the head and face turn to the opposite side. This is accomplished by a rotation of the Atlas on the Axis to the side opposite the lateral bend and this is the typical position seen in the torticollis victim (Ill. Intro-1). This peculiar posture has been reported being observed by physicians going back into the 19th century. This Atlas rotation on the Axis can be construed by some to be a subluxation. However, there is no articular locking or fixation in this articular positioning. The patient can readily turn their head to the side it is facing quite pain free and this requires a freely moving Atlas. BUT, they cannot turn their head toward the opposite side (the side of lateral bend) without severe pain. Turning the head the way that it is facing, toward the opposite side of the lateral bend, would ease the stress on the capsular ligament of the (open) subluxated facet. However, rotating it toward the side of the lateral bend is painful if not impossible. This motion would aggravate the stretch stress of the articular capsule surrounding the open facet of the subluxated vertebra, Axis or below.

Pain conclusions

The subluxation in itself is not painful, the stress that it applies to the surrounding ligaments, tendons, muscles, and neurological structures is the cause of the pain. In determining these pain areas we should focus our primary attention on the synovial membranes of the vertebral facet joints. They are, as I've said before, irrefutably capable of eliciting much pain upon stress. Chiropractors historically have palpated these sore spots on the spine. The patient often exclaiming, "that's it Doc, how did you know it was there?" Yes, we've always been able to lay our hands upon the spine and locate these inflamed facet capsules. Many instruments, too numerous to mention, followed the development of the Neurocalometer by B. J. Palmer. All of these instruments were able to read the heat elicited by the inflamed capsular membranes (capsulitis). As reported in my text, TORTIPELVIS[16], surgery was developed and used by Dr. S. Rees to denervate the capsular ligaments, thus eliminating the pain of the subluxation. The brilliant neurosurgeon and author, Dr. C. Norman Shealy, advanced this technic to the point where today he merely injects phenol to denervate the capsules thus eliminating the use of a knife. Both surgeons, through their research, have indicated that the major pain of the subluxation is due to stress on the capsular ligament of the facet joint. This surgery, to my knowledge, has not been performed in acute torticollis, it is my understanding that it has mainly been used in chronic low back and cervical syndromes that often display neurological symptoms. It is also interesting to note that as the result of this surgery, neurological symptoms such as sciatica and brachialgia often disappear. Remember now, they have not changed the position of any vertebra. What then has caused the nerve irritation that produced the neurological symptoms?

Today it is well recognized that inflammatogentic products

from the stressed capsular ligament irritate the nerve root. The swelling of the articular capsule also alters the dimensions of the intervertebral foramina, undue rotation causes the posterior inferior border of the superior vertebral body to approximate the inferior articular pedicel of the vertebra below further compromising the foraminal dimensions. These multifactorial aspects lead to what is rightly referred to chiropractically as the vertebral subluxation complex. When such subluxations become chronic, radicular pain and nerve root compression syndromes appear. (see pages 255-273) The aforementioned rhizolysis surgery pioneered by Dr. S. Rees and later by Dr. C. Norman Shealy may reduce the capsulitis through denervation and halt the inflammatory process that would irritate the nerve. However, the vertebral malposition remains the same and most certainly pathological consequences will follow. Certainly the more conservative approach of spinal adjustment is to be preferred. Restoring the normal vertebral position removes the causes of nerve root compression and normal function is the result. So, as Hippocrates said, "Look well to the spine for the cause of disease." We must look well to the subluxated facet for the cause of the pain in vertebral subluxations. The painful facet is the **open** facet. The job of the chiropractor is to determine the direction of thrust needed (through x-ray and palpation) to close the **open** facet. That subluxations exist between two segments must not be forgotten by the chiropractor. Correct the malposition, one to the other, before concerning yourself with the acute curvature; even if it calls for adjusting into the concavity of the curve. X-rays taken **after** the correction of the acute subluxation become a necessary part of the patient evaluation to determine the initiating causes of the acute episode and to determine future adjustic considerations to reduce said causes.

The adjustment preferred by the author is a spinous pull move. On the next page, (Ill. VIII-10) you see the classic rotatory involvement found in this subluxation. **The pull move pulls the spinous towards the side of the open facet thus closing it. As the spinous is pulled, the thrust also lifts the vertebra on its inferior side allowing the shifted nucleus to resume its normal central position. The combined "pull" and "lift" releases the articular lock of the subluxation.** This is not the common rotatory cervical **manipulation** wherein the patient's mandible and occiput are used as levers.

This is a **specific** spinous pull **adjustment** that corrects the rotation of the subluxation and also addresses the disc wedge.

AXIS SUBLUXATION TORTICOLLIS

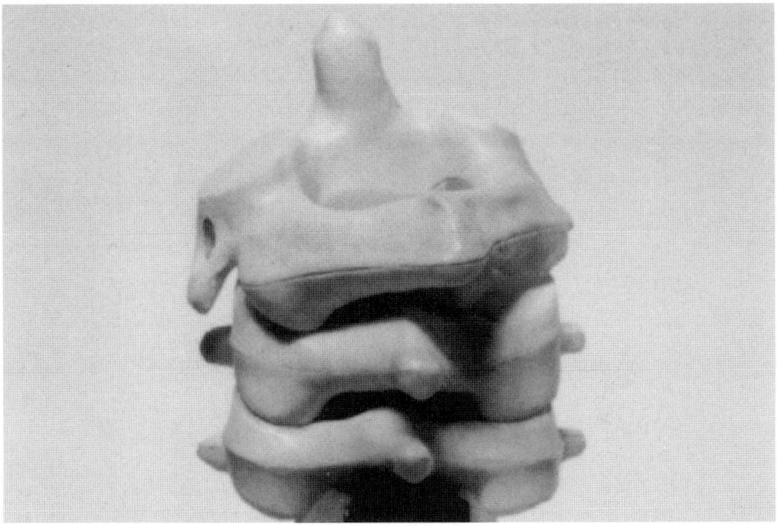

(Ill. VIII-10) On the illustration above, the Axis is rotated body left, spinous right (Gonstead PRS). The facet is separated –"open"– on the left. The spinous pull move, described in the next chapter, pulls the spinous from right to left thus closing the open facet. It is the author's opinion that the swollen capsular membranes and the resultant nerve root irritation, are the major cause of the pain syndrome in torticollis.

The next chapter describes the author's favored adjustments in the correction of this subluxation, but I want to emphasize the point that the adjustment of this subluxation must be specific if you are to gain the results reported in this text. The common rotatory move is, in the author's opinion, a deplorable non-specific manipulatory procedure, the time is past due for such procedures to be dropped from the chiropractor's armamentarium of corrective adjustic technics.

WOODCARVING, TORTICOLLIS

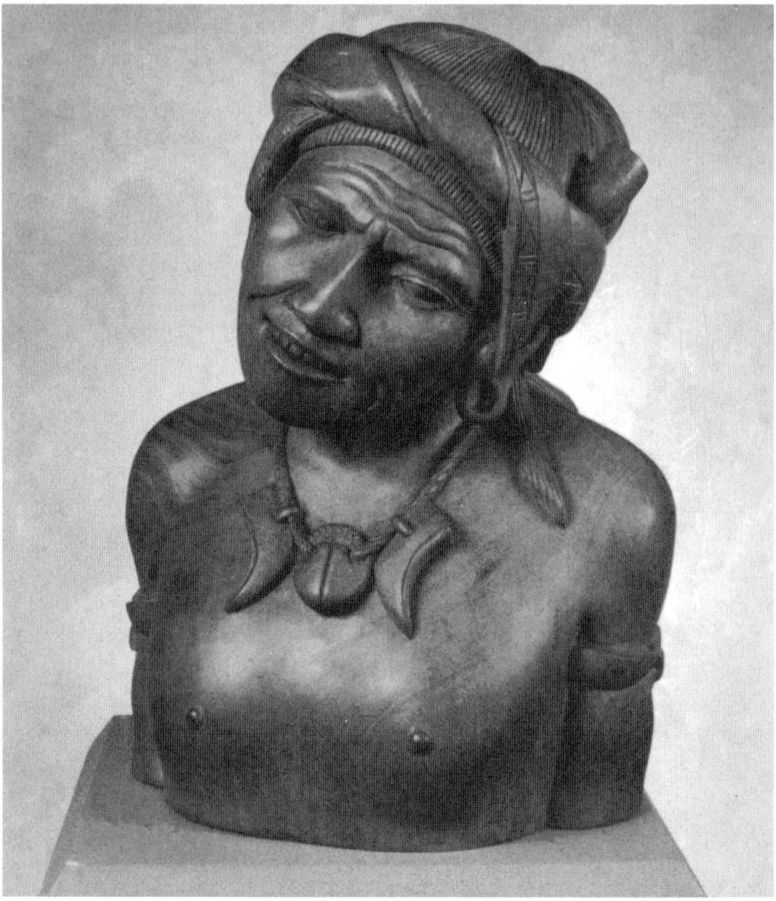

(Ill. VIII-11) The left lateral torticollis displayed on the Bali wood carving above, could well be caused by the subluxation illustrated on the next page.

The anguished face of the victim of torticollis, portrayed on the Bali bust above is a fitting end to this discussion on the pain of torticollis. The reader, by now, should thoroughly understand the mechanical misalignment of this disc block subluxation. The adjustic correction must not only consider the rotational factor but the disc wedge and shift of the nucleus pulposes must also be addressed. Read on now as we focus on the adjustic correction of torticollis.

CHAPTER IX
THE ADJUSTMENT

I Lateral Torticollis
II Anterior Torticollis
III Anterior Lateral Torticollis

We will now take examples of acute torticollis subluxations to explain the adjustment.

I Lateral Torticollis

In this subluxation, as explained in previous chapters, a disc wedge will be found creating lateral vertebral tipping. The vertebral body immediately above this disc wedge will be rotated away from the wide side of the disc wedge in relation to the vertebra immediately below.

ACUTE LEFT LATERAL TORTICOLLIS

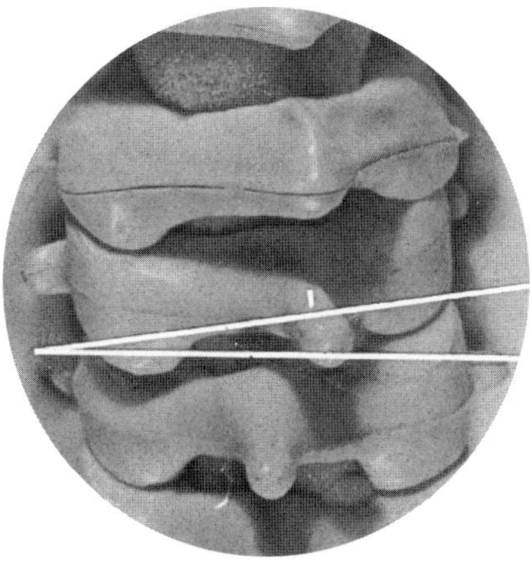

(Ill. IX-1) Left lateral torticollis - 3rd cervical spinous right-body left. The 3rd cervical is tipped inferior on the left, its vertebral body rotates to the left separating the facet joint. The author refers to this as the **open** facet.

On the specimen above notice how the right facet of the 3rd cervical slides up on its inferior partner. This is the wide side of the disc wedge, the side of the nuclear shift. The change of the fulcrum of support has created an inferiority on the left and thus the body of the 3rd cervical rotates to that side. The facets between 3rd and 4th cervical (on the left) are **open** and the joints capsular ligament is under considerable stretch stress.

TYPES OF ADJUSTMENTS

1. **The Spinous Pull and Lift Adjustment**
2. **The Transverse Thrust Adjustment**
3. **The Transverse Thrust Spinous Pull Adjustment**

1. The Spinous Pull and Lift Adjustment

The rationale for the use of this adjustment rather than a direct laminal cervical, or pedicel facet contact thrust, is that it is the least painful of contacts. Any direct contact to the facet area of the involved vertebra is painful, both on the concave and convex side of the lateral bend of the cervical spine. This is due to the acute disc wedge subluxations articular lock causing constant stretch stress to the strained capsular ligaments of the facet joints. The capsular ligament of the facet joint on the wide side of the disc wedge is stressed because the range of motion is at its articular limit. However, this facet joint is not separated and the joint surfaces are pressed firmly together. As a result of the contra-rotation between the two segments, the facets on the narrow side of the disc wedge are separated and the articular capsule is under a marked degree of **stretch stress**. (Ill. IX-3) This is the subluxated facet.

With the patient sitting let us analyze the subluxation in regards to the malposition of the facets. For example, in left lateral torticollis, the patient cannot tip his/her head to the right due to the nuclear shift creating a physiological lock (disc block subluxation). If you ask the patient to rotate his/her head to the right, they can usually do this in limited fashion as this movement would tend to close the separated left facet joint.* But, if you ask the patient to rotate their head to the left, it causes more pain as it separates the facets on the left side even more.

So, with the position of the patient's head tipped to the left, the patient can rest their head with reasonable comfort in the adjustor's right hand (Ill. IX-2). Tell the patient that you will not rotate their head in the painful way, but only in the way they can turn it (right). The spinous pull contact is not painful, and the pull of this contact will reduce the rotation of the segment and close the open (separated) facet. With the pull, the adjustor's hand lifts the segment up on the inferior side thus allowing for the nucleus to assume a more central position. The articular capsule on the convexity of the curve is also relieved of stress. The combination of the pull and lift effectively reduces the subluxation and often produces an instantaneous relief of

*Remember the patient's head is already turned somewhat away from the lateral bend. This posture is assumed by the patient as it would favor the closing of the facet joint on the narrow side of the disc wedge.

symptoms. Immediate reduction of the distortion is seen in most cases of torticollis when the adjustment is delivered correctly. The "lift" part of the adjustment comes into play near the end of the rotary pull. The finger contact on the spinous process first pulls down upon it; but as the thrust progresses it pulls it through an arc until at the end of the thrust it is lifting the spinous process up.

THE SPINOUS PULL AND LIFT CONTACT

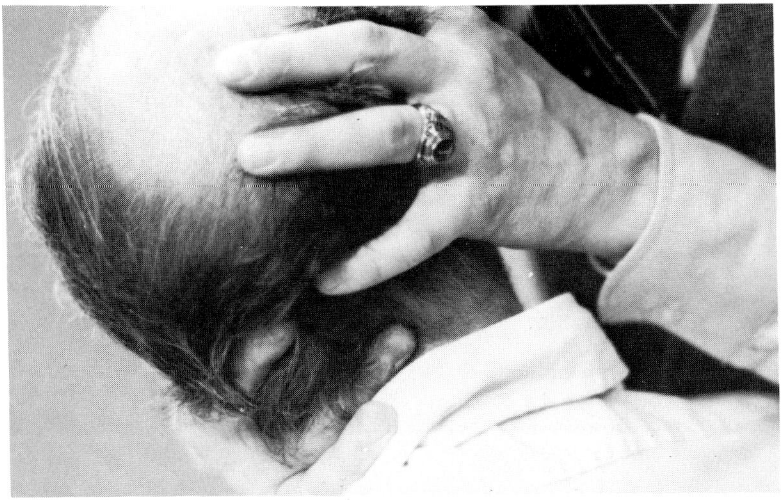

(Ill. IX-2) The Spinous Pull and Lift contact, left lateral torticollis. The adjustor's finger tip, nail point 5, (page 93) wraps around and grips the spinous of the subluxated vertebra. The palm of the same hand supports the weight of the patient's head; this allows the cervical musculature to relax.

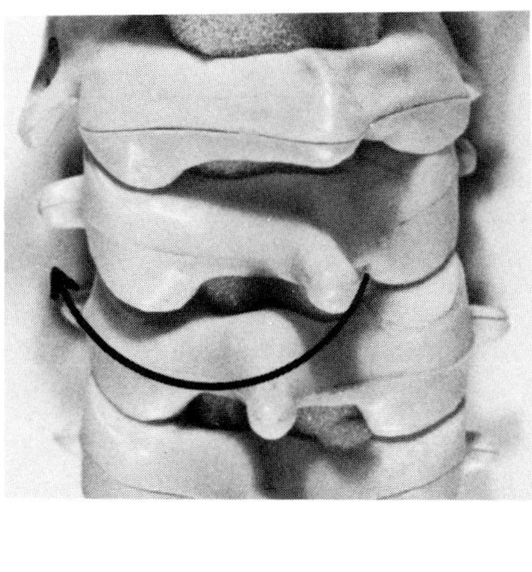

(Ill. IX-3) The arrow indicates the line of drive of the thrust. The pull is actually a directional arc that pulls the spinous process laterally to close the facet, and then lifts the vertebra to close the disc wedge. It could be described as a scooping type motion.

THE SPINOUS PULL AND LIFT STANCE
Lateral Torticollis

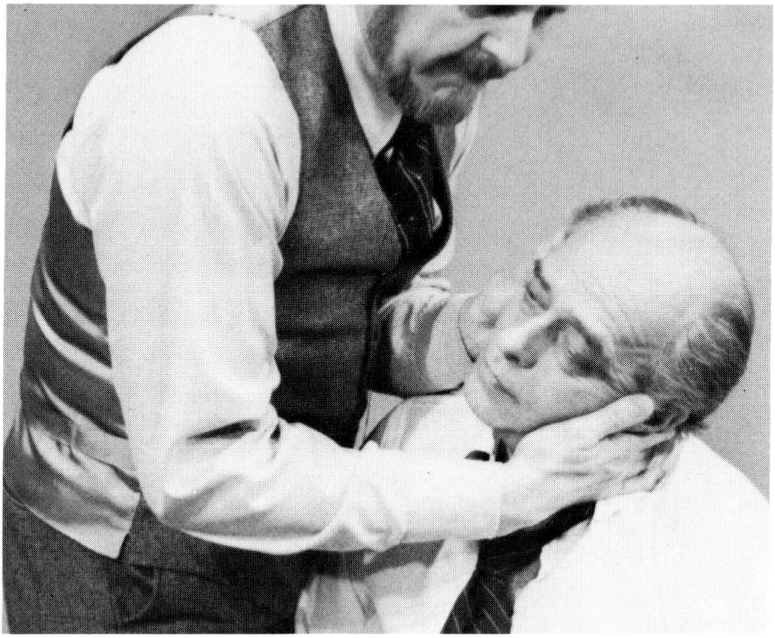

(Ill. IX-4) The patient is told, "press your head into my hand." To make sure the patient understands which hand you mean, tap the patient's head with the free pointer finger of your adjusting hand. This also takes the patient's mind off the situation and helps in the relaxation of the cervical spinal muscles. Remember they are **not** in spasm but are only under a splinting type contraction endeavoring to hold the head erect. Once the patient really allows you to support their head, there is an immediate reduction in the muscle tension. The doctor's adjusting arm must be free to move through an arc. The stance must be one that allows quick reflex movement ... speed in this adjustment is very important and **do not recoil!** When the adjustment is completed (Ill. IX-5 C) allow your grip on the patient's head and neck to relax allowing them to accept the lack of your support gradually. This is what I mean by **no recoil**, do not release the head and neck instantaneously, slowly release your support of the patient's cervical spine. As I said before, oft times the torticollis position is entirely gone or at least greatly reduced immediately after the adjustment.

THE SPINOUS PULL AND LIFT THRUST
Lateral Torticollis

PRESS A

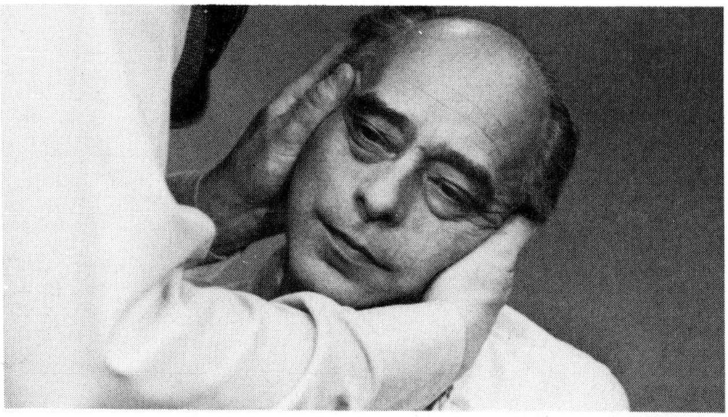

PULL B

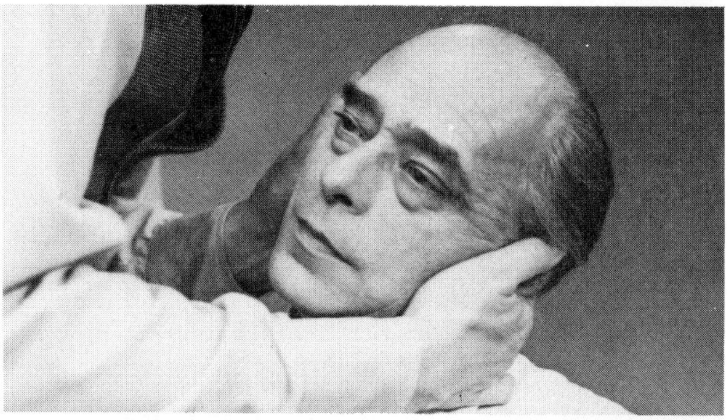

LIFT C

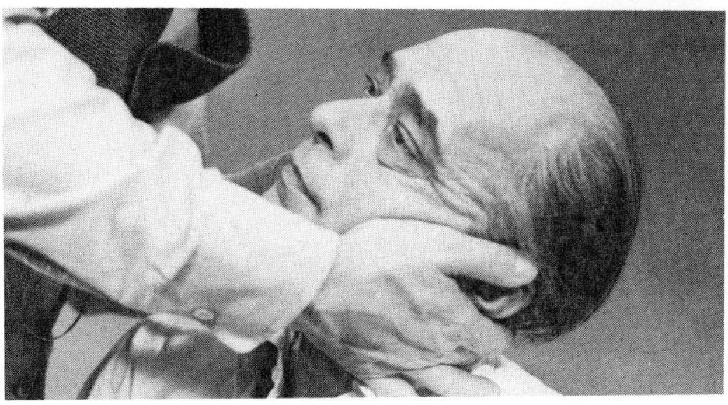

(Ill. IX-5) The patient will be able to lay their head comfortably in the doctor's hand, (A) as this is the side the head and neck are bent to. With a little persuasive talk the patient will actually let the weight of their head fall into the doctor's hand and **this relaxed state is imperative for the adjustment** to be made possible. In

the case of an unusually tense patient, ask him/her to press their head into your hand and immediately upon feeling the pressure initiate the thrust. Pull the spinous laterally to close the facet (B), lift the vertebra up to close the disc wedge (C).

2. The Transverse Thrust Adjustment

We will now describe and explain the transverse contact and thrust for the same left lateral torticollis. The disc wedge is open to the right, the nucleus is shifted from its central position to the right creating the lock or disc block subluxation. The vertebral body immediately above this disc wedge is rotated away from the wide side of the disc wedge in relation to the vertebra immediately below. This rotation opens the facet on the left. The adjustor's thrust must close the facet and improve the rotary malposition. The force must also raise the vertebra up on the inferior side to allow the nucleus pulposus to draw back towards its (proper) central position. This contact is more painful as it necessitates contacting the area of facetal swelling and inflammation. Try to stay off the facet and on to the transverse process. This contact can be made with the thumb or with the lateral aspect of the index finger - see Ill. IX-7 and IX-8 for a description of each contact.

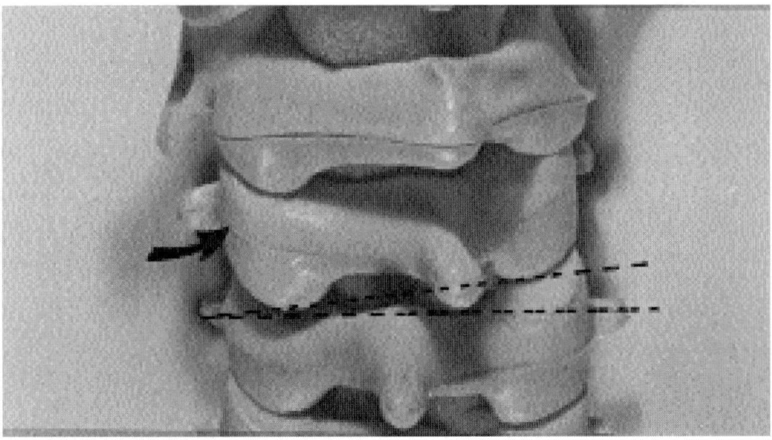

(Ill. IX-6) The thrust must close the facet - thus the line of drive must be from P to A. Near the end of the thrust the vertebra should be lifted up on its inferior side (the narrow side of the disc wedge) as the arrow indicates.

THE TRANSVERSE CONTACT
Left Lateral Torticollis

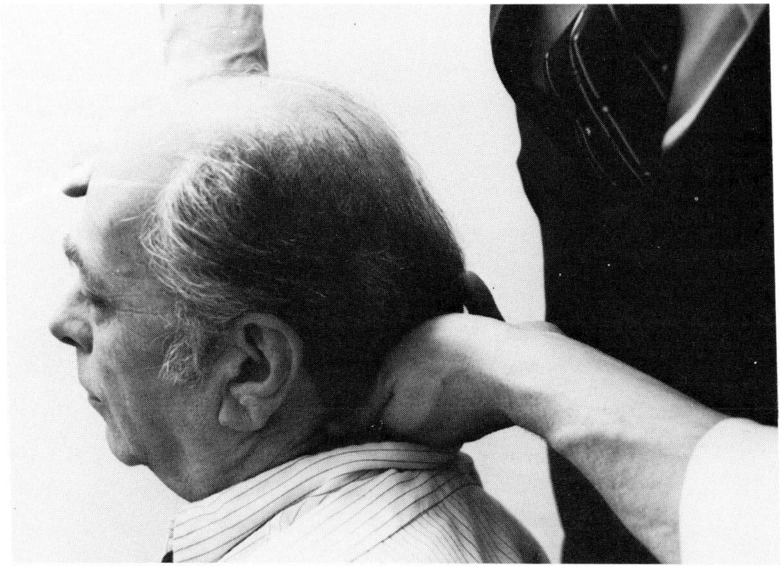

(Ill. IX-7) Thumb Contact (nail point 9).

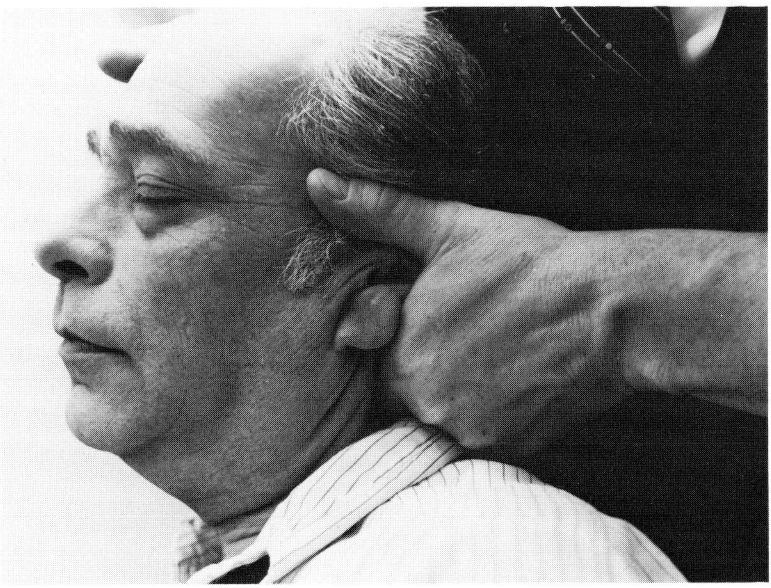

(Ill. IX-8) Index Finger Contact (nail point 7).

THE TRANSVERSE CONTACT, STANCE AND THRUST
Left Lateral Torticollis

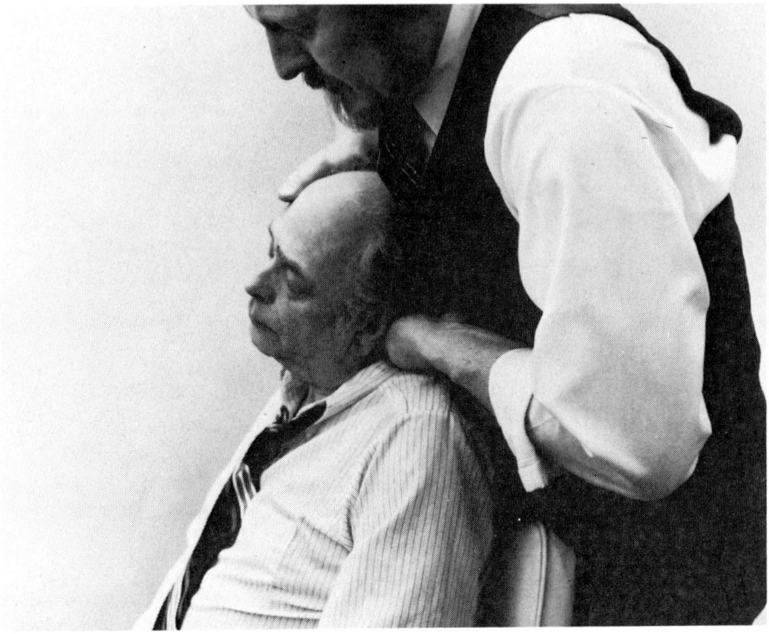

(Ill. IX-9) If at all possible the patient should rest their head in the adjustor's nail (adjusting) hand, if the patient can rest his/her head against the adjustic hand (or the doctor's chest) it is easier for them to relax. In the illustration above the doctor is supporting the patient's head against his chest. The author's cervical chair can be leaned back and raised (hydraulic or electric) so the adjuster can deliver the inferior to superior line of drive necessary in this adjustment. The rotation of this subluxation **plus the inferiority** must be addressed. The adjusting arm's elbow should be lower than the vertebra to be adjusted. The objective is to close the open facet and lift the vertebra up in one smooth scooping action. High velocity is a necessity.

For a doctor who is tall, the ability to raise the cervical chair is an important consideration. The Lloyd Table Company produces Dr. Barge's cervical chair. Again, I must emphasize, **never recoil** in **any** adjustment given in torticollis. The rule is hold the final position for a moment and then **softly,** slowly remove your support.

THE TRANSVERSE THRUST

The art of delivering this thrust is commonly taught in most technics in the chiropractic profession. It is variously known as the T.M. (thumb move), thumb thrust, the Gonstead Thumb Thrust, etc. I would have to believe it is as old as chiropractic itself and early on it had the unfortunate name of the Cervical Break Adjustment. It is very difficult to show this thrust in a sequence of pictures. The action of the doctor's "nail" hand drives the facet from P. to A. (closing it) and then lifts the vertebra up on this same side to reduce the disc wedge thus allowing the nucleus to return to its normal central position.

In this text I have often used the terms "nail hand" and "nail point." I know I am using old Palmer vernacular and can be accused of using antiquated terms; however, this terminology is unique to our profession, it was developed by our founding fathers. A mark of any profession of real substance is the existence of its own lexicon, and I feel we should cherish and retain our own rather than parrot that which has been developed by others. Besides that, naming the anatomical location of each hand contact is cumbersome indeed and thus a numerical classification **is** appropriate. Below I have reproduced a chart known as contact points - nail points. Throughout the text I will refer to this chart in regards to contacts. For those not familiar with the term "nail hand," it simply refers to the hand that makes the contact in the spinal adjustment.

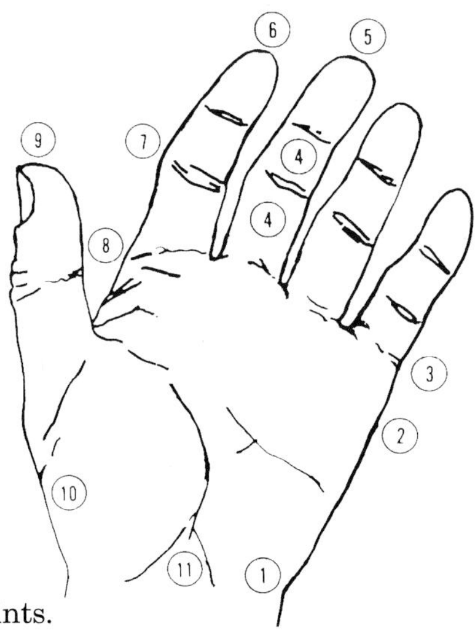

(Ill. IX-10) Nail Points.

3. The Transverse Thrust Spinous Pull Adjustment

This is actually a combination of a thrust and pull adjustment. With palm up, the adjustor's finger (nail point 6) pulls the spinous, the thumb (nail point 9) contacts the transverse area, as the thrust is delivered it must **scoop up** the vertebra to give the lift necessary for nuclear repositioning. Individual capabilities and dexterity of the adjusting doctor must always be kept in mind. It is folly for some to try to absolutely mimic the adjustic thrust of another doctor. Various contacts and thrusts are described in this text. I have used them all with good success in torticollis.

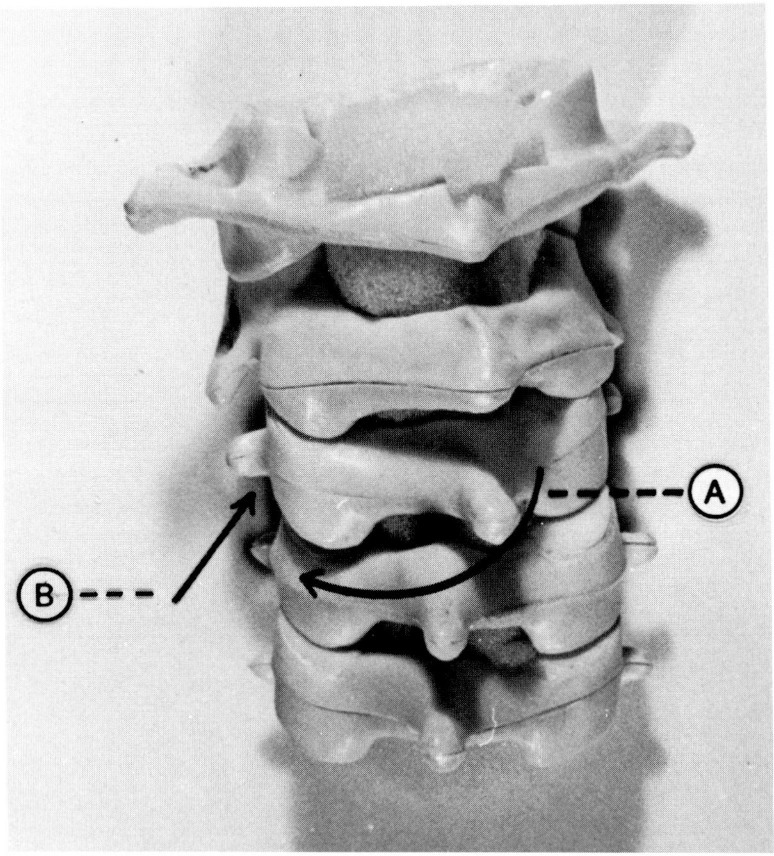

(Ill. IX-11) Arrow (A) indicates the finger contact - arrow (B) the thumb contact. Nail point 6 and nail point 9 respectively.

The Transverse Thrust Spinous Pull Contact
Left Lateral Torticollis

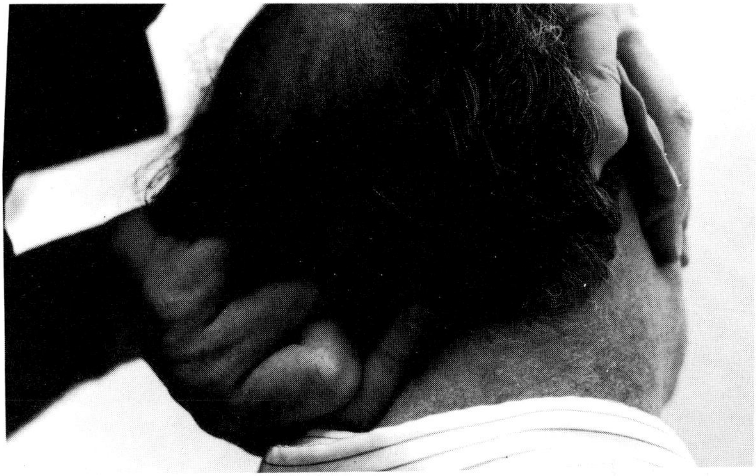

A

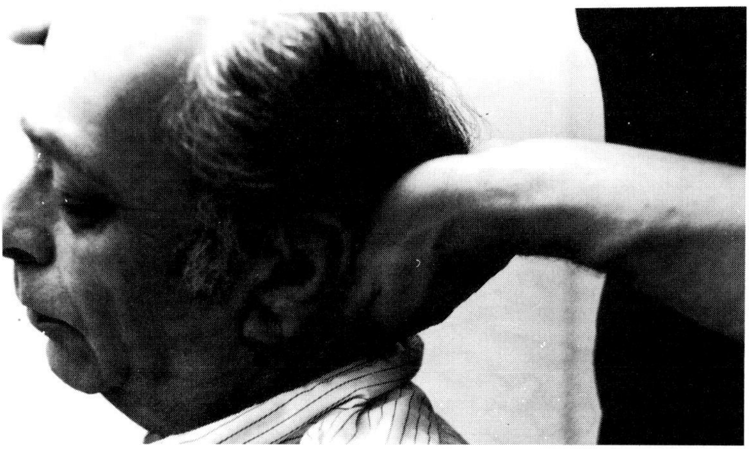

B

(Ill. IX-12) The palm of the adjusting hand is supporting the head, the index finger pulls the spinous, (A) the thumb contacts the transverse process (B). A combination of contacts very effectively used by many D.C.s. The thumb helps close the facet, the finger first pulls the spinous laterally, but then lifts it up to eliminate the disc wedge. This lift draws the nucleus back into its normal central position in the disc space and frees the "block" it has created in its lateral malposition. Be sure to get "under" this thrust, it must lift the subluxated vertebra up at the end of the adjustment; and again **no recoil** - release slowly.

THE TRANSVERSE THRUST SPINOUS PULL STANCE AND ADJUSTMENT
Left Lateral Torticollis

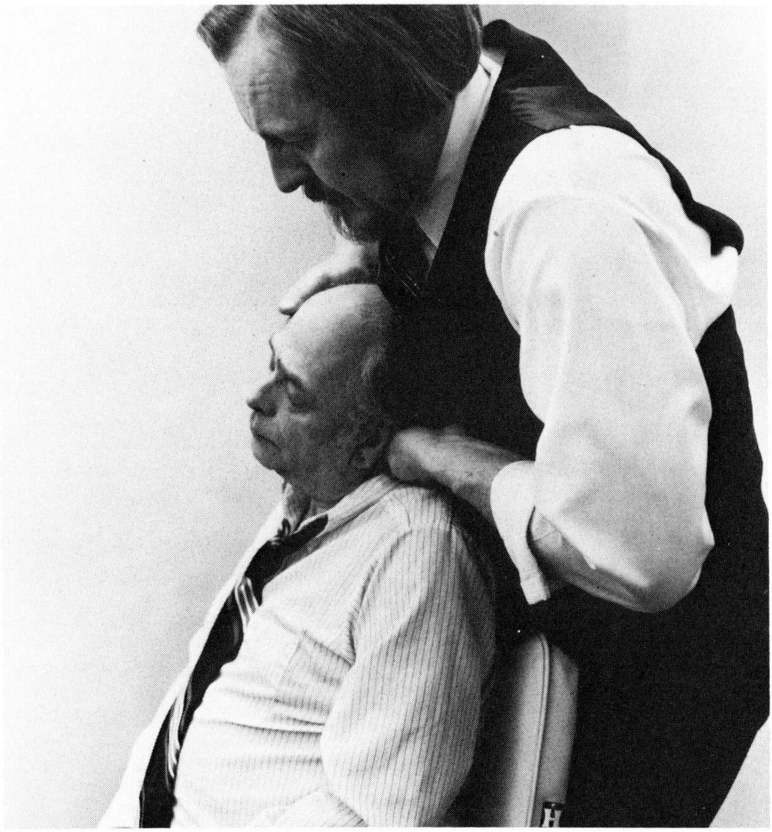

(Ill. IX-13) The doctor is in back of the patient and somewhat on the side of the patient's head tilt. The patient is told to rest their head in the doctor's adjusting hand. Tell them to press their head into your hand and when you feel them do so initiate the thrust. Speed is necessary, this is the so-called high velocity thrust.

As mentioned before, a cervical chair that can be raised up facilitates the doctor's comfortable stance as the adjusting hand's elbow should be **below** the articulation to be adjusted. You must close the facet and **lift** the vertebra **up** on the inferior side of the disc wedge. After the thrust **do not** release the patient's head quickly, **there is no recoil in this adjustment!**

THE TRANSVERSE THRUST SPINOUS PULL ADJUSTMENT

Left Lateral Torticollis

PRESS

A

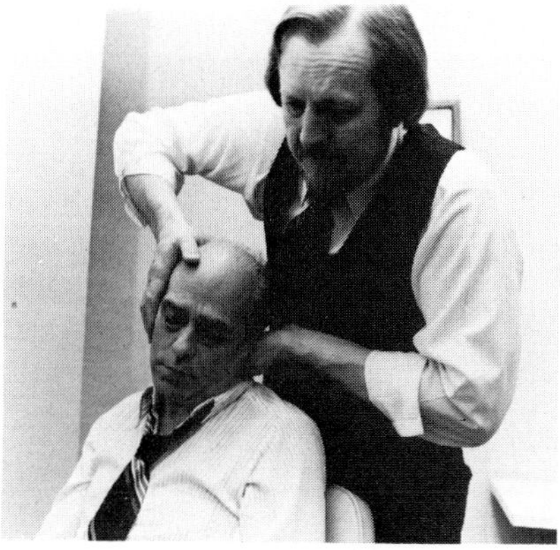

PULL

B

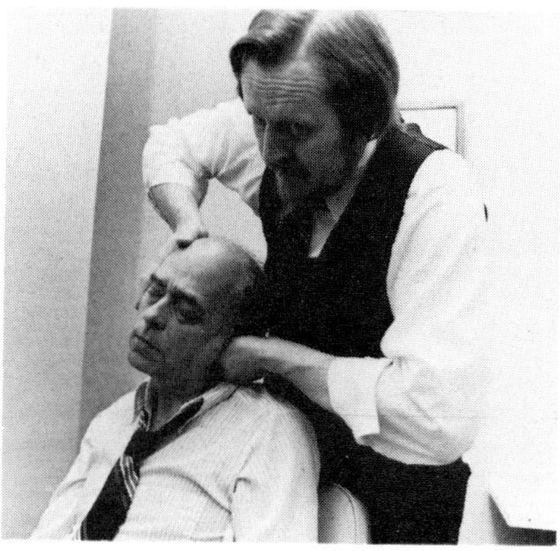

LIFT

C

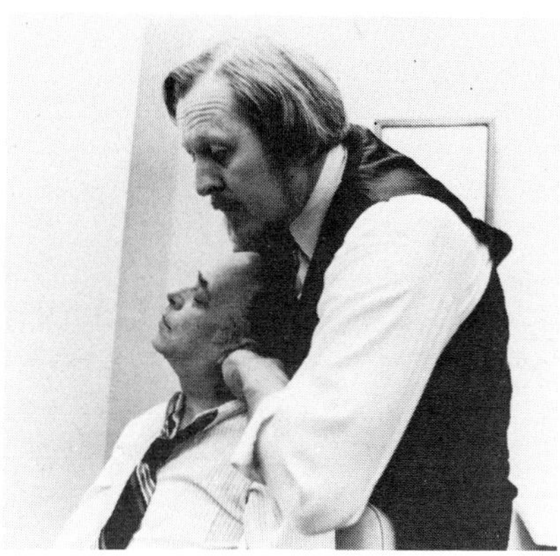

(Ill. IX-14) The patient's head should rest in the doctor's adjusting hand. This is quite easy to accomplish as the doctor's hand can be palmed up against the patient's occiput (A). Close the facet (B). Lift the vertebra up to close the disc wedge (C).

II Anterior Torticollis

Now let us turn our attention to the subluxation of anterior torticollis. Four major analytical factors exist in this subluxation.

1. A flat, or reverse wedged, cervical disc.
2. The vertebra immediately above this disc wedge is tipped inferior on its anterior aspect raising its spinous process superiorally.
3. The facet articulations are stressed in an open state due to the malposition of the subluxation.
4. There is a posterior shift of the nucleus pulposa in the disc space creating a disc block subluxation.

ACUTE ANTERIOR TORTICOLLIS

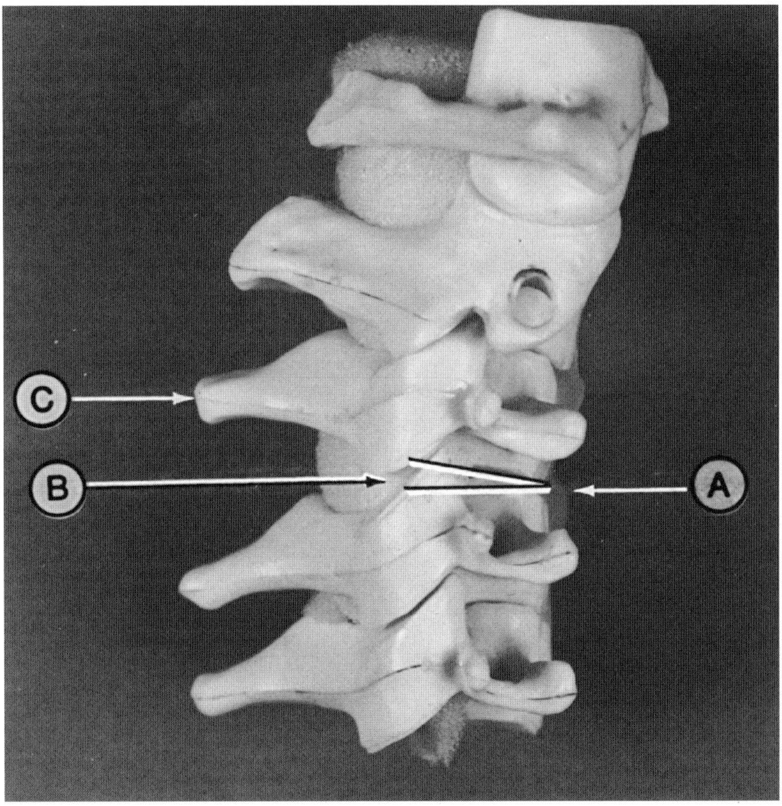

(Ill. IX-15) A - Disc Wedge open to the posterior
B - Open Facet — bilateral
C - Superior Spinous

THE ADJUSTMENT
ANTERIOR TORTICOLLIS

We adjust this subluxation in two different ways:

1. The posterior Cervical Thrust Adjustment (For mild cases of anterior torticollis).
2. The Spinous Pull Adjustment (the preferred adjustment).

Anterior torticollis is simplicity in itself, a one direction subluxation. However, to some chiropractors, this acute disc lesion subluxation's muscular rigidity and evident pain often brings qualms of indecision as to the adjustment. Some are prone to use modalities, heat, and rest to allow time for Innate's adaptation and partial correction of the subluxation; they then will proceed to adjust after the severe, acute phase has passed. This is not advisable as the subluxation may become chronic and more difficult to correct. Why wait when a simple adjustment will bring quick relief and a more speedy, full recovery?

Sometime in the late 1950s, Dr. W. Frederic Keck of Bronx, New York, sent out a descriptive booklet[24] on some of his pet procedures. In this booklet he described a pillow for delivering the posterior cervical thrust.

This writer had experimented with the headpieces of adjusting tables for some time, trying to make them compatible to the posterior cervical thrust. The pillow solved the problem. The pillow is necessary because the adjustable mechanism, and paper roll rod, are not deep and soft enough on most adjusting tables for the amount of the depth used in a posterior cervical thrust. However the pillow developed by Dr. Keck was not very uncomfortable to the patient's neck and larynx.

After much experimentation the author developed a posterior cervical adjustment pillow that facilitates the use of this thrust perfectly.

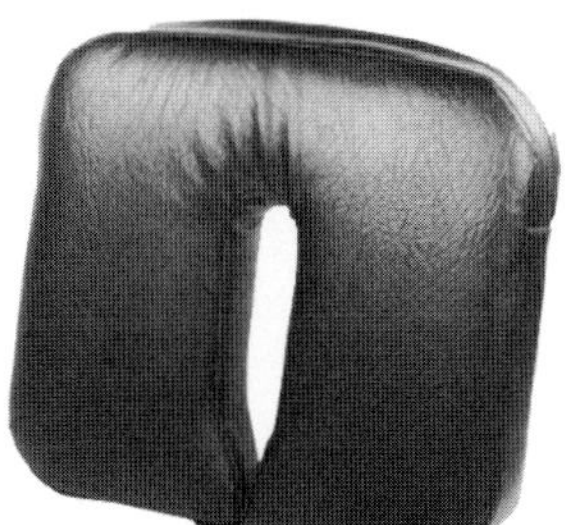

(Ill. IX-16) The Barge Cervical Adjustment Pillow.

The pillow on the above illustration has a center aperture situated differently from the original Keck pillow. The face slot is placed lower down on the pillow so the lower portion of the pillow will not cause discomfort to the anterior aspect of the patient's neck and larynx. If the patient's face is very wide the strap on the bottom of the pillow can be opened to produce a wider face slot. The density of the foam is such that it provides comfort to the patient's face yet is firm enough that when the thrust is delivered the adjustic force is not absorbed by the pillow but moves the vertebra.

1. The Posterior Cervical Thrust Adjustment, Anterior Torticollis

(To be used only in mild cases of anterior torticollis)

Anterior torticollis is indeed a painful condition and most often the patient cannot assume the prone position on the Hi-Lo table or on any prone stationary type adjusting bench. After the acute phase of this condition has been resolved, then the posterior cervical thrust can be applied very constructively to facilitate full correction of the subluxation or subluxations involved in this condition.

The posterior cervical thrust can also be used as a specific P to A and rotational directional adjustment in many other subluxations other than torticollis and will be a useful tool in the chiropractor's armamentarium of specific adjustic thrusts to apply to the subluxations of the cervical spine. I have found it to be indispensable in my own practice and I commonly carry this pillow on my journeys chiropractically as I seem lost without it when called upon to adjust the cervical spine. The line of drive is determined by the lateral x-ray and may be applied from inferior to superior along the plane lines of the facet, or (most commonly) straight P to A or superior to inferior as in the adjustment of anterior torticollis that I will now describe. In this thrust we are endeavoring to drive the spinous of the involved vertebra inferiorly; thus, in torticollis, **the line of drive in this adjustment is from superior to inferior.** In the dynamics of the thrust the kyphotic state of the cervical spine is driven anteriorly, opening the disc space on the anterior; thus allowing the nucleus to return to its normal central position in the disc space.

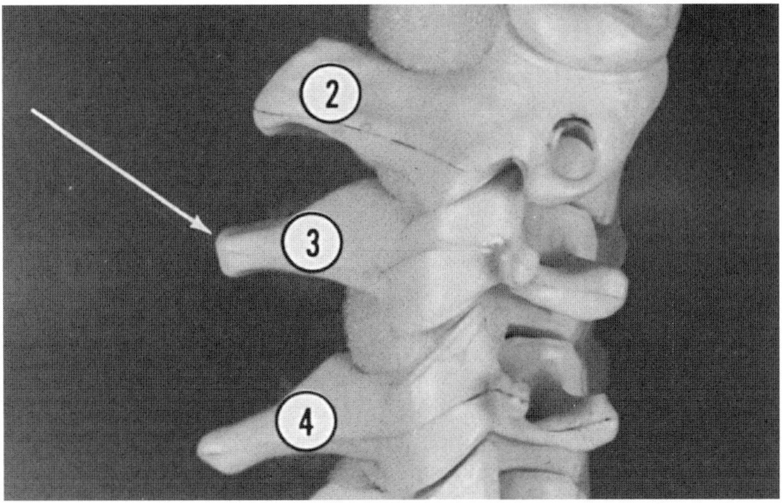

(Ill. IX-17) The arrow indicates the line of drive of the thrust. The contact used by the adjustor can vary. Two that the author has used and taught successfully are shown on page 103.

POSTERIOR CERVICAL THRUST
Patient Position

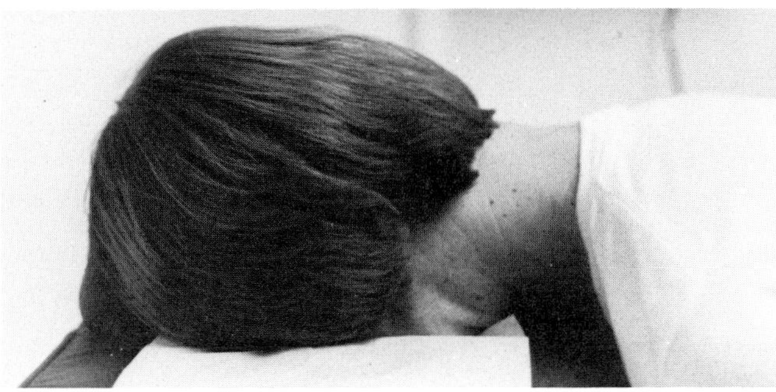

(Ill. IX-18) **The pillow is placed on the headpiece of the Hi-Lo Table and the patient's face placed in the pillow before the table is reclined.** If the patient complains of severe pain going down on the Hi-Lo, **do not use this adjustment.**

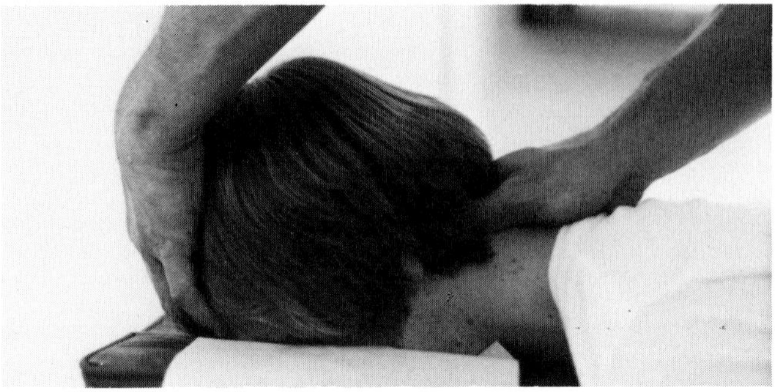

(Ill. IX-19) You cannot successfully adjust this subluxation if the patient retains the chin down posture. Once the weight of the head is relieved from the neck by lying down on the table, the patient can usually raise his/her chin up a bit. By placing one hand under the patient's forehead and the other on the patient's occiput, the doctor may ease the patient's head back and chin up.

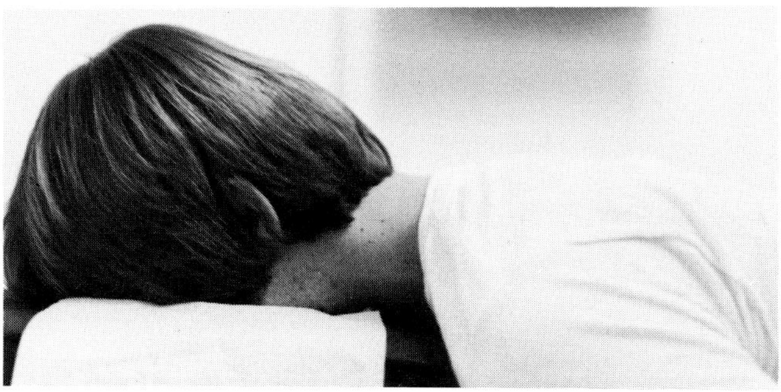

(Ill. IX-20) With the patient's head tipped up so that the cervical spine is at least flat (and not reverse curved) the posterior cervical thrust can be delivered.

POSTERIOR CERVICAL THRUST
Contact

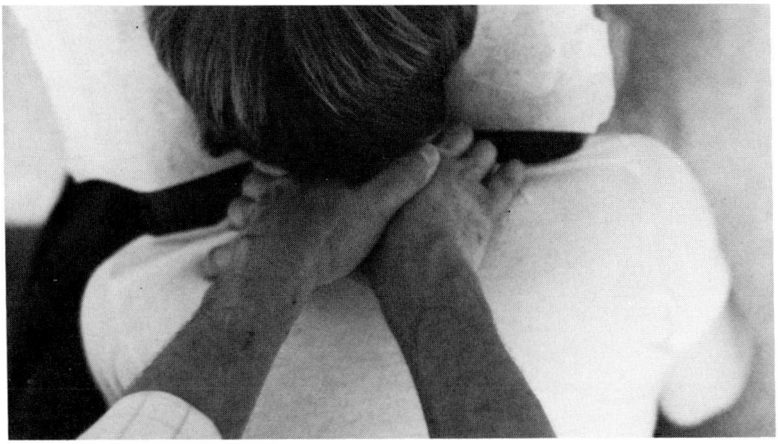

(Ill. IX-21) Hand Contact. This contact is best when some laterality, or rotation, is present in the segment to be adjusted. Either hand can exert more force to add directional correction for laterality and/or rotation. The contact is nail point 8, contacting the lamina on **each side** of the vertebra.

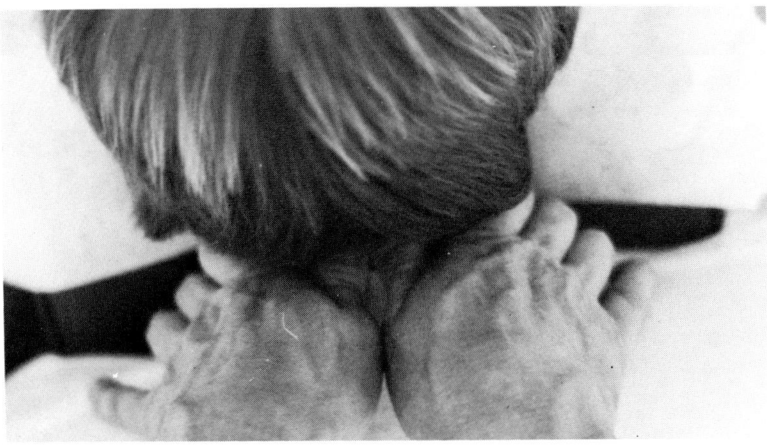

(Ill. IX-22) Thumb Contact. This contact is most effective when straight posterior to anterior line of drive is indicated, or when adjusting a straight posterior vertebra not necessarily torticollis. The contact is nail point 9, directly on the spinous process or on the lamina on **each side** of the spinous process.*

* When rotation is involved in the subluxation, directional force is applied in the thrust to correct the rotation.

THE POSTERIOR CERVICAL STANCE AND THRUST

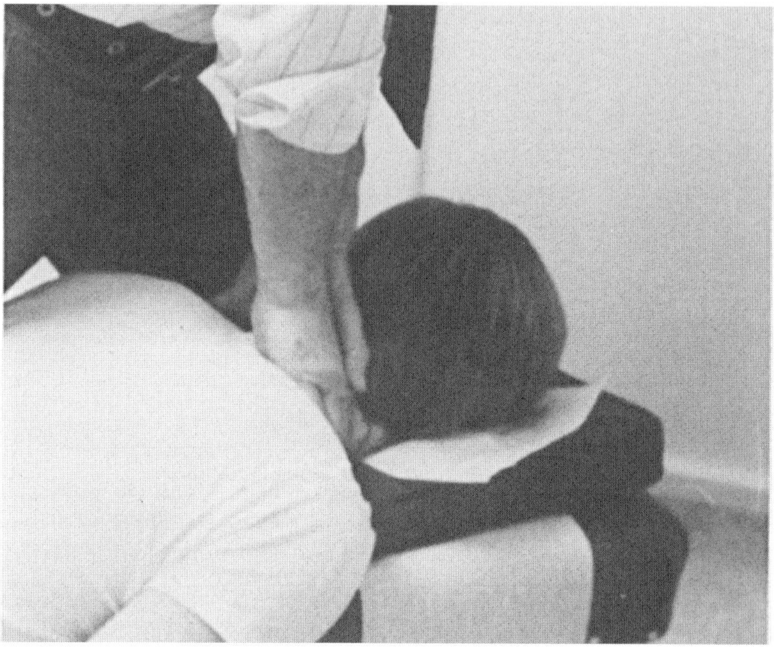

(Ill. IX-23) The stance for this thrust is illustrated above. The contact used here is the hand contact as illustrated on Ill. IX-21. Notice the line of drive is superior to inferior. Let me emphasize here again that rotation of the vertebrae can be addressed by applying more force on the side of vertebral rotation. Nail point 8 contacts the laminae near its pedicel junction and a derotating force can be directionally applied more forcefully on one side than on the other.

By turning a patient's head slightly to the side of spinous process deviation, nail point 8 can actually contact the spinous and the spinous can be used as a lever to correct rotation along with retropositioning. The variable uses of this thrust will become apparent to the chiropractor once he/she becomes proficient in its use. For retrolisthesis alone it is invaluable. It should rarely, however, be used on the Atlas as it would tend to strain the transverse ligament of this vertebra. Lateral x-rays are a must in the determination of the line of drive of the posterior cervical thrust, all spinal adjustments should be specific.

THE POSTERIOR CERVICAL THRUST

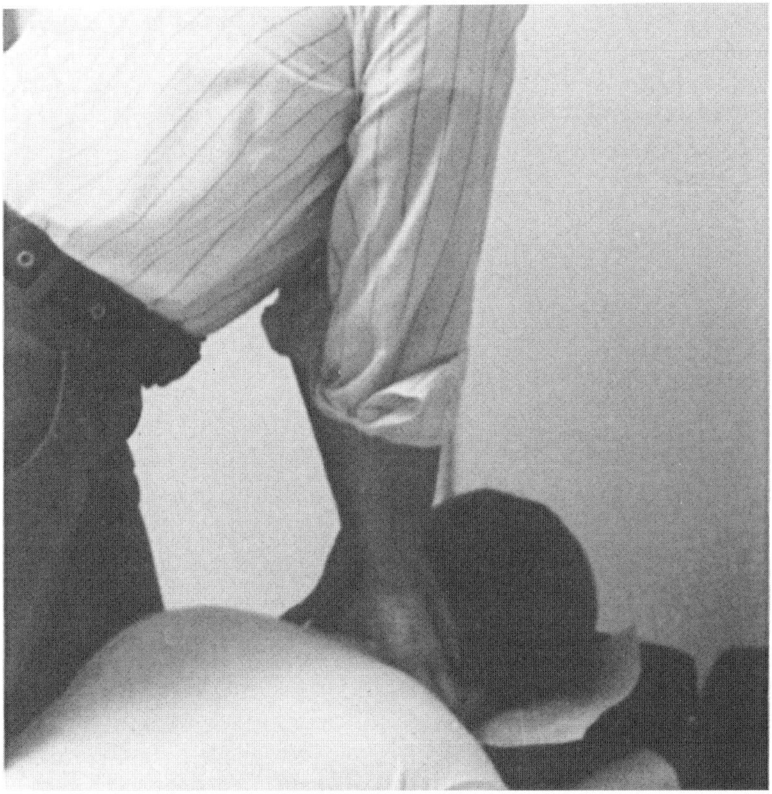

(Ill. IX-24) Notice the doctor's shoulders are dropped somewhat - the elbows are not bent. The thrust is accomplished by a contraction of the pectoralis and triceps combined with a mild body drop. Do not recoil as abruptly as in the toggle recoil, also do not hold at the bottom of the thrust; allow a **slow** recoil to exist thus producing a **soft** return to normal. **If the contact or the initial pressure causes undue pain do not use this thrust in torticollis.** Again I must state that in severe anterior torticollis this thrust **is not** advisable. It is excellent to use once the severe acute subluxation has been reduced by a sitting cervical adjustment. Also, **do not** adjust the vertebra sitting and then immediately thereafter use this thrust, wait a few hours or until the next day to adjust the subluxation again and only if necessary. **It is not a treatment, it it a correction!**

2. The Spinous Pull Adjustment

Severe cases of anterior torticollis simply cannot lie down on the Hi-Lo table due to pain. In these cases, the pull move is very effective, using a spinous pull from posterior to anterior. Ask the patient which side they can best tip their head. If this side is the left, then use the right hand as it will be most comfortable for the patient. If he/she can tip their head easier to the right, then the use of the left hand is called for. Your stance should be from the front of the patient. (Ills. pages 107, 108, 109, 111)

I personally have become so adept at the pull adjustment that I prefer it in the majority of cases. But in all adjusting, the D.C. should use the moves in which he/she is most dexterous, as long as the directional correction of the subluxation is addressed.

Once a thorough understanding of the malposition is achieved, the problem becomes clear and the adjustic technic can be altered to suit personal capabilities. In training numerous chiropractors, throughout my many years of practice and teaching, I have found the spinous pull adjustment to be not only the easiest to teach in the correction of this disc lesion subluxation, but also the most comfortable for the patient.

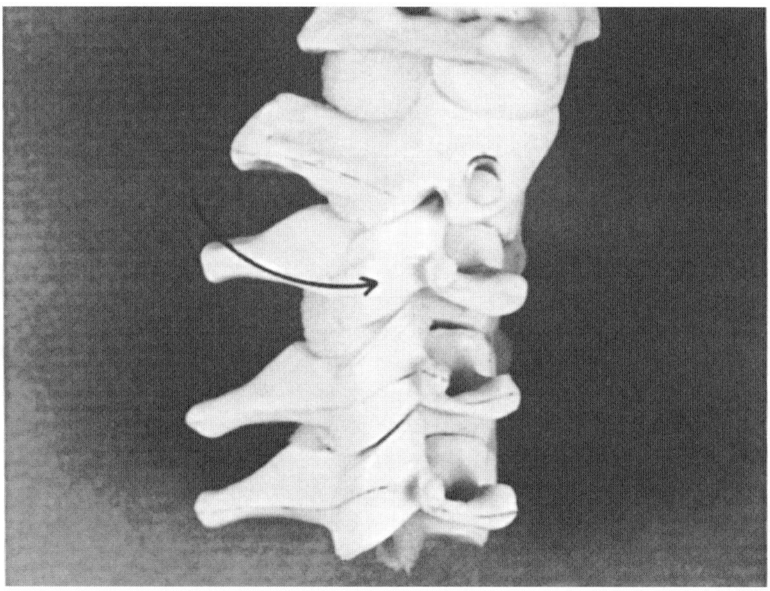

(Ill. IX-25) The line of drive is the same as in the posterior cervical thrust. The patient is now sitting, but the problem is the same and thus the line of correction remains identical.

THE SPINOUS PULL CONTACT
Anterior Torticollis

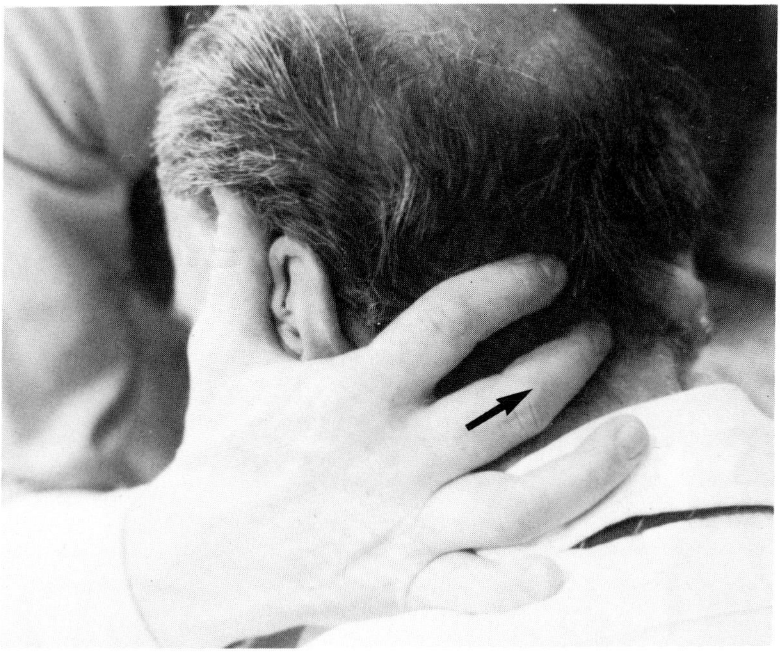

(Ill. IX-26) Notice how nicely the chiropractic index finger can contact the spinous process (nail point 5). The cervical chair is tilted back to facilitate doctor patient positioning, see (Ill. IX-30, page 111).

Throughout this text I have stated that I prefer the spinous pull adjustment in torticollis. The chief reason for this is that it is the most comfortable contact for the patient. The patient will willingly lay their head into your hand thus facilitating relaxation of the cervical musculature. The doctor's nail hand can actually feel this relaxation. At the optimum moment, when the doctor feels this relaxation, he/she can move the vertebra. If the patient is having difficulty "letting loose" so to speak, just ask them to press their head into your hand, and when the pressure is felt initiate the thrust. When you ask the patient to "press your head into my hand," tap them on the occiput with the pointer finger of the adjusting hand. This lets them know which hand you mean and also gets their mind off the pending adjustment.

THE SPINOUS PULL STANCE
Anterior Torticollis

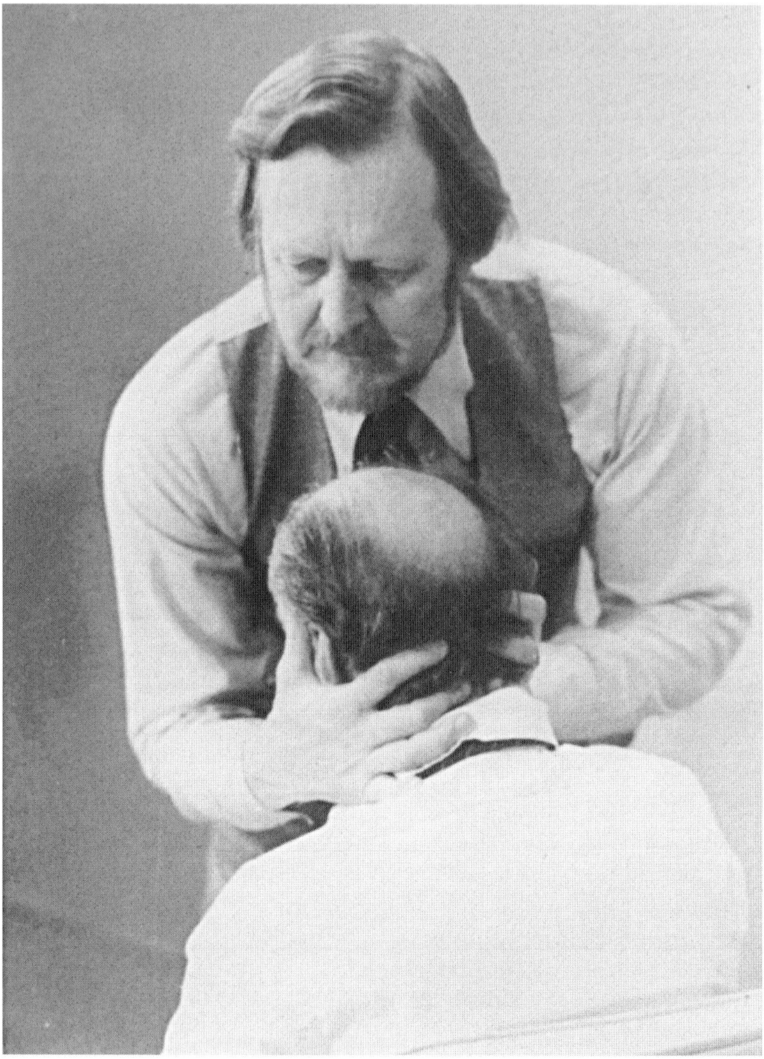

(Ill. IX-27) Using the spinous pull contact the doctor can easily grasp the spinous of the involved vertebra. The stance should be in front of the patient. You must be able to pull the spinous down and finally lift the vertebra up to separate the vertebral bodies on their anterior aspect. See page 113, (Ill. IX-32 A-B-C) for information on doctor/patient placement.

THE SPINOUS PULL THRUST
Anterior Torticollis

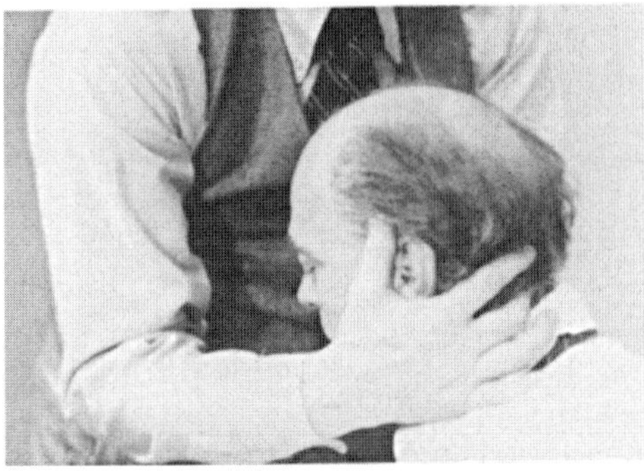

PRESS A

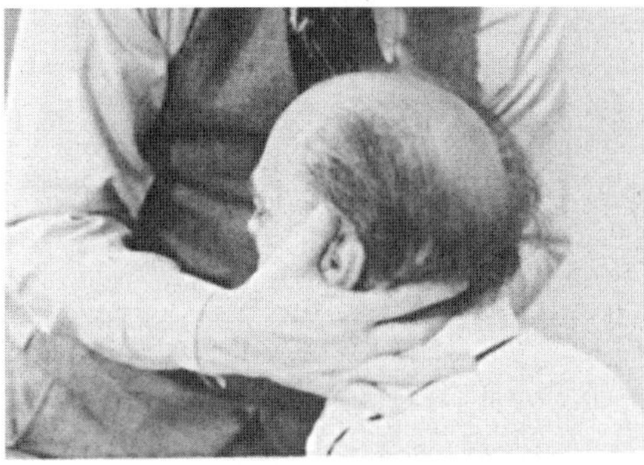

PULL B

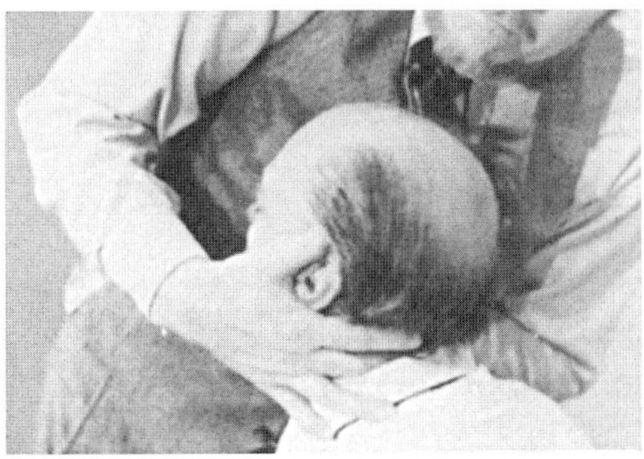

LIFT C

(Ill. IX-28) In illustrations A, B, and C the lift (scooping action) of this thrust can be seen. In Ill. (A) the contact, note the patient's head is tipped forward in a mild state of anterior torticollis. In Ill. (B) the doctor has initiated the thrust bringing the spinous process down. In Ill. (C) the lift part of the thrust separates the vertebral bodies on their anterior aspect allowing the nucleus to shift anteriorly to a more normal position. Remember in anterior torticollis there is a *posterior nuclear shift*. You must separate the bodies of the involved vertebrae on their *anterior* aspect to allow for the return of the nucleus to normal position.

III Anterior Lateral Torticollis

This condition, as the name implies, is a combination of both anterior and lateral torticollis. The nucleus has shifted both posteriorly and laterally in the disc wedge and thus the patient's head is held to one side and also bent forward. The degree of rotation and lateral disc wedge can be objectively seen in the amount of lateral bend of the neck. The degree of posterior disc wedge is indicated by the forward tipping of the patient's head. Your A.P. and lateral cervical x-rays will pinpoint the subluxation, **sometimes two vertebrae are involved**.

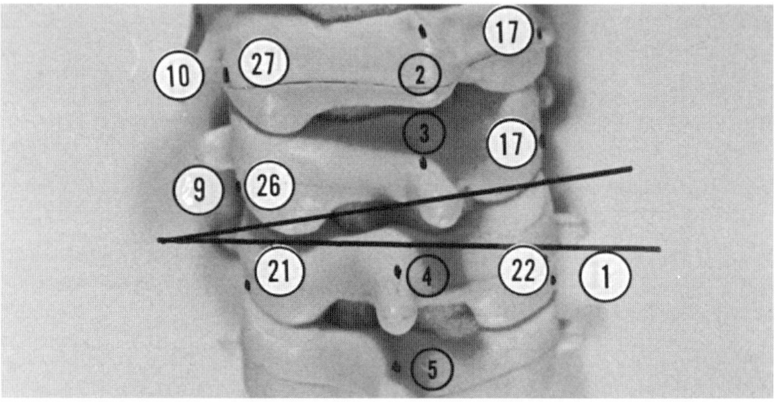

(Ill. IX-29) The spinous of C 4 is somewhat superior indicating the posterior nuclear shift of anterior torticollis. C 3 is obviously in a state of lateral torticollis, note the contra-rotation between the segments and the "open" facet on the narrow side of the disc wedge.

Anterior lateral torticollis is usually the most severe. Following the concept of the kyphosis preceding and producing the tendency for torticollis it is easy to see how, at times, the nuclear shift can be both posterior and lateral. Because of the position of the head and neck, the contact for the transverse thrust adjustment becomes more difficult. The lateral bend of the neck also makes the use of the "Keck" pillow impractical. Thus the Spinous Pull and Lift adjustment is most proficient in the correction of this multi-directional disc block subluxation. The contact finger actually first brings the spinous down, then to one side, lifts the vertebra up on that side and also lifts the vertebra up on its anterior aspect. However, with the transverse thrust and spinous pull adjustment the finger can also pull the spinous and thus some doctors prefer this thrust. Page 112 illustrates both contacts.

THE SPINOUS PULL STANCE
Anterior Lateral Torticollis

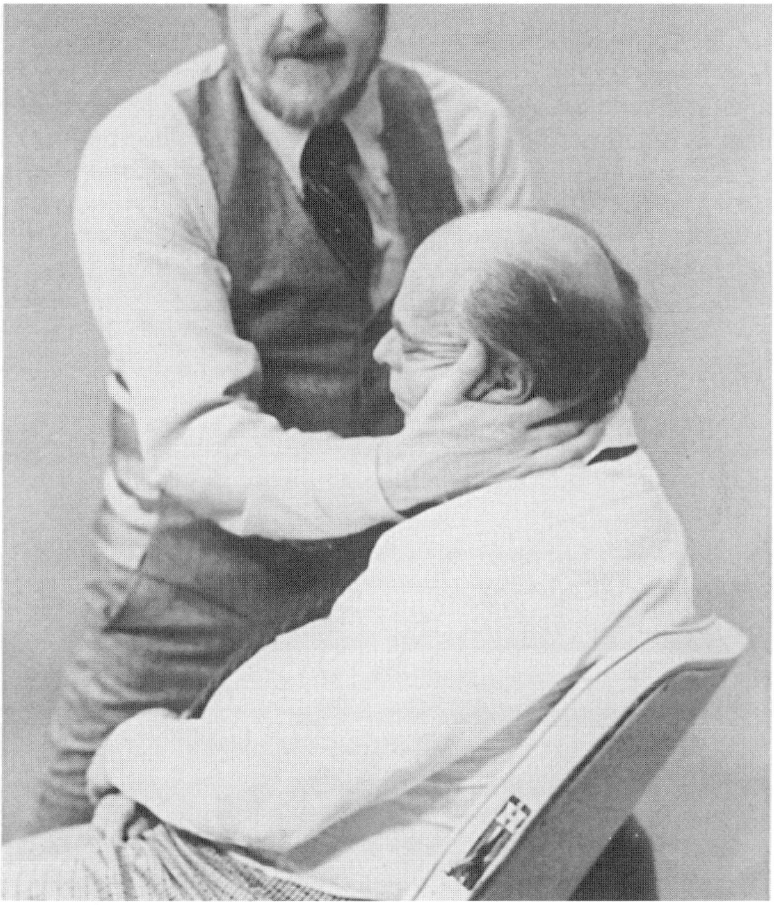

(Ill. IX-30) In the illustration above the chair is tilted back to facilitate better doctor/patient position. The doctor assumes a position somewhat in front of the patient. This position should be modified in respect to the subluxation. (See page 113, Ill. IX-32 A, B, C) The doctor's stance should not be stiff. He should bend his knees and assume a posture for poised muscular action. The thrust must be quick and the vertebra must be brought through a complete corrective movement, do not recoil.

Again, high velocity is necessary but the amplitude, the length of the pull, is short. A high velocity, low amplitude thrust.

THE SPINOUS PULL THRUST
Anterior Lateral Torticollis

The line of drive to correct this subluxation must take into consideration the rotation of the vertebra and the disc wedge. I prefer the pull and lift adjustment in these cases, the position of the stance can be modified to favor the rotational factor. The more rotational correction necessary, the more the doctor moves to the side opposite the vertebral body rotation. The more the posterior disc bulge is involved the more the doctor moves in front of the patient. Ill. IX-32 A, B, and C. The thrust must pull the spinous process down and to one side, then as this action is near completion the lift begins. The vertebra must be lifted not only on its inferior lateral edge, but also its *anterior body aspect* to correct the posterior and lateral nuclear shift.

When two vertebrae are involved, the transverse thrust spinous pull adjustment is very effective as the two vertebrae can actually be individually contacted. Nail point 6 can effectively pull the spinous of one vertebra while nail point 9 thrusts the other.

A 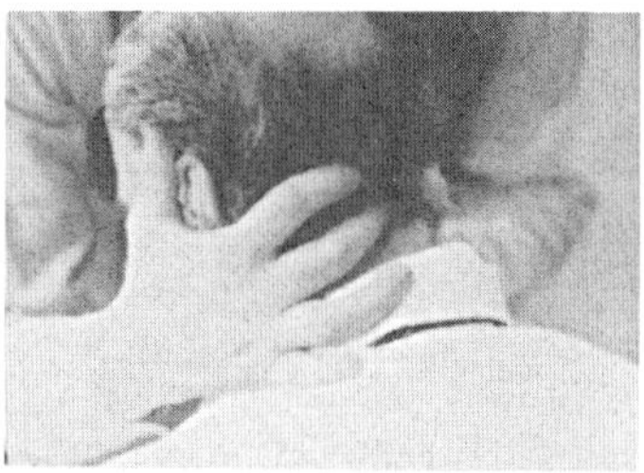

B 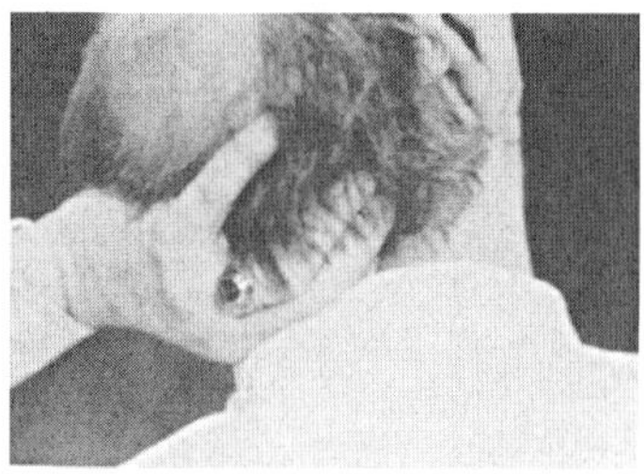

(Ill. IX-31 A and B) A - indicates the contact for the pull and lift, B - the contact for the transverse thrust spinous pull. In both illustrations we attempt to show how the adjustor's contact can pull the spinous inferior, lateral, and then with a scooping action lift the vertebra to allow for the nucleus to shift toward its normal central position in the disc space.

(A) When using the spinous pull thrust we refer you to pages 107, 108, 109, anterior torticollis; and pages 87, 88, 89, lateral torticollis. The elements of both are involved. The Spinous Pull and Lift thrust is the author's preferred adjustment for anterior lateral torticollis.

(B) The transverse thrust spinous pull adjustment contact is described on pages 95, 96. On page 97 the thrust is illustrated, but remember in anterior lateral torticollis that in addition to lateral nuclear shift the nucleus is also shifted posteriorly.

DOCTOR/PATIENT POSITIONING
Anterior Lateral Torticollis

Using the spinous pull adjustment the doctor positions himself to accommodate the line of drive necessary for the correction of the subluxation. If the subluxation has very little posterior nuclear shift and shows more lateral shift and rotation, the doctor then positions himself to the side of the patient. (A)

If lateral shift, rotation, and posterior nuclear shift are involved to an equal degree the doctor moves more toward the front of the patient. (B)

If posterior nuclear shift is the main involvement, the doctor, again, moves more in front of the patient. (C)

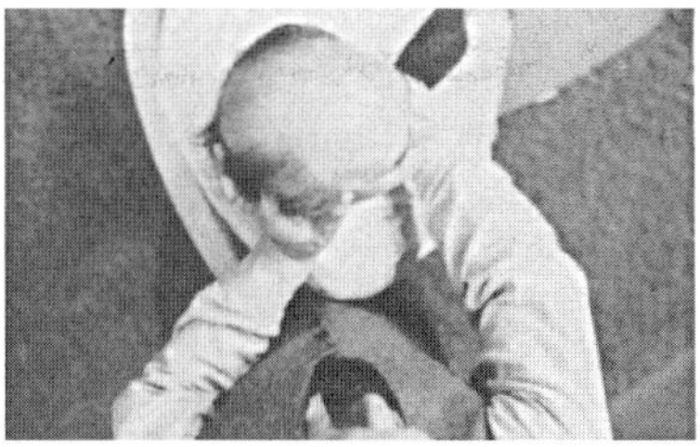

(A) Anterior Lateral Torticollis, mainly lateral involvement.

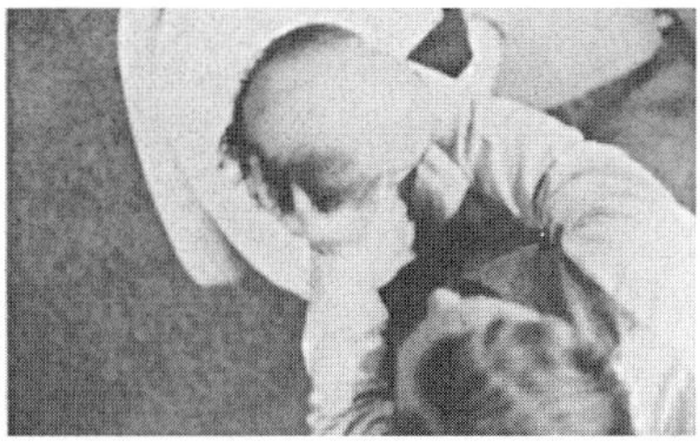

(B) Anterior Lateral Torticollis, both lateral and anterior involvement are equal.

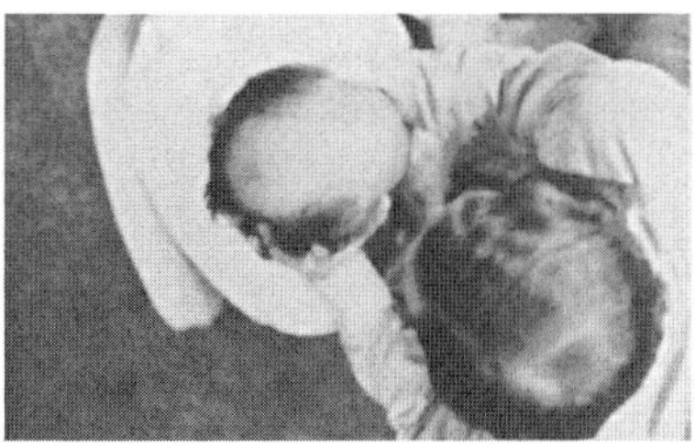

(Ill. IX-32)

(C) Anterior Lateral Torticollis, mainly anterior involvement.

Author's Note

The adjustic illustrations in this chapter, concerned with lateral and anterior lateral torticollis, all illustrate left lateral involvement. (The patient's head is tipped to the left.) The adjustic procedures are, of course, reversed for right lateral torticollis.

CERVICAL CHAIR

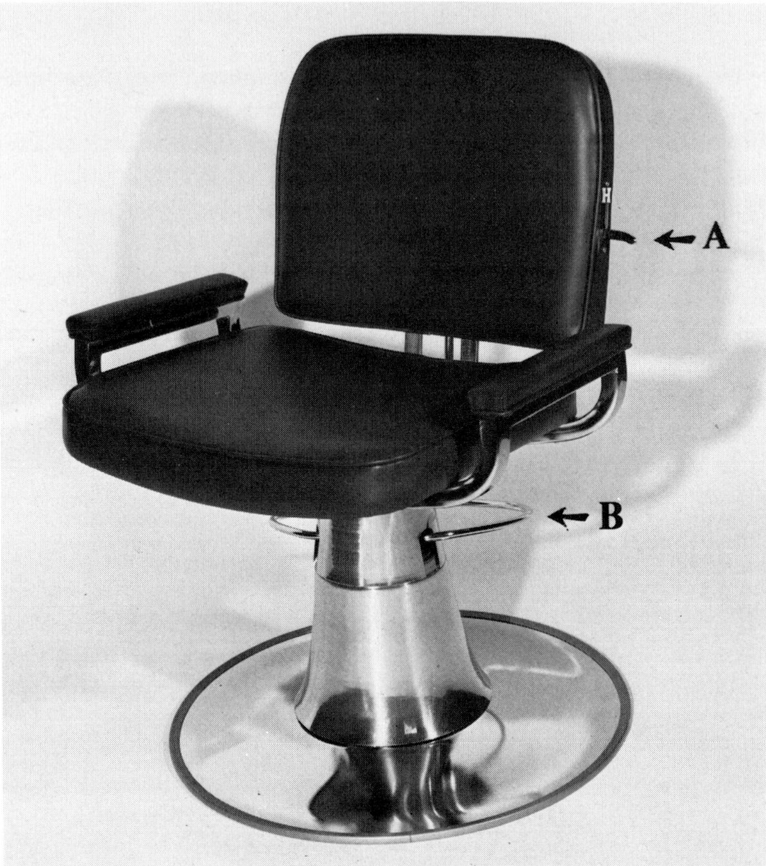

(Ill. IX-33) In order to facilitate proper doctor patient positioning for the adjustment of torticollis it is advantageous to use a cervical chair. The chair pictured is one developed by the author. As the back rest is tilted backward (activated by lever - A) the patient's position is more favorable for the posterior to anterior pull of the adjustor's thrust. The patient also finds it easier to lay his head back into the adjustor's hand if he is allowed to recline somewhat. Note on page 111 how the patient is leaning back, thus allowing his neck to assume a position wherein the line of drive can be more easily accomplished by the doctor. Without this positioning the doctor would have to crouch for proper alignment to the patient. Whenever possible the patient should be positioned to the doctor's natural stance.

This chair's hydraulic base also allows the doctor to raise, lower, or rotate the patient. The pump ring (B) is activated by pressure from the doctor's foot thus allowing 'hands free' operation. The author's adjusting tables and cervical chairs are available from the Lloyd Table Company, 120-122 West Main Street, Lisbon, IA 52253.

The adjustment of torticollis described in this chapter does elicit some very brief pain. The patient's response is an "oof-aah" type reaction. Initial pain, but immediate relief is felt and herein lies a problem. The relief is commonly so profound that patients are prone to immediately try to test their neck's turning capabilities. DON'T LET THEM! Tell them not to test their neck, but keep it still and warm, wrap a scarf around it or a piece of flannel. The velcro fastening soft cervical collar is of definite value. (Ill. IX-34) It immobilizes and stabilizes the patient's neck, keeps it warm and helps secure the adjustment. I recommend its use for patients who will not be cautious with cervical movement, and in all cases of trauma. Patients can also be told that moist heat may help. Go home and put a hot, moist pack on your neck for 20 minutes every two hours. But do not let them lay on a heating pad all night. In my opinion, dry heat in itself is contra-productive and all night use is extremely fatiguing to the cervical musculature. Heat used before the adjustment can aggravate the condition. Traction is contraindicated as it only aggravates the kyphotic problems which are usually present in these cases. The inflammation already present due to the capsular strain is compounded by heat and traction. Only after the articulation is relieved of its stress by an adjustment can heat be of any benefit.

Be reminded that the transverse thrust adjustment for this subluxation delivers its force into the concavity of the curve. In many disc block subluxations, be they lumbar or cervical, this line of drive is necessary. The use of the rotary lift move pulls the spinous from the convexity toward the concavity and thus has a more positive effect on the acute curvature. All cervical thrusts lack the disc contact used in the lumbars and described in VOL. I, TORTIPELVIS.[16] This multi-directional type thrust is difficult to achieve cervically. However, the lift effect of the Spinous Pull and Lift adjustment compensates for the lack of disc contact.

It is sometimes necessary to adjust the patient two, even three times the first day if they will **not hold** their adjustment; (waiting a few hours between adjustments). Check them again the next day, then wait two days - **check** twice a week the next week, once the next week, then wait two weeks, then one month. I prefer to post x-ray the patient when I feel that the adjustment has fully achieved correction. When you **check** the patient adjust only when necessary. The adjustment is made to facilitate correction not to manipulate the joint, it is not a treatment. If predisposing spinal factors have initiated the attack, (as post x-rays often indicate) explain them to the patient and tell them what course of adjustic care is necessary for full correction of the problem. This is good case management and a positive patient relationship is developed. Predisposing factors in torticollis are discussed in Chapter XI.

A careful case history will record prior events that may indicate chronicity, and the patient should be carefully questioned regarding episodes of minor "stiff necks" brachial symptoms, occipital and sinus headaches, etc. Remember, patients do not relate such symptomatology to vertebral subluxations and such discussions will increase their understanding of the far reaching effects of vertebrtal subluxation. Furthermore, it brings forth in the patient an appreciation of the total benefits that can be derived from chiropractic care. Often in such discussions with patients, as I discuss the sympotomatology related to the patient's vertebral subluxation complex, the patient will exclaim, "oh you can help that, my friend has that problem" - and so you see the effect such discussions can have on patient referrals.

When the case history does indicate a past history of so-called "minor" stiffness or "common" neck ache, headache, or backache, set the stage for post x-ray studies after the acute episode has been resolved. For instance, "Mrs. Jones you have related to me that you have had occasional stiff necks and headaches prior to this nasty attack of neck pain. Now the x-rays I have taken of you show your spine in a very bent and crooked condition due to this attack; as soon as we straighten things out I want to retake the x-rays to find out just what predisposed you to this problem, you don't want to suffer this anguish again, now do you?" This is just good doctoring, and it leads to increased patient understanding, patient confidence, appreciation and referrals. But I digress and I cover such discussions thoroughly in my text, VOL. IV, "ARE YOU THE DOCTOR, DOCTOR?"[25] Back to torticollis and the use of the cervical collar.

CERVICAL COLLAR

The cervical collar is recommended by the author in severe cases of torticollis. Patients tend to try to test their neck for free movement immediately after an adjustment. This collar prevents them from doing so. The patient should be cautioned **not to test their neck**. If they do so and resubluxate themselves (as is often the case) immediately after the adjustment, **do not try to immediately adjust them again!** It is almost always contra productive. Wait two to three hours before again endeavoring to adjust the vertebra.

CERVICAL COLLAR

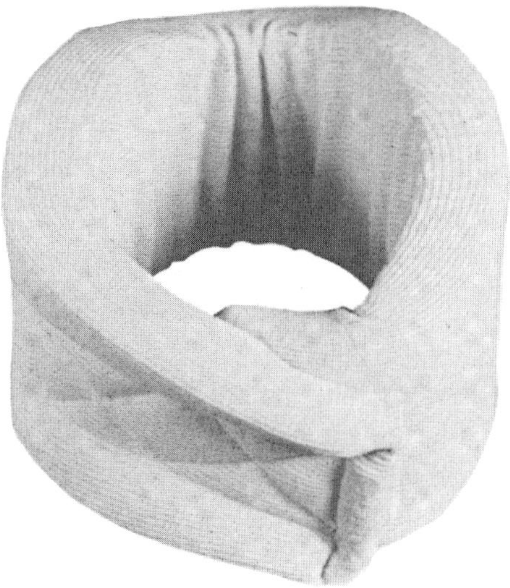

(Ill. IX-34) The soft cervical collar with velcro fasteners is a vast improvement over the more rigid types. This collar stops a patient from trying to test their neck for movement. It adds warmth and security and is a definite aid in more severe cases of torticollis.

The Emergency Case

The doctor of chiropractic is often called upon to help in an emergency situation wherein the public is aware that his/her expertise can be of benefit. I have found that I will be asked most commonly for help in backache, tortipelvis, intercostal pain, headache, and torticollis. Usually the chiropractor faced with such a situation has no way of x-raying the case, and thus faced with a torticollis problem, the D.C. must function somewhat in the dark, so to speak.

So it is up to you, Doctor, will you be willing to risk your reputation, chiropractic's reputation for that matter, on this type of case? Well, if you're on the Island of No-doc-ta, or in a backwoods camp on a fishing trip, or at a motel and the desk clerk calls you at 11:00 p.m. and asks you to help Mrs. Jones in room 13, you may elect to provide help for the person in pain. After all, humanitarian concepts dictate to us to help when we can.

Following the rationale presented in this text, let us examine Mrs. Jones who is confined to her chair with heat on her excruciatingly painful neck. They heard you mention you were a chiropractor at the Sky High Lounge last night. You were relaxing on a trip you felt would free you from such cases. Mrs. Jones browbeat her husband into asking the hotel clerk if any doctors were registered and sure enough you had forgotten, by habit, the Dr. . . or D.C. had been written adjacent to your name. Oh well, "that's the joys of motoring," my late father would say. Mrs. Jones, of course, is a hypersensitive complainer, wet handkerchief, red-eyed, quivering in all the anguish she can muster. You question her and her husband carefully. "No, there has been absolutely no trauma, possibly just a draft has caused the problem." O.K., no trauma, she's approximately age 40, and they've stated she has no chronic diseases, so let's get on with it, doctor.

Now, reflect upon the malposition of the subluxation as described throughout this text. Mrs. Jones' neck is laying on her left shoulder. Listing? Body rotation left, spinous right - disc wedge would be **wide** to the right (thus right nuclear shift). The facet would be **open** on the left, on the side the head is tipped to, the side of vertebral incline. Her head is held somewhat forward, listing posterior nuclear shift, spinous superior. O.K., you have your listing and thus you determine your line of drive. Classic anterior lateral torticollis. You palpate and find the rotated spinous and open facet. Ah, yes, it's Axis, "the big handle." You stand on her right side, reach around her face, and have her lay her head into your hand. "Now rest your head in my hand, Mrs. Jones. Remember now, as I've said, you'll feel a little 'snap' - but I'm not going to force you to move your head in the way you cannot move." "Oh, Oh no!… I can't stand it, No-no … ." "Just press your head into my hand a little." - Snap - Scream (the maid rushes to the door). "Now doesn't that feel better? Now **don't** test your neck. I'll send Mr. Jones out for a cervical collar. You stay right here and relax until he gets back." You exit, already your wife has packed and you move across town and this time you register as *Mr.*

Seriously now, your results will be fine, you've adjusted according to a proper listing **and** you **will** check her the next morning now won't you, Doctor! You have given first aid care and justified your profession's need for existence. However, I must repeat, such emergency procedures should only be used in true emergencies. I need not remind doctors today of the consequences of malpractice proceedings.

Case Management

The management of acute pain syndromes, always presents special problems and torticollis is no exception. To say the least, this is a very painful condition. It must be remembered by the doctor that the spine is in a state of anatomical lock ... the disc block subluxation. Muscle spasm is not causing the tortuous position of the cervical spine and thus heat application has little positive effect before spinal adjustment. After the adjustment moist heat can provide some relief to the strained muscles, but it is of limited value unless the subluxation has been corrected.

One of the most difficult problems faced by the person afflicted with this condition is the inability to support the weight of their own head when leaning backwards to lie down. Both rising and reclining to and from bed is difficult indeed. After first sitting on the bed a patient will find that they can slowly tip to one side or the other; by laying down first on one side, they may then support the back to their head with their hands and roll over to a supine position. The pillow may have to be quite high to support their head and **if possible** a cervical pillow can be used so that the convexity of the pillow encourages the return of the normal lordotic curve of the cervical spine. **But**, it should not be used unless it is **comfortable**! (Ill. IX-35)

If at all possible a torticollis case should have someone on hand to help when reclining and rising from bed. It is best to allow the patient to support the back of **his/her own head with one hand** while extending the other for help in rising. In this way they can personally control the support necessary for comfort.

As the patient improves they must be continually cautioned not to test their neck for mobility. Such twisting and turning can cause a relapse of the disc block subluxation. A cervical collar, as stated before, is very helpful in this problem, it offers stability and support while limiting the patient's movement. Frequent rest is necessary during recovery and the patient is to be encouraged to lie back in a recliner for frequent periods of rest. Fatigue of the cervical spinal musculature must be avoided.

Unless one has suffered the discomfort of this disc lesion subluxation it is difficult to appreciate the amount of pain involved and the doctor should be sure to advise the patient's family that this is, indeed, a very painful condition. There truly is nothing funny about it and the sympathy and help of family members can be a helpful aid in promoting early recovery.

FREQUENCY OF ADJUSTMENTS

As I've stated before it may be necessary to adjust the individual twice the first day, on rare instances even three times, then check them the next day and if needed, adjust again. Check them each day until the adjustments hold, then you may elect to see them every other day, then once a week until the patient completely recovers. Chronic pain and minor restriction is a sign of chronic malposition and re-x-raying is indicated. Minor states of misalignment can lead to chronic adaptive distortion therefore post x-rays are important. Underlying spinal distortions can and will often cause a relapse.

CERVICAL PILLOW

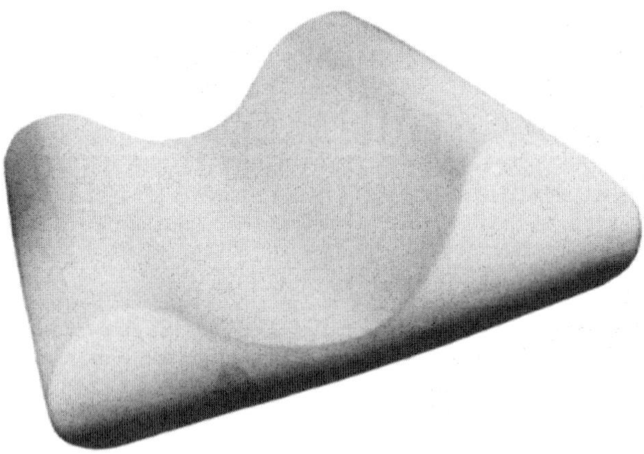

(Ill. IX-35) Pictured above is the cervical pillow referred to by the author. The patient may choose the high or low side of the pillow to suit their comfort. Do not use in torticollis unless the patient finds its use definitely comfortable.

PATIENT EXPLANATION

It is important that the patient understands that you are thoroughly aware of his/her pain and its cause. I am in a habit to first briefly explain the vertebral malposition and my x-ray findings. Then standing next to the patient, on the side opposite the lateral bend of the neck, I reach around the patient's head and face and place my hand around their neck much like the illustration shown on (IX-5, A) page 89. At this time I am not endeavoring to contact the vertebra but simply applying support to their head. I then say to the patient, I know exactly how you feel Mrs. Doe, you can press your head into my hand can't you? The patient tries and says, "yes doctor." But you can't tip it the other way can you? The patient tries a little but immediately states, "Oh no I can't do that doctor."

I then say to the patient, while I turn their head slightly **away from** the lateral bend — "You can turn your head to this side can't you Mrs. Doe?" "Oh yes doctor, that does not hurt much at all." But you can't rotate it this way can you? (you rotate the head **slightly** towards the lateral bend) "No, no, doctor, please don't do that to me."

"You see Mrs. Doe, I know exactly what you can and cannot do. I will not force your head in a direction that is painful. You will hear a little snap in your neck when I adjust the vertebra, so don't let that startle you." Now you proceed to make the spinous contact, once you have the contact established you are ready to make the adjustment. "All right Mrs. Doe, just relax and press your head a little bit into my hand like you did before." She presses, you initiate the pull and lift adjustment. She may elicit a little expression of pain or surprise. You hold your position, no abrupt recoil, you ease your hands from her neck, she exclaims, "my that feels better doctor." At this time you admonish her not to **test** her neck but just keep it still, and you go on to explain your regimen of care.

With this technic of patient management you have explained your knowledge of their dilemma; the patient should have complete confidence in your competence to handle this very painful condition so that they will relax and thus facilitate the adjustment.

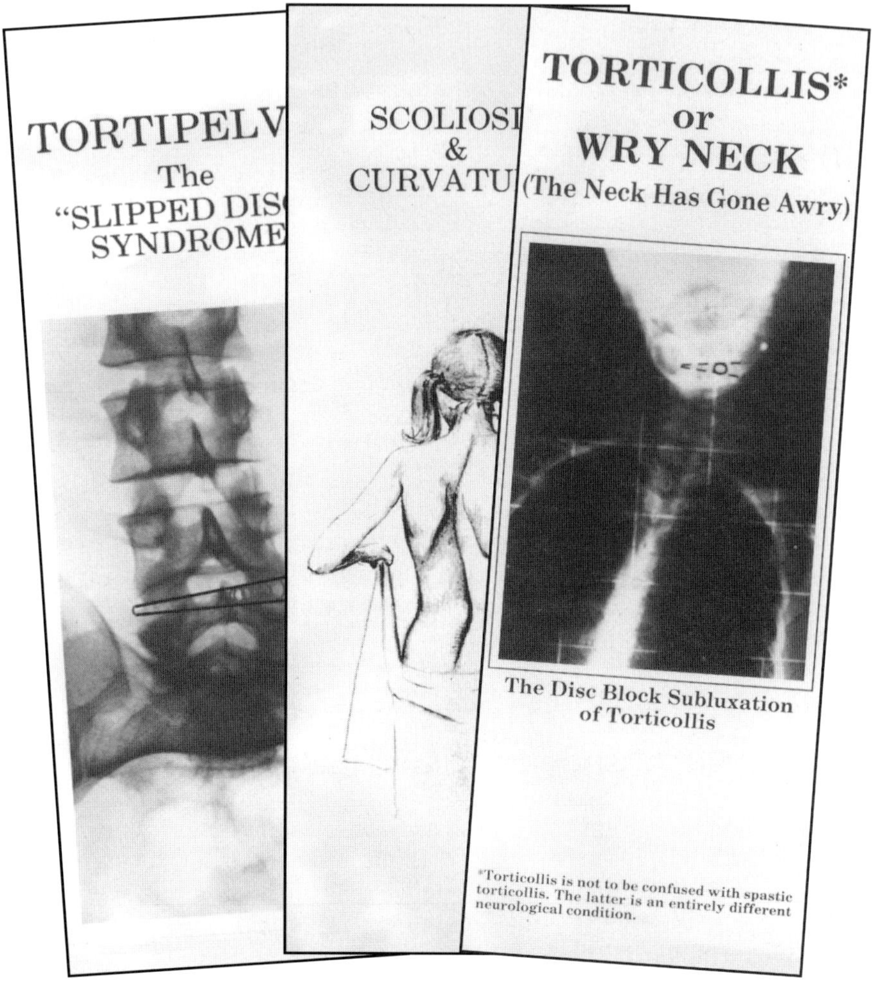

(Ill. IX-36) The author has written a patient brochure that explains the torticollis subluxation in layman terms. Readers interested in information on this and other patient brochures written by the author, contact the publisher; Barge Chiropractic Publishing, Inc., 322 Cameron Aveune, LaCrosse, WI 54601.

CHAPTER X
UPPER CERVICAL SPECIFIC
ITS
APPROACH TO TORTICOLLIS

Introduction by Fred H. Barge, D.C., Ph.C.

As chiropractic evolved in the early 20th century, many differing technics were developed for the adjusting of vertebral subluxations. Schools vying for students would often tout their technics, and advocates of each one would develop courses for chiropractors to receive advanced education. Dr. H. B. Logan developed a technic and opened a college utilizing its concepts. Willard Carver and C. S. Cleveland Sr. also founded colleges based on technics. The Clevelands followed the Meric system of spinal adjustment and the Cleveland Colleges still feature this technic today. But of all the various chiropractic technics, the one that created the most controversy and the most intense research was the one created by the "Developer of Chiropractic," B. J. Palmer; he referred to it as "Upper Cervical Specific," or "H.I.O." (Hole In One). This technic was proclaimed by B. J. to be the ultimate correction in respect to subluxation. B. J. stated that the major subluxation in the human spine, the only true subluxation that could interfere with "mental impulses," was at the level of Occipital Atlanto Axial Articulations. His research clinic used, almost exclusively, this approach to chiropractic adjusting; seldom was a vertebra below 3rd cervical ever adjusted. Outcome assessments were researched and documented in numerous disease syndromes. Body function was monitored with the use of a full complement of laboratory procedures employing medical physicians to do the laboratory tests. To say the least the results were impressive, I myself interned in his clinic in 1954 and can attest to many a remarkable recovery that occurred under strictly upper cervical care.

It is not the intent of this text to go into an indepth discussion of upper cervical specific technic, this author was fully trained in its concepts and I still use this excellent technic along with a goodly number of others in my practice. It is hopeful that this brief explanation of the technic's history will serve to enlighten the reader.

The upper cervical specific practitioner adjusts the upper cervical subluxation according to its specific listing regardless of the level or malposition of the torticollis subluxation. They would hold that this is the "major" (or primary) subluxation and the torticollis subluxation is simply a manifestation of the incoordination caused by the major. With this observation I now turn your attention to a chapter written by one of the most renowned upper cervical practitioners in the chiropractic profession, Dr. E. L. (Bud) Crowder, D.C. Ph.C. Now retired from 38 years of involvement in the Palmer School of Chiropractic and later the Palmer College of Chiropractic. He was personally trained and tutored by B. J. Palmer, and one of his adjusting doctors in the B. J. Palmer Research Clinic. He was the last director of the Research Clinic before it was closed by Dr. David Palmer in 1961; he continues to practice today.

Dr. Crowder is a master in the use and teaching of the toggle recoil adjustment. I take pride in the fact that he was my teacher. For the toggle recoil approach to torticollis I turn to the words of the good doctor himself.

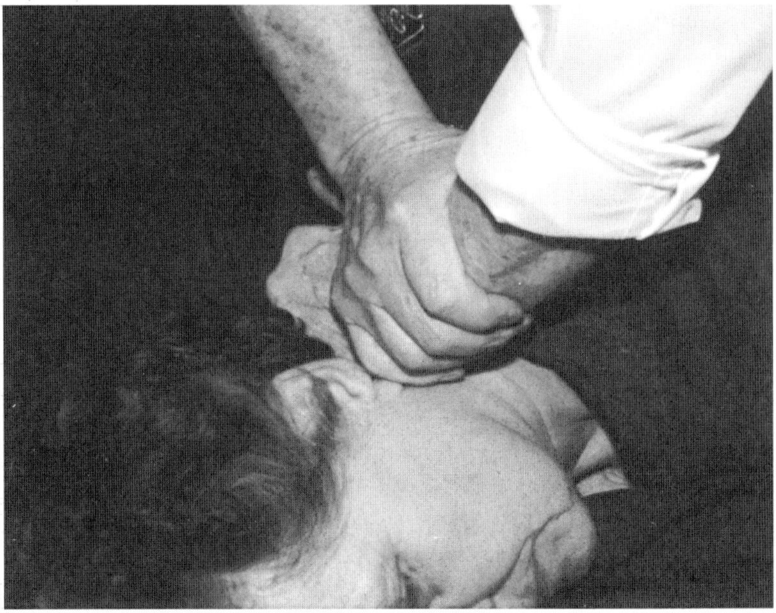

(Ill. X-1) The master of the toggle recoil, the hands of Dr. E. L. Crowder; Axis, Spinous Left, Pisiform contact. Side Posture Table, Lloyd Table Company.

Toggle Recoil And Torticollis

E. L. Crowder D.C. Ph.C.

"Toggle recoil and torticollis are sister dinosaurs but neither are likely to become extinct. Although toggle recoil is not obsolete it is somewhat passe among today's contemporary adjusting technique fads. The toggle technique is, however, very traditional and is a highly effective procedure in the chiropractic management of torticollis.

"Intervertebral insufficiency and torticollis references are legend in the history of spinal disorders. Explicit drawings, pictures, and descriptions of the pain are strikingly the same in most texts. Even recommended care and management has changed very little.

"Methods of maneuvering the spine have always received center stage attention with the nearly ever-present warnings to consider surgery only as a last resort.

Intervertebral Instability

"The spine is a chain of interacting segments with normally understood function. The individual parts are expected to reliably complement each other in health. It is also common to expect unfavorable interaction in the presence of wear and tear, trauma and disease.

"Even intervertebral instability has the neurological component of cause and its inevitable effect on the pathological outcome. Our professional and intellectual understanding would be enhanced by analyzing or diagnosing the conditions as *Neurological Intervertebral Instability*. Corrective and repair functions are impossible without an adequate nerve supply and uninterrupted pathway connection with the brain. Beware the subluxation and its interfering influence!

"Variances of structure and function of the motor segment will have serious consequence and are the nature but not the primary cause of instability. In assessing the torticollis spine, look carefully for integrity of the disc. As the largest and main retaining restraining unit of the entire motor segment the disc is paramount to intersegmental integrity.

"A loosening in the motor segment is the most common form of insufficient performance. **Schmorl and Junghanns,** in reference to vertebral instability: "In its early stages, in the presence of usual strain, this loosening is compensated for by the muscles. This takes place within the framework of unconscious and well-adjusted spontaneous reflex mechanisms."

"Latent instability lies in wait for a special event to transform the quiescent inefficiency into a recognizable performance weakness which may very well be **torticollis.**

The Dilemma of Assessment

"In cases of torticollis the chiropractor is confronted with the dilemma of assessment, the challenge of correction and the quandary of determining an expected outcome (prognosis).

"Case history is more than information about the wry neck, it is intimately connected to the subluxation. Determining the probable cause of the subluxation can be translated into an assessment of prognosis which touches the senses of the patient and the professional sensibilities of the chiropractor.

"It is tempting to connect recent trauma with an acute episode of torticollis and to promise a quick uncomplicated recovery. Torticollis (wry neck), as so many other functional disorders are, is frequently acute manifestations of the chronic underlying cause. Acute manifestations are usually self-limited episodes that were triggered by stress in one or more of its many forms. Trauma, fatigue, emotional and chemical stressors are categoric examples capable of overwhelming a response system limited by subluxation.

"Subluxations are frequent culprits in limiting the ability of the response system to produce sufficient coping to offset the invasive nature of the stress. Torticollis can be and is frequently systemic; that is, systemic in its production and systemic in its toxic by-products. The gradual onsetting wry neck or the recurrent torticollis should be viewed as chronic or as having a more complex etiology than merely mechanical. This is a compelling reason to determine the exact nature of the subluxation complex.

"Disoriented function is the nature of this malady caused by the subluxation. Postural distortion, muscle spasm and pain complicate an assessment of a specific subluxation complex with substantial certainty. X-ray studies of the torticollis neck are important. (Ill. X-2)

"Associated spinal misalignment exaggeration can confuse definition of the primary subluxation listing needed for side posture toggle recoil upper cervical management of the torticollis neck.

"Static palpation, motion palpation, and visual observation aid in confirming the nature and extent of the distortion. Fortunate is the patient who has had previous chiropractic care with a precise subluxation analysis determination. The primary subluxation complex will usually prevail and adjusting the established major can be expected to produce most effective positive results. It is usual to observe the torticollis distortion configuring to the subluxation complex mechanics. If the situation is so observed it gives added security in using the established major. Even so a detailed history and examination are necessary.

SPECIFIC UPPER CERVICAL ANALYSIS

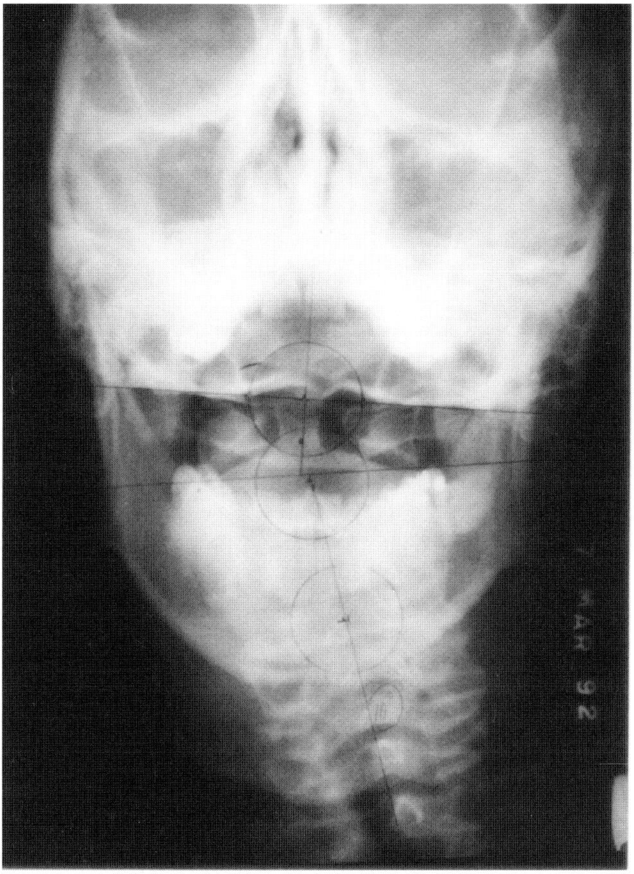

(Ill. X-2) Dr. Crowder's upper cervical analysis.

"If the established subluxation configuration and torticollis distortion do not conform, further investigation, further examining and added information is required. Trauma or systemic factors of sufficient intensity may cause to change the mechanics and the major subluxation complex. The listing will then be suspect.

"If the torticollis patient presents without previous and reasonably recent chiropractic spinal x-ray assessment, the protocol for procedure will change. The distortion specifics of lateral tilt, rotation and flexion or extension will be helpful in the final determination of major listing; *only helpful—not absolute!*

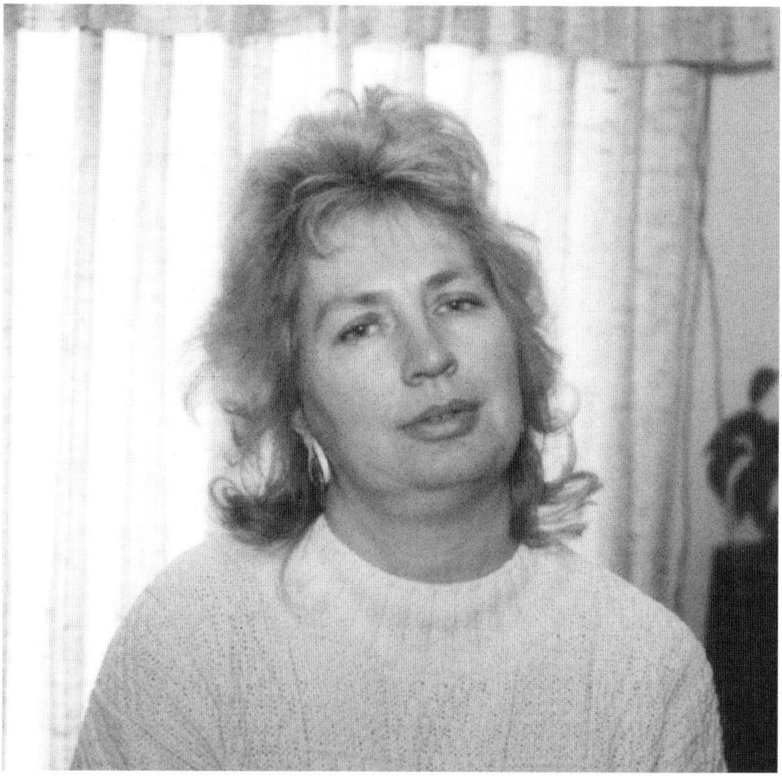

(Ill. X-3) Dr. Crowder's patient above, displays the typical presentation of a person in torticollis. The head is tipped to the right and the face is turned to the side opposite of the lateral bend. This posture has been observed in clinical texts going back into the 19th century. Both Dr. Crowder and I agree that the distortion is a guide to the listing of the subluxation.

"A wise, experienced and critical x-ray survey is always necessary when assessing the newly presenting torticollis case.

"X-ray findings of exaggerated segment rotation and laterality are the rule. The greatest misalignment might not, in fact, usually does not, equate with the major subluxation to be adjusted. The gross misalignment distortion distracts from its cause! The gross misalignment distortion usually **follows** the major **subluxation's** mechanical component!

"Careful history and survey for trauma is crucial for a proper clinical assessment and outcome prognosis.

The Challenge of Correction

"Correction is more complex than adjusting the subluxation of a wry neck. Correction takes place after the adjustment. Time is important in any process, but perhaps it is the most important factor of physiology and healing. Monitoring the subluxation signals is helpful and quite critical in judgement of case progress and calculating prognosis.

"If left unexplained, symptoms will be the patient's measure of results, even if relief is spontaneous and without any intervention. It is dangerous to the patient and an injustice to chiropractic when the explanation is ignored by the patient or not given by the chiropractor.

"The dynamics of this neuro-vascular-musculo-skeletal disorder play out in a predictable and orderly fashion. If these dynamics are misunderstood or ignored the accumulating effects are far-reaching and can be systemically destructive.

"Establish the primary cause with substantial certainty, adjust the major and understand the orderly nature of healing to provide a guide for prognosis.

"'Will it hurt?' 'I can't move!' 'Don't touch my neck!' All are immediate and overwhelming concerns of the torticollis patient seeking relief from the stabbing disabling pain in the neck. It is of little consolation trying to assure the patient your procedure will be painless. Even the biggest toughest bruiser will be brought to his knees with an acute torticollis. The same for 'Wispy Nellie' except more tears.

"Side posture on an adjustable headpiece table is well suited to a proper patient posture for the adjustment. (Ill. X-4) Getting the patient placed on the table, in side posture, is often the greatest challenge. Be patient with the torticollis neck in all preparations. Proceed slowly and with appropriate instructions, the patient will find the easiest route!

"With the head and all its weight fully supported on the headpiece, the torticollis distortion will, for the most part, disappear or be greatly minimized.* This neutral undistorted cervical posture is desired and quite necessary for specific adjusting as in **all** toggle recoil specific subluxation corrections. (Ill. X-4 & 5)

PATIENT PLACEMENT
SIDE POSTURE ADJUSTING TABLE

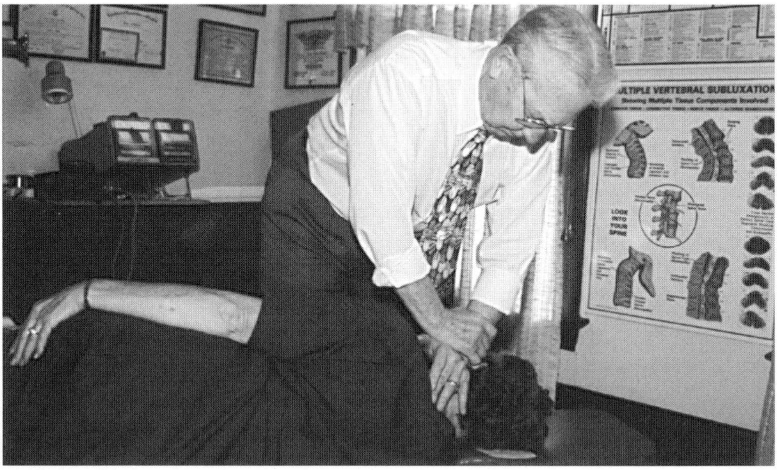

(Ill. X-4) The toggle recoil contact and stance, Atlas adjustment. Nicholas Table, Lloyd Table Company.

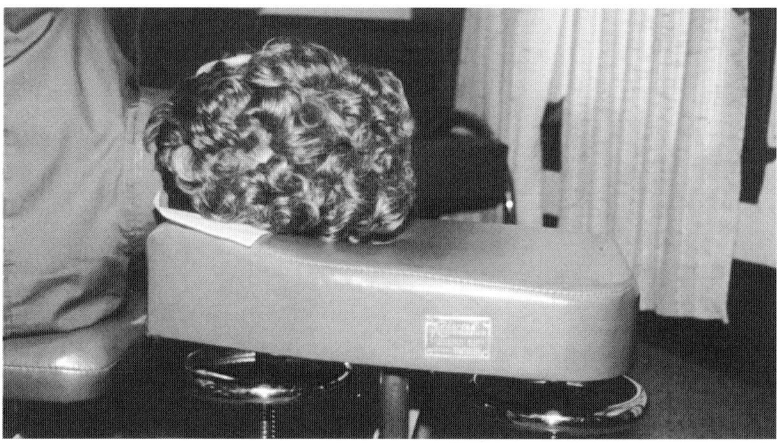

(Ill. X-5) The adjustable drop headpiece, Nicholas Table, Lloyd Table Company.

* Dr. Crowder's and my observation concur, once the patient's head is supported properly, muscular contractions and distortion is minimized.

"With the head completely supported on the headpiece and the lower shoulder firmly and squarely placed on the table, (Ill. 6, 7, 8) the cervical region can be tested for appropriate adjusting condition. A mild and gentle test of general movement of the neck by the chiropractor should be painless. (Ill. X-9 next page).

*Specifically set the headpiece elevation and angle to properly conform to the primary subluxation profile.(Ill. X-5, 6, 7, 8)**

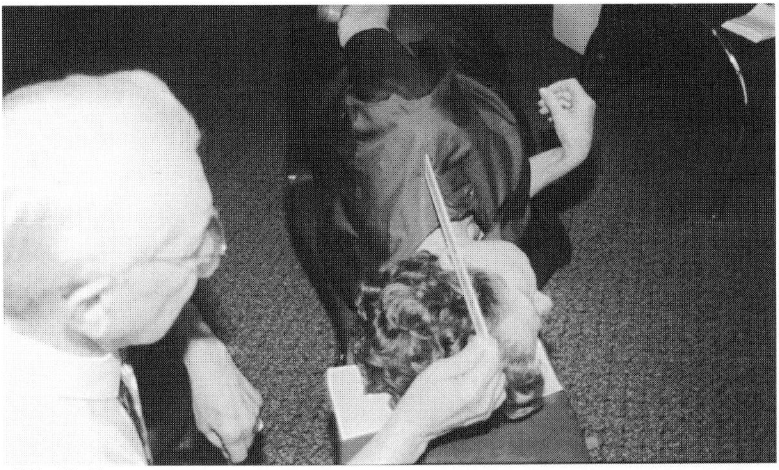

(Ill. X-6)

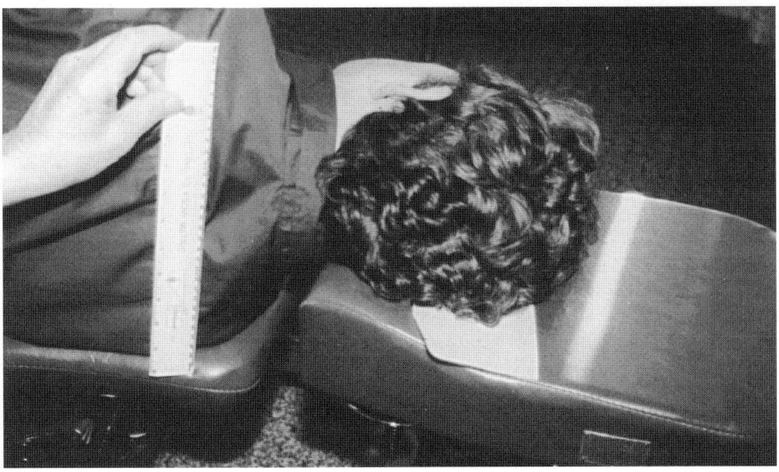

(Ill. X-7)

*Mrs. Mary McCubbin, printed with patient's permission.

PATIENT PLACEMENT

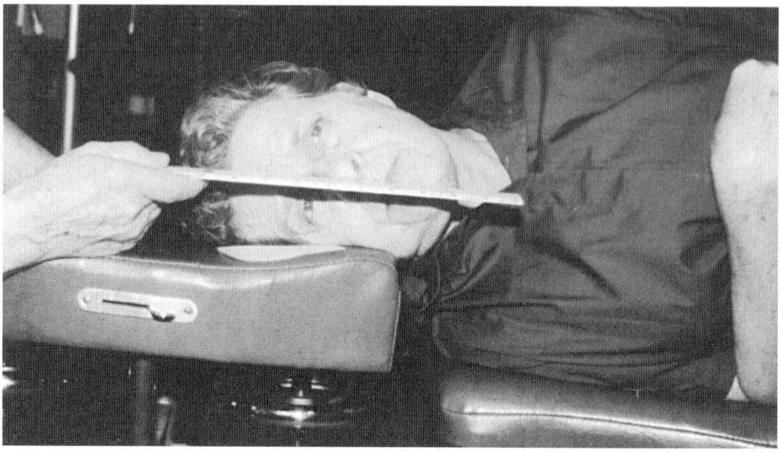

(Ill. X-8) Proper and relaxed patient placement is necessary in the toggle recoil adjustment of torticollis. As Dr. Crowder stated, "The distortion will, for the most part, disappear or be greatly minimized" - with proper support by the headpiece.

TEST THE PATIENT

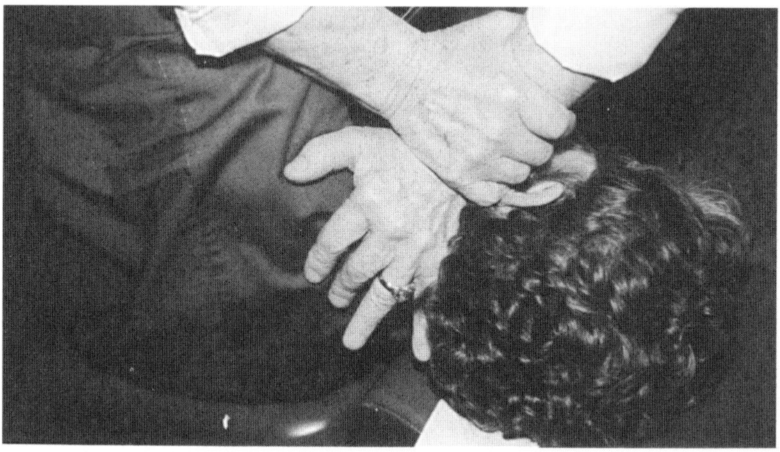

(Ill. X-9) As Dr. Crowder explained on page 131, "the cervical region can be tested for appropriate adjusting condition. A mild and gentle test of general movement of the neck by the chiropractor should be painless." The doctor takes the contact (in this case, Atlas) with the pisiform (nail point 1), and he/she tests by applying gentle pressure - again, it **should be painless**.

"Adjustors with a heavy contact are reminded of the tension reaction of the patient. *In torticollis the heavy contact is especially contraindicated. The patient will contract and tense directly proportionate to the weight and pressure of contact.*

"Toggle recoil adjusting is precise in contact, angle, depth and speed.

"The cervical region should not bow or distort under the toggle to any degree greater than the earlier "painless" test for proper table position. Properly delivered, and incisive precision toggle recoil is fundamentally painless to the torticollis neck.

"The next and immediate step is rest to permit function to reorient from the torticollis spasm. A few minutes on the adjusting table, then the patient can carefully move to the upright posture. Let the patient do it to prevent pain and spasm, until they can be moved for better rest.

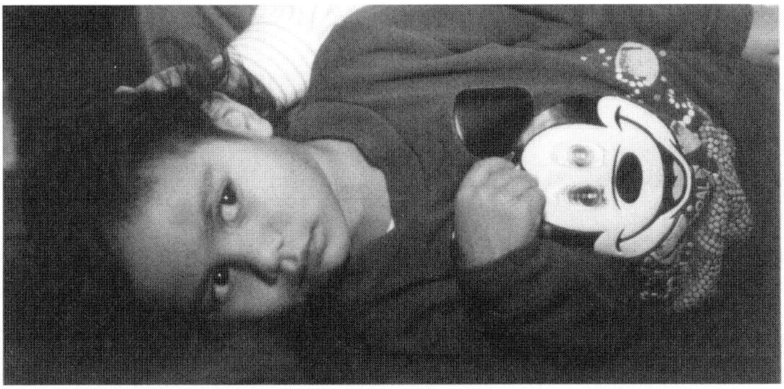

(Ill. X-10) Juvenile torticollis* is common in the chiropractically unattended.

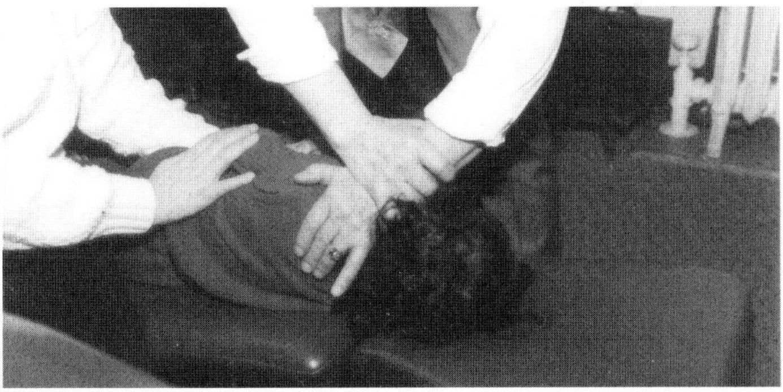

(Ill. X-11) Toggle recoil adjustment does not stress the spasm of torticollis.

*Printed with parental permission, Mr. & Mrs. John Trujillo, patient Jasmine Trujillo, age 4.

"Unencumbered time is necessary for the innate energies of the body to reorient the bizarre physiology of torticollis. Twenty minutes of recumbent rest in the office will usually allow initial stabilization, then the patient can get to an environment more conducive to an undisturbed recumbent two hour rest.* *Unencumbered means no therapeutic infringements during this functional reorientation of physiology time. No heat, no ice, no medicine—no therapeutics!*

The Expected Outcome

"Judging the outcome and prognosis will immediately remind any caretaker of torticollis that health care is an inexact science. Even so, the chiropractor has an advantage over other health providers by knowing, monitoring and attending to the principal cause of torticollis.

"Vertebral function insufficiency is a frequent co-partner of torticollis. The chiropractor should at all times be attentive to the neurologic component of the subluxation and have particular knowledge of the body's own healing mechanisms. True restoration is incomplete in the sense of normal anatomical conditions or with a return to complete performance efficiency when there is subluxation interference. Without doubt the body's own healing tendency is directed at a pain-free state and partially at the achievement of certain statics without healing in the anatomical sense. The changes are compensatory, adaptative and usually at the expense of successful restoration of full normal vertebral health and function.

"Even in apparent sudden onset acute causes of subluxation-deficit torticollis it is common to experience several weeks to several months of measurable instability. **Smorl & Junghanns** warns of the sequelae produced deficit of the spinal cord pathways based on pressure produced by intervertebral instability.

"The innate energies of the patient must adapt, correct and heal through the value and nature of tissue and material available for the acute or chronic, traumatic or systemic demand.

"Fortunately in chiropractic protocol there are reliable landmarks and functional road signs for outcome judgement.

"In chiropractic protocol we first look to the signs of the subluxation and for substantial certainty that our procedure of cor-

* I heartily agree with Dr. Crowder, rest after an adjustment is imperative. In all of the chiropractic clinics that I have developed resting facilities (cots) are available for all patients

rection was effective. The functional signs of the subluxation can be considered the window to the innate energies of the patient. So the chiropractor's subluxation testing and correction assessment is a reasonably reliable benchmark of outcome. If the innate energies are sufficient to stabilize the disfunction of the corrected subluxation it is reasonable to calculate general functional reorientation within the material value of the torticollis neck.

"If the chiropractic tests are reliably related to the functional profile of the subluxation they can be used with substantial certainty in prognosis of torticollis.

"'Correct the subluxation to correct the torticollis!'"

With these words, Dr. Crowder ends this chapter, I echo a strong affirmation. Torticollis **is** a subluxation. Upper Cervical Specific adjusts what it determines to be the major and this may be the Atlas but then too it is often determined to be the Axis, as I commonly hold to be true. I concur with most of Dr. Crowder's observations and I too often use the toggle recoil adjustment. I have also developed a special toggle recoil table for my specific upper cervical work, it is illustrated and explained. Those interested may contact The Lloyd Table Company for information. (Ill. X-13)

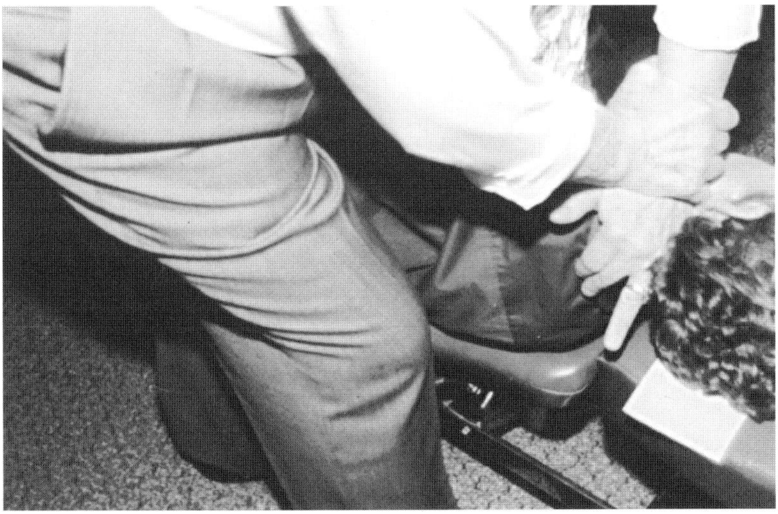

(Ill. X-12) Dr. Crowder's contact and stance for an Axis spinous left adjustment. This is the same contact and stance used by the author for this adjustment.

BARGE SPECIFIC
Impulse Table

*Built on The Nicholas Toggle Table**

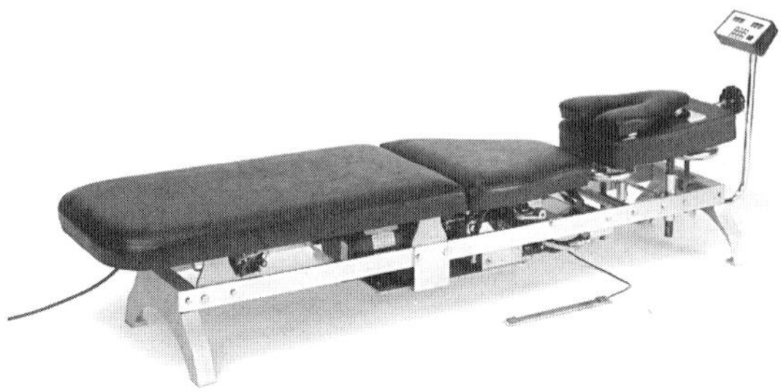

(Ill. X-13) **The Barge Specific Impulse Table** combines the best of two worlds. This advanced adjusting table eliminates the three greatest human variables in toggle recoil adjustment, speed, force and depth. And, unlike other adjusting instruments, the Impulse Table allows the doctor *'hands on'* control.

The doctor simply applies the contact, line of drive and tissue pull to produce the proper adjustment. Triggered by a selectable amount of force controlled by the table's electronics or by a convenient switch under the doctor's heel, **the headpiece drives upward** instantly as fast as 1/20th of a second. The height of the spring resistant chest cushion *'self adjusts,'* so the patient's spine may be maintained in the most desirable position. A lever locks the cushion into position.

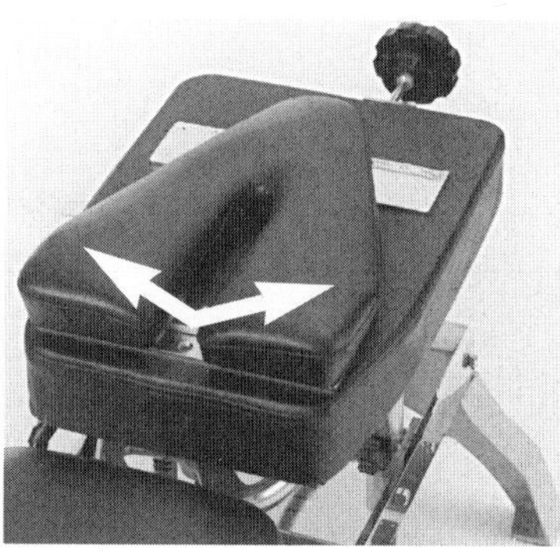

(Ill. X-14) Headpiece pivots sideways to correct for superiority or inferiority of upper cervical vertebra.

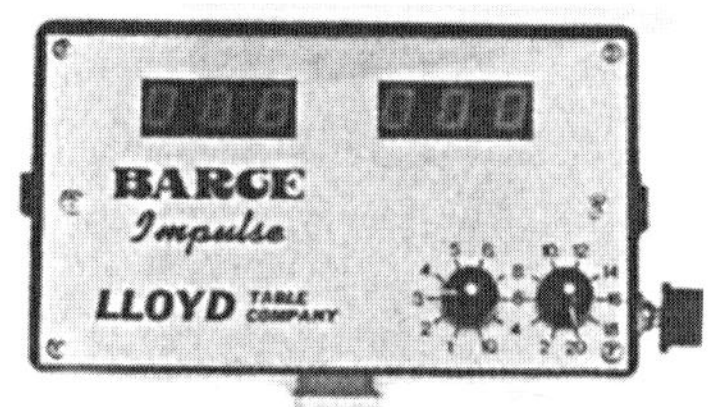

(Ill. X-15) An electronic programmable control box, with a visual digital readout, displays adjustable thrust force on the left window when the button on side is momentarily pressed. The ultimate force used during the adjustment is displayed on the right.

* Contact The Lloyd Table Company for information on the Impulse Table.

I was taught by B. J. Palmer and Dr. J. Clay Thompson, the Palmer/Thompson Drop Headpiece* was introduced to the profession during my time as a student at P.S.C. (1951-54). Before the drop headpiece, the B. J. Research Clinic used the solid headpiece side posture toggle recoil table and prior to that a toggle was delivered with the head turned to one side on the knee chest table. With the event of the Palmer/Thompson Drop Headpiece, developed by Dr. J. Clay Thompson, B. J. boldly announced the discontinuance of the other methods as this new table was heralded as the latest state-of-the-art advancement in the upper cervical technic of the toggle recoil. I believe B. J. would make a similar announcement today after he had seen, investigated, and used the new Impulse Table. (Ill. X-13)

You see B. J. Palmer simply **did not** condone "adjusting guns"** and they were as plentiful then as they are again today, he insisted that the chiropractic adjustment was a "hands on art!" The Impulse Table is an advancement in the toggle recoil concept that he would appreciate, it controls the three most critical variables of the toggle recoil adjustment, namely, speed, depth and force, and yet it is a "hands on" technic with the doctor in full control of the adjustment. I began working with the concept of the Impulse Table in the late 1970s, by 1981 the first prototype was created. In May 1981, I was granted a U. S. Patent on the adjusting table. You see, I was continually vexed by the problem of teaching the toggle recoil adjustment to chiropractors who attended my seminars. If the doctor had not learned the technic in chiropractic college, it was difficult indeed to teach them the technic in the time constraints of continued education programs. Thus, the development of the **table that thrusts** concept. This concept still allows the doctor to apply the "hands on" approach. The doctor determines the contact, line of drive, force, torque and recoil. The table simply thrusts **up** a given increment of an inch ($^1/_{16}$ to $^1/_8$ inch) at a speed no human can duplicate.

SPEED

The table provides a variable speed setting from 1 second to a 20th of a second.

* The headpiece dropped approximately $^1/_4$″ when the chiropractor applied the adjustic thrust. The resistance of the drop was controlled mechanically and adjustable.

** Adjusting instruments that apply the adjustic thrust.

It has been said that the most accomplished toggler thrusts at $^{3}/_{10}$ths of a second. Physical reflexes cannot match the speed of this table!

DEPTH

The second greatest variable in the toggle recoil adjustment is depth. Oft times I have heard an adjustor say, "I don't believe I went deep enough." The Impulse Table drives up as the doctor applies force down. The depth, which in this case is the drive, can be set from $^{1}/_{16}$ to $^{1}/_{8}$ of an inch.

FORCE

The final variable in the toggle recoil is the force. The Impulse Table can be set to thrust at any force desired from 4 to 20 pounds and higher. The doctor simply sets the headpiece to thrust at the specific weight of force desired and when the doctor's hand applies the desired weight to the vertebra to be adjusted the headpiece responds with the thrust. For those who want the lightest possible force, or those who wish to self trigger the headpiece, a foot switch placed under the doctor's heel will initiate the impulse/thrust.

MULTIPLE THRUSTS

I have often seen chiropractors adjust with two to three consecutive thrusts. To say the least, this requires the utmost dexterity and cannot be done with the drop headpiece table. The Impulse Table can be set to deliver one to ten thrusts in a row, as fast as the doctor desires.

TORQUE

The doctor can provide torque to the adjustment by using tissue pull. Furthermore, the headpiece rotates and can be set in a rotated position to favor the torque.

RECOIL

The table recoils instantaneously, the doctor can withdraw as fast as he/she desires. The recoil is controlled by two factors, the table, which is a constant, and how rapidly the doctor releases his/her force.

DIGITAL READOUT

The table's digital readout mechanism will give the approximate amount of force in pounds that was delivered to the patient by the impulse adjustment; thus a convenient record of force applied can be kept by the doctor.

To sum up the effectiveness of this table let me say that I personally have 'cleared'* many a difficult case with the use of the impulse adjustment. It is absolutely painless and most commonly when a patient is adjusted on this table they prefer to be adjusted the same way again. Children are not afraid of this table, once the drive mechanism is demonstrated to them, they prefer the adjustment to a traditional toggle recoil.

My first mechanisms were powered by compressed air which made the use of a bulky compressor necessary. Then I turned to Dr. Lloyd Steffensmeier for advice, he assured me the table could be produced hydraulically and thus ensued a period of some eight years of mechanism and prototype development. The table is now perfected.

Dr. E. L. 'Bud' Crowder has adjusted on this table. Dr. John Hofmann of Michigan insisted on having the first Impulse Table and it has been in use in his office for over five years. Drs. Harley and Vickie Gilthvedt of Auburn, Washington, also use the technic and recommend it highly. Proven in practice at my own clinic since 1981, you can be assured that with this table the patient receives the same quality adjustment regardless of the fatigue or dexterity of the practitioner.

Dr. Lloyd Steffensmeier and myself have spent many years perfecting the Barge Impulse Table. By eliminating such variables as speed, depth and force, but yet leaving the practitioner in full control of line of drive, force, torque and recoil, it provides the chiropractor with the best technology available for upper cervical adjustments.

For information on the demonstration or purchase of the Barge Impulse Table contact Lloyd Table Company at 1-800-553-7297, or write Lloyd Table Company, 102-122 West Main Street, Lisbon, IA 52253.

* Achieved adjustic correction.

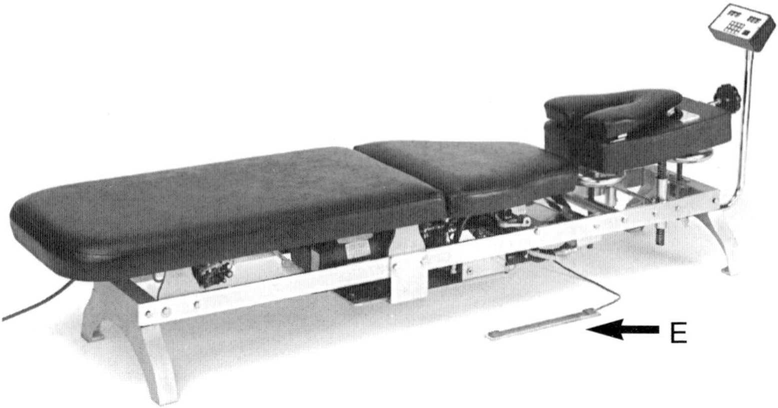

(Ill. X-16) The Impulse Table is based on the frame and adjustable mechanisms of the tried and true Nicholas Toggle Recoil Table.

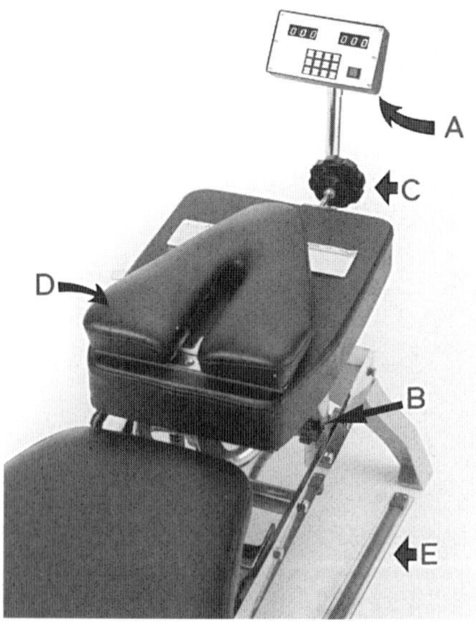

(Ill. X-17) (A) Indicates the digital readout instrument panel. The speed, number of thrusts and weight to be applied to initiate the impulse thrust, are set by the doctor. The display also indicates the amount of force applied to the patient after the thrust has been delivered. *(B)* Sets the depth (drive) of the impulse/thrust. *(C)* Releases the head rest, *(D)* to allow it to be rotated to the desired position. (Ill. X-14) *(E)* The moveable foot switch that allows the headpiece to be triggered by the doctor's foot for the ultimate in lightness of the impulse/thrust.

CHAPTER XI
INITIATING & PREDISPOSING FACTORS

Initiating Factors

1. Muscular Chill
2. Occupational Hazards
3. Trauma

1. Muscular Chill

"Man, the creature with the naked neck." We are prone to ignore this area of our body when it comes to clothing. Perhaps we should wear our hair down to our shoulders. At any rate, the human neck is subject to drafts and chills more than any other part of the spine. Thus, fans, air-conditioners, drafty rooms, riding in a car with the window open, etc. all can chill the cervical musculature. Patients, when questioned as to the cause of their torticollis attack, will often relate a draft as the only possible cause of their problem. Living in the north country as I do, I can recall many torticollis cases in early spring evidently brought on from driving with the car window open. It is not so much the chill factor itself as it is the disproportionate chilling of the neck created by drafts, fans and circulated air. This one-sided type chilling seems to create an incoordination in muscular function, thus leading to the torticollis subluxation.

2. Occupational Hazards

In my section of the country there are many farms. Farmers turn their heads to look back over their right shoulder to observe tractor-drawn equipment. When pulling haybalers and field equipment this strain can become quite constant. Many are the cases of torticollis that evolve from this occupational hazard. Construction workers using air hammers, typists looking constantly one way at copy, draftsmen bending their necks forward over the drafting board; all are examples of occupational hazards that lead to attacks of torticollis.

3. Trauma

Chiropractors can all relate cases of trauma-caused torticollis. Five of the most common traumatic type origins are:

1. Whiplash
2. Sports Activities
3. Heavy Lifting
4. Reaching
5. Fetal Delivery

1. WHIPLASH — The classic car accident neck injury. Again I must repeat the plea for x-raying all cases of torticollis. In whiplash injuries it is of utmost importance. Avulsion fractures, compression fractures, and facet dislocations all can evolve from such injuries. Most commonly, however, torticollis comes on a day or two after the whiplash injury. X-rays will reveal the exact level of vertebral involvement and any of the aforementioned complicating factors.

2. SPORT ACTIVITIES — Wrestling, football, soccer, and most body contact sports can initiate an acute attack of torticollis. These injuries should be handled with the same respect as whiplash injuries. Fractures and dislocations are always suspect.

3. HEAVY LIFTING — When lifting is done using one arm more than the other, or when turning or moving a heavy object with the arms, torticollis can result. Inordinate strain can be reflected up into the neck producing the torticollis subluxation. Such occurrences seldom involve the complications of fractures, etc., that direct force injury can produce. *If muscles, ligaments and tendons are injured, prognosis is slowed considerably. More frequent adjustments are called for and care over a long period of time may be necessary.*

4. REACHING — Extending one's arm and shoulder to reach for an object, i.e., like reaching for a coffee cup high in a kitchen cabinet. This type of reaching strain can initiate an attack of torticollis.

5. FETAL DELIVERY — Mishandling during delivery (or soon after) can cause torticollis in the newborn. Not only from my own experience, but that of the other doctors in my clinics, I can say that infant torticollis is quite common. Objectively the baby will favor one position with their head and neck or be unable to turn their head in one direction as well as they can to the other. This may be one reason why babies will lay with their heads only one way thus causing malformed cranial development. Palpation of the infant's cervical spine reveals the swollen facets, and deviated spinous process. X-rays are difficult to take of infants, but with the equipment of today they can be very worthwhile in the deter-

mination of this subluxation. However, as before stated, the child's restriction of movement and cervical spinal position indicates the listing of the subluxation, palpation verifies the listing and locates the vertebral level. (See pages 117, 119, The Emergency Case.) Chapter XIII goes into detail on adjusting infants with torticollis.[7]

Predisposing Factors

1. Kyphosis
2. Scoliosis
3. The Righting Reflex

Regardless of the circumstances or activities that initiate a torticollis attack, predisposing factors are usually present. Of course, trauma can be the direct cause without predisposition, but most torticollis cases relate no traumatic incidences. In these cases the spine developed problems that allowed this subluxation to occur. Chapter IV of this text describes the development of the cervical kyphosis. This distortion places the nucleus of the disc in a weight-bearing position that it was not intended to bear. The nucleus than acts as the fulcrum of support to the superior vertebra, and by shifting from its normal central position in the disc space causes the disc block subluxation of torticollis. Thus a major predisposing factor for this disc lesion subluxation is curvature.* When this is the case trivial movements such as reaching, or minor drafts or chills may be all that it takes to precipitate a sudden attack of torticollis. Dr. Crowder explains this in his words in Chapter X.

The two types of curvature that most commonly predispose the spine to the disc block subluxations are kyphosis and scoliosis.

1. Cervical kyphosis, this reduction of the normal cervical lordotic curve has been thoroughly discussed in this text and the reader by now should understand how the nuclear shift, both lateral and posterior, is made probable by the kyphosis. (Ill. XI-1)

2. Scoliosis, the rotational weaknesses and disc wedges of the adaptive curves of this complex curvature predisposes the spine to the torticollis subluxation. Most commonly scoliosis and kyphosis are combined in the adolescent spine. The author's conclusions on the cause of the idiopathic rotatory scoliosis are covered in VOL. III, SCOLIOSIS. However, at

* Curvatures; Dorland's Medical Dictionary (25th edition) C., deviation of the spine from its normal direction or position; see kyphosis, Lordosis, scoliosis.

this point, I would like to say that uncorrected disc block subluxations of both torticollis and tortipelvis can be the cause of adolescent scoliosis and they should never be neglected. Early correction prevents the adaptive curves that can create the scoliosis.

FULL SPINE X-RAY
Cervical & Lumbar Kyphosis

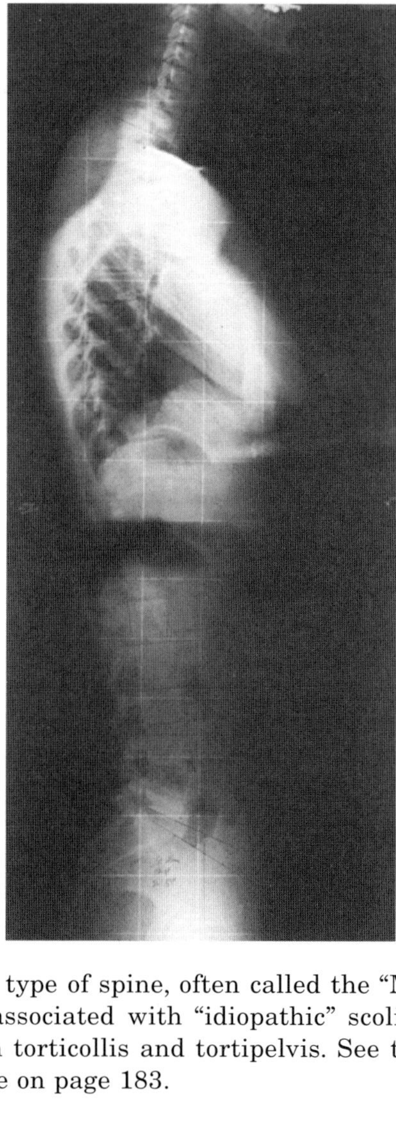

(Ill. XI-1) This type of spine, often called the "Military Spine," is frequently associated with "idiopathic" scoliosis and acute attacks of both torticollis and tortipelvis. See the A.P. view of this same spine on page 183.

In youth a lumbar scoliosis can initiate attacks of cervical torticollis. Chiropractic adjustic correction of the acute torticollis subluxation will eliminate symptoms, but the child will have reoccurring attacks. The adaptive strain on the dorsal and cervical spine from the lumbar scoliosis is creating the problem. Correction, or balancing of the lumbar curve, will prevent reoccurring attacks of torticollis. In all cases of non-traumatic torticollis in youth, one must suspect curvature and/or scoliosis. 14x36 x-ray studies should be taken after the resolution of an acute torticollis attack to determine preexisting spinal problems.

On the next four pages I show x-rays that dramatically illustrate the effect of torticollis on the spine of a young adult female. So although scoliosis can be a cause of torticollis attacks, the torticollis subluxation can lead to spinal adaptations which in turn create scoliosis. Early detection of such problems and chiropractic corrections will prevent chronic spinal distortions that we find so evident when x-raying adults.

Spinal x-rays and chiropractic analysis should be included in all physical examinations given to children. To bring this to light and gain public acceptance for chiropractic's preventive measures in curvature, is one of the great challenges facing this generation of chiropractors.

The young lady, age 15, whose x-rays are shown on the next four pages, was a neighbor of mine. She had been having occasional so-called "stiff necks" and when this attack of torticollis came on they called me. It is often our practice, in childhood torticollis, to take a 14x36 A.P. and lateral x-rays. We have found that most cases of non-traumatic torticollis (in youth) have problems in the lower spine. Analysis of the x-ray (Ill. XI-2), on the next page, reveals a minor nuclear shift and disc wedge between C 4 and C 5 but a major disc wedge with 3mm contra-rotation between C 3 and C 4 - C 3 is the torticollis subluxation.

Notice the acute scoliosis created by this acute disc block subluxation. (Ill. XI-3 page 147). But look at the 4th and 5th lumbar. The fourth lumbar is grossly wedged and the 5th is anomalous; there also is a 6mm right leg deficiency.

Three adjustments solved this torticollis subluxation. Twelve days later the x-ray (Ill. XI-4) was taken. The lumbar problem and lack of total spinal balance is easily seen on Ill. XI-5. A sacral base x-ray was taken (T.S.B.) as explained on pages 160-165. The sacrum was substantially low on the right. Subsequent wedging of 4th and 5th lumbar has overcompensated and created an inferiority on the left. The left leaning tower scoliosis creates a lack of spinal balance and thus cervical strain and resulting torticollis. This patient could well have developed more distortion and even scoliosis without chiropractic care. Lumbar adjustment restored balance to this young lady's spine and her cervical problems ceased. She remained under my personal care until her spinal growth ceased. As stated by Dr. Crowder in Chapter X: "Juvenile torticollis is common in the chiropractically unattended."

Remember, in most cases of torticollis spinal change has occurred that predisposes the person to this peculiar disc block subluxation. A patient may only relate that while shampooing, she tipped her head forward to rinse her hair and sustained an attack of torticollis. Pre and post x-rays commonly reveal a chronic kyphosis, proving that the predisposition existed before the attack.

LATERAL TORTICOLLIS
Before

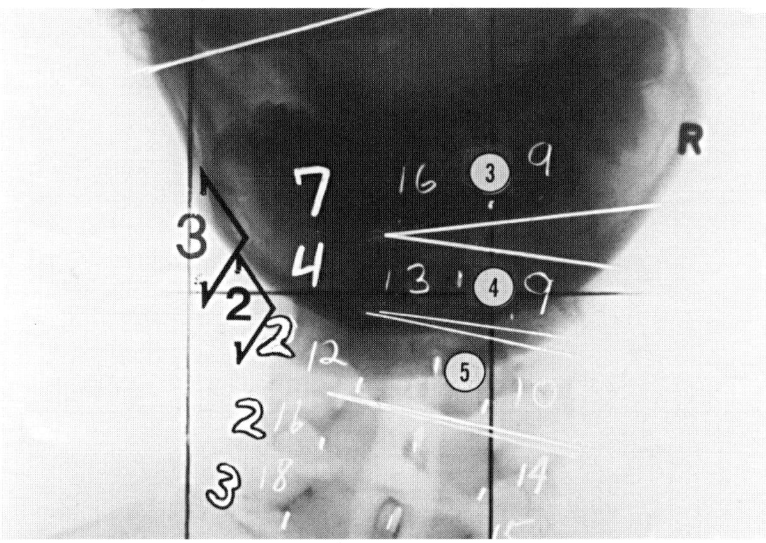

(Ill. XI-2) This is a close-up of the cervical subluxation seen on Ill. XI-3, next page. Notice the minor involvement and nuclear shift between C 4 and C 5. The major subluxation exists between C 3 and C 4. The 3rd cervical is rotated 3mm body left in relation to C 4, that is **away** from the open side of the disc wedge. C 3 is the major subluxated vertebra.

ACUTE TORTICOLLIS SCOLIOSIS
Before

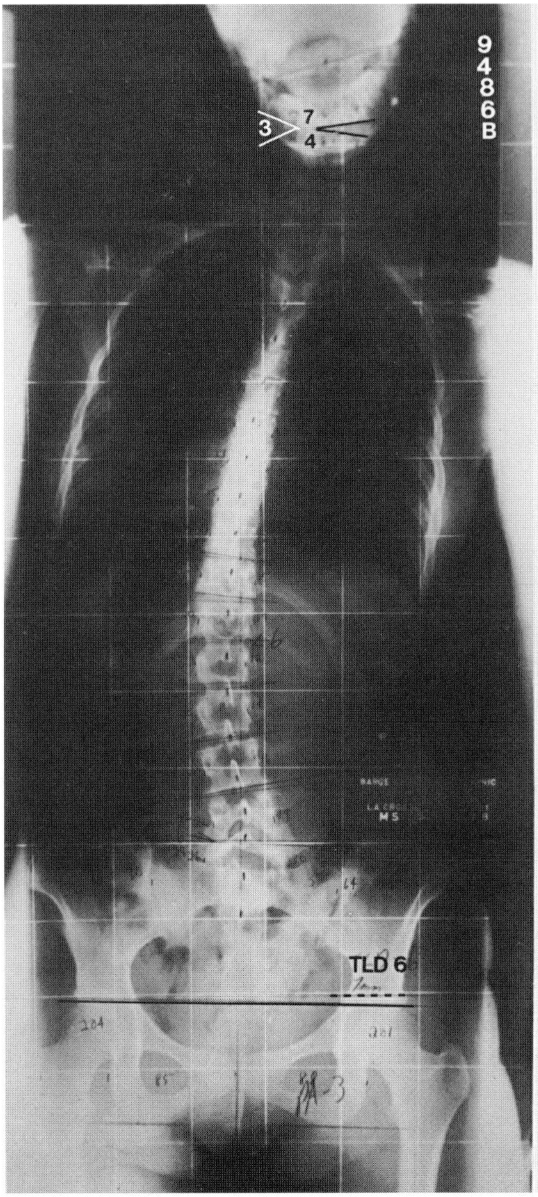

(Ill. XI-3) The scoliosis during the acute attack of torticollis, see page 145, 146 for the explanation.

LATERAL TORTICOLLIS
After

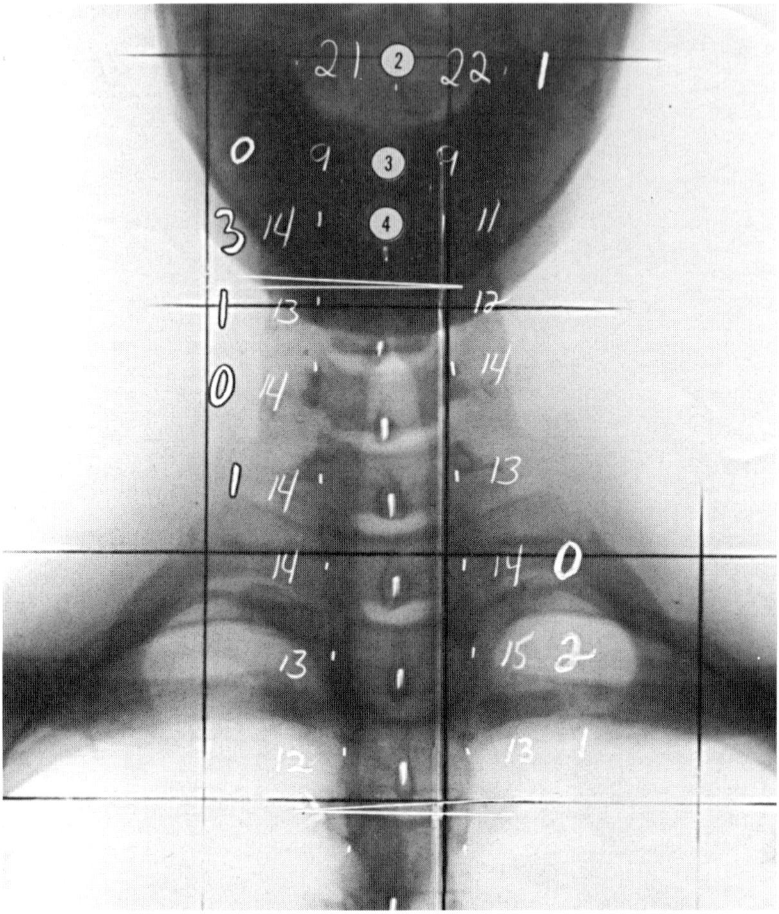

(Ill. XI-4) Twelve days later, three adjustments between x-rays and the cervical spine is quite normal. Remember that total spinal balance must be achieved to stop reoccurring attacks of torticollis. The cause of faulty spinal balance can be supragenic or infragenic. Forces below such as unilateral sacral inferiority, anatomical short leg, lumbar disc block subluxiation, all can combine to necessitate spinal adaptations and curvatures. Forces above can cause faulty spinal balance due to a disturbance in the righting reflex which can be improved through upper cervical adjustment. For a complete discussion of these factors consult the author's text SCOLIOSIS, VOL. III[21], a brief overview is given in this text, pages 160-171.

SCOLIOSIS
After Adjustment

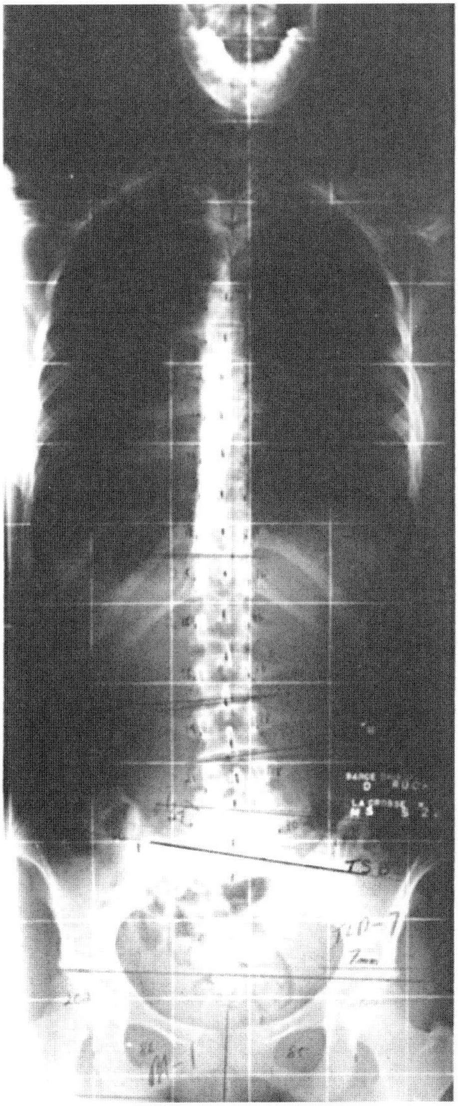

(Ill. XI-5) The same scoliosis as on (Ill. XI-3) after chiropractic correction of the torticollis subluxation, see page 145 & 146 for the explanation. The sacral base line TSB on the above x-ray was derived by taking a 14x17 sacral base x-ray. See page 160.

SCOLIOSIS
Prone to Torticollis
Before

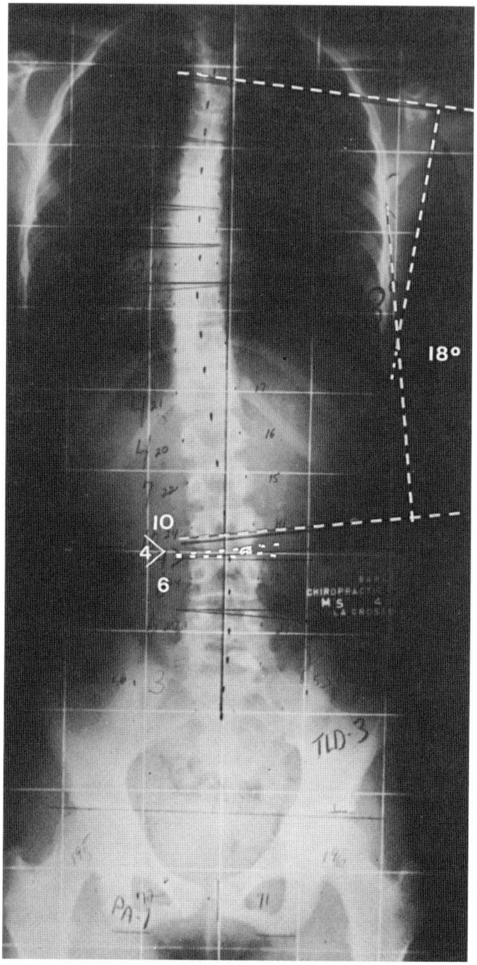

(Ill. XI-6) A chronic 3rd lumbar tortipelvis subluxation created the curvature in this young lady of 14 years. Note that the 3rd lumbar is rotated 4mm away from the open side of the disc wedge. For those interested in this subluxation I refer you to VOL. I TORTIPELVIS.[16] Lack of spinal balance in curvatures is prone to produce torticollis. Not visible on this x-ray is a torticollis subluxation of the Axis, for a close-up of this subluxation see Ill. XI-8 page 152.

SCOLIOSIS
Prone to Torticollis
After

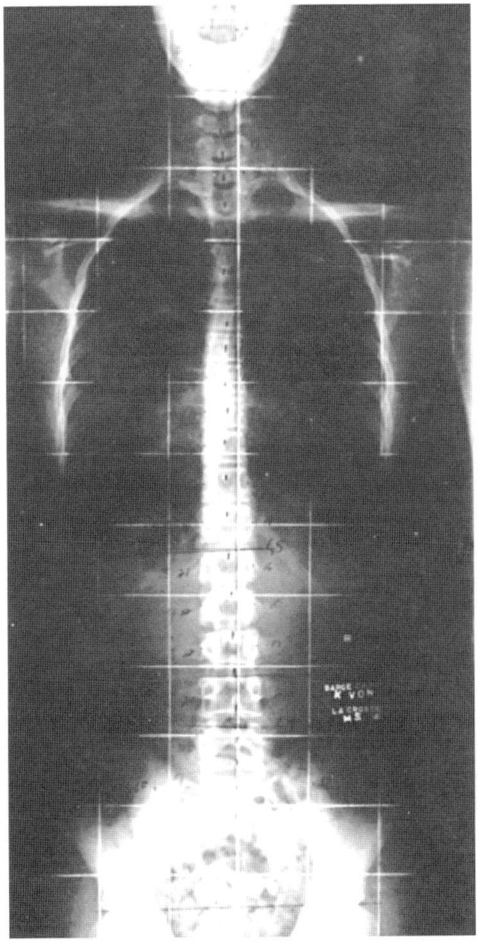

(Ill. XI-7) Here is an x-ray of this same young lady one year later. The scoliosis on the opposite page is prone to torticollis. The lumbar disc block subluxation created the scoliotic curve, the cervical spine endeavoring to achieve balance develops disc wedges that are prone to torticollis. Full spine x-rays should be taken of all youthful torticollis cases. Three adjustments solved this young lady's acute problem. (Ill. XI-8 & XI-9) Adjustment then followed throughout the next year for overall correction of the scoliosis.

LATERAL TORTICOLLIS
Before

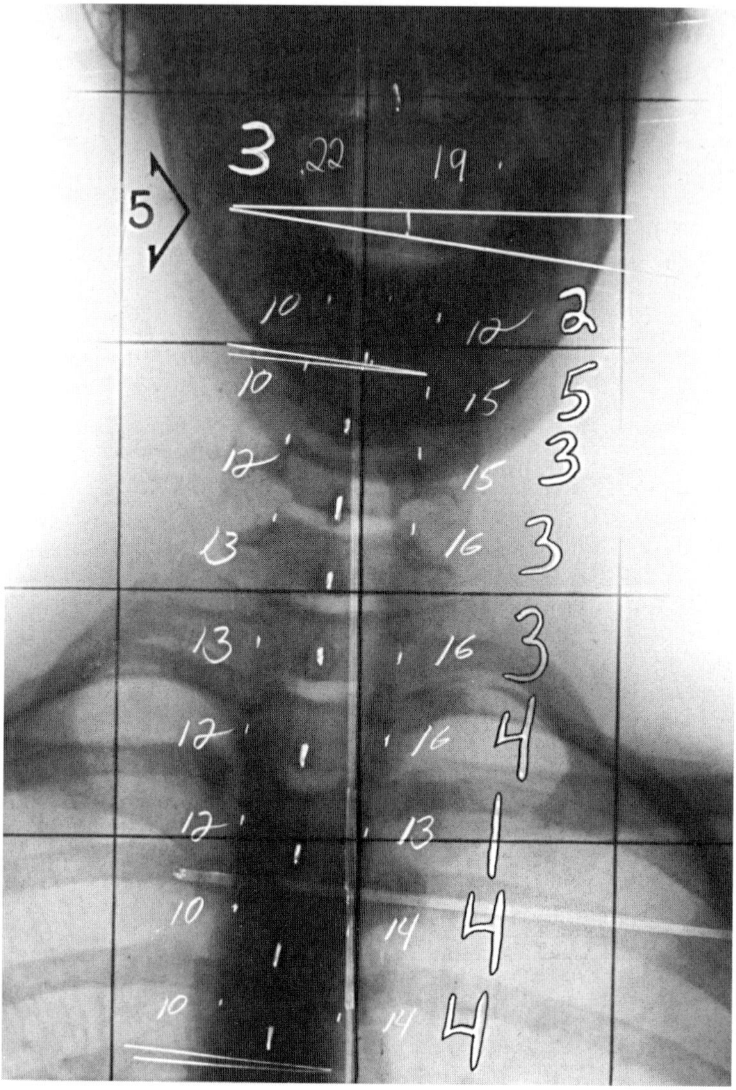

(Ill. XI-8) A close-up of the acute torticollis subluxation shown on Ill. XI-6 page 150. The 3rd cervical is rotated 2mm body right, the Axis is rotated 3mm body left *away from the wide, (open), side of the disc wedge*. A 5mm contra-rotation exists between C 3 and C 4. Now look at the next page.

LATERAL TORTICOLLIS
After

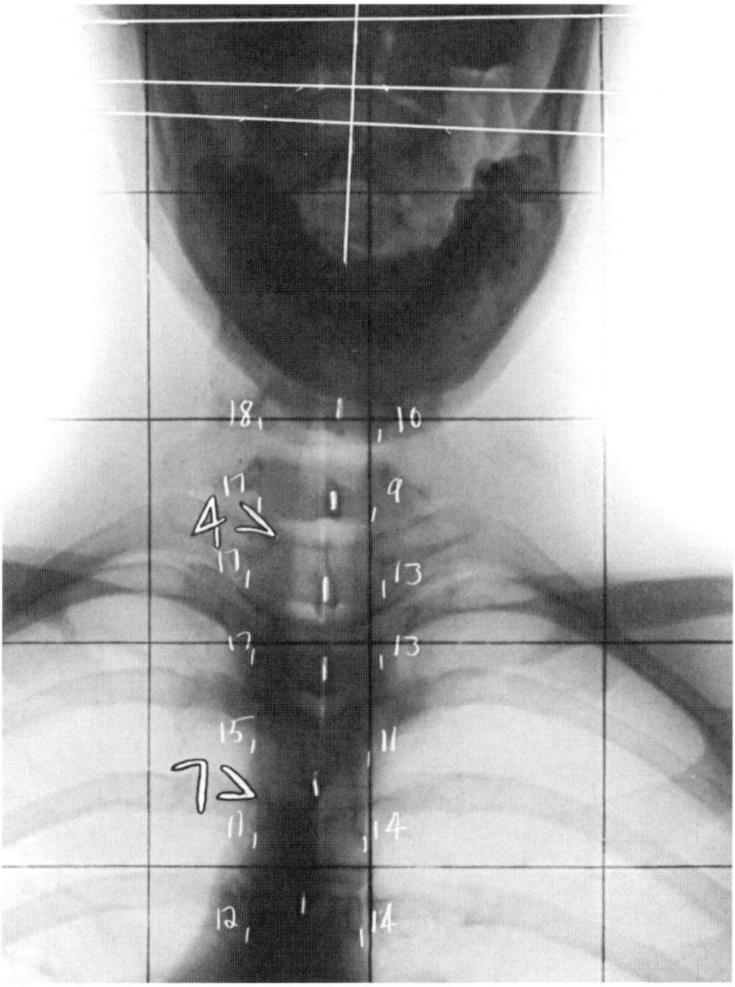

(Ill. XI-9) After two adjustments this patient was quite well. The third adjustment completely solved the acute problem. Full spine correction was then undertaken to eliminate the curvature. Our adjustic and symptomatic report sheets indicated that objectively the curvature was gone on the eighth visit. Careful surveillance followed for one year with another set of x-rays taken then. See the full spine view on Ill. XI-7 on page 151 for the complete correction of this problem.

ANTERIOR LATERAL TORTICOLLIS
Before

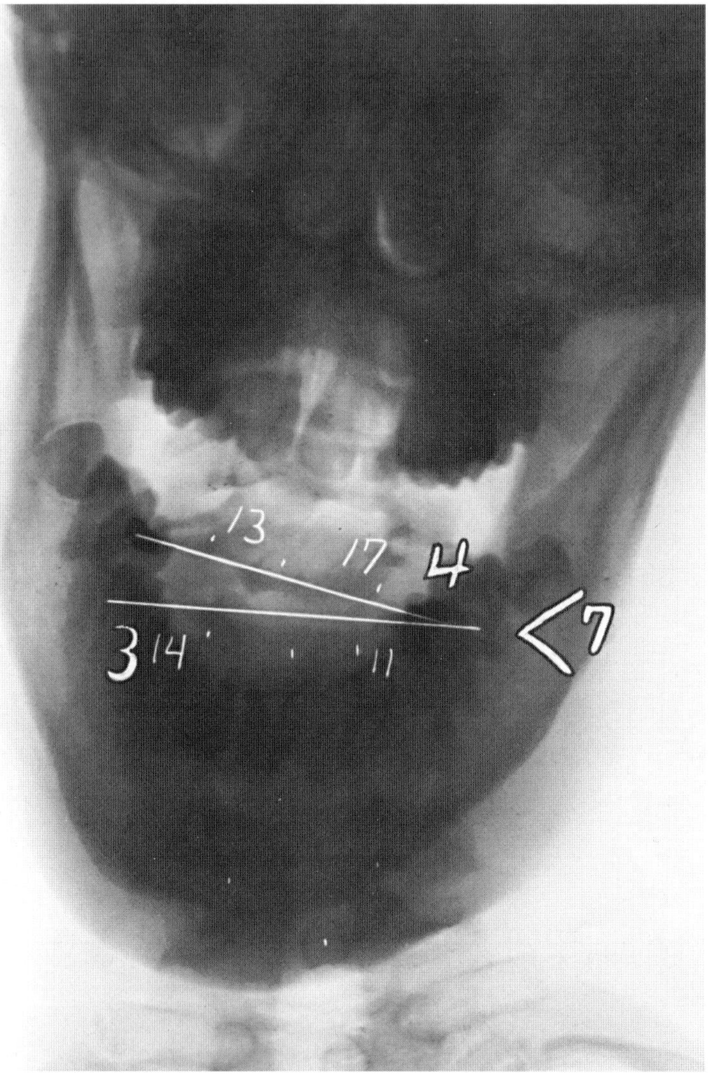

(Ill. XI-10) The x-ray above, and on the next five pages, is of a young man, age 14, who sustained an attack of anterior lateral torticollis playing football. The subluxation is C 3* with contra-rotation 7mm away from the open side of the disc wedge. The lateral x-ray is on page 156.

* Do not mistake the image of the tooth for the odontoid on this x-ray.

ANTERIOR LATERAL TORTICOLLIS
After (Eight Days)

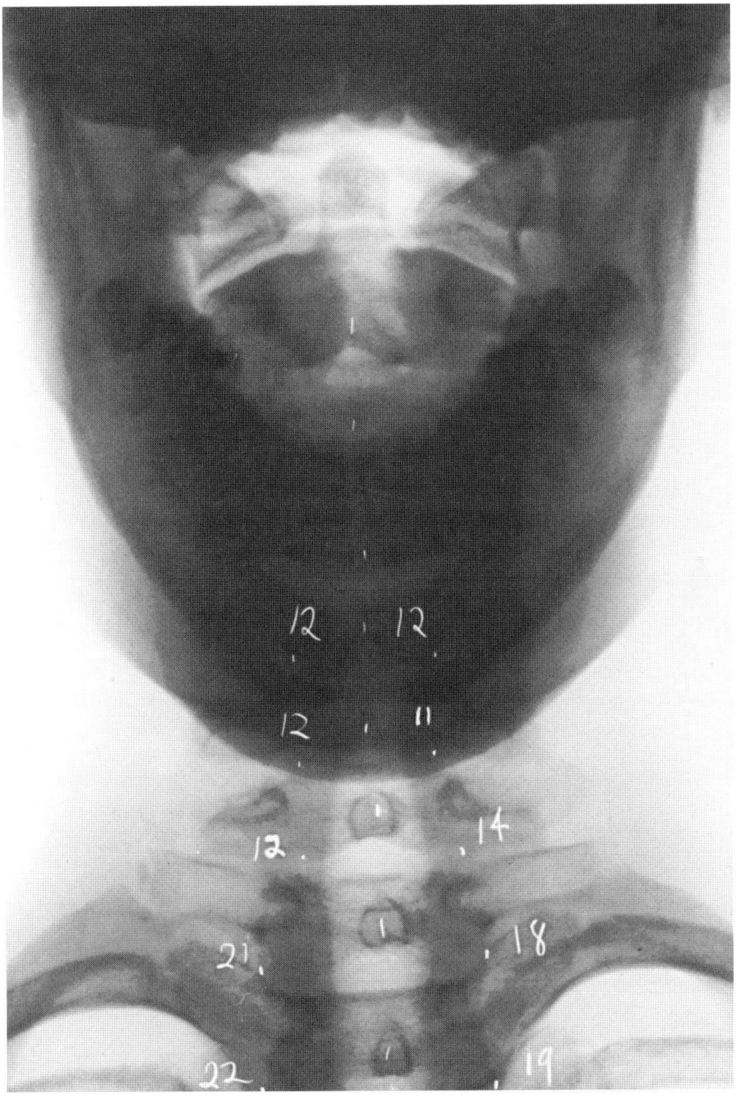

(Ill. XI-11) Eight days between the x-ray above and (Ill. XI-10) on the opposite page. Three adjustments accomplished the reduction of this subluxation. The laterals follow on the next three pages. The lateral of this x-ray is on page 157.

ANTERIOR LATERAL TORTICOLLIS
Before

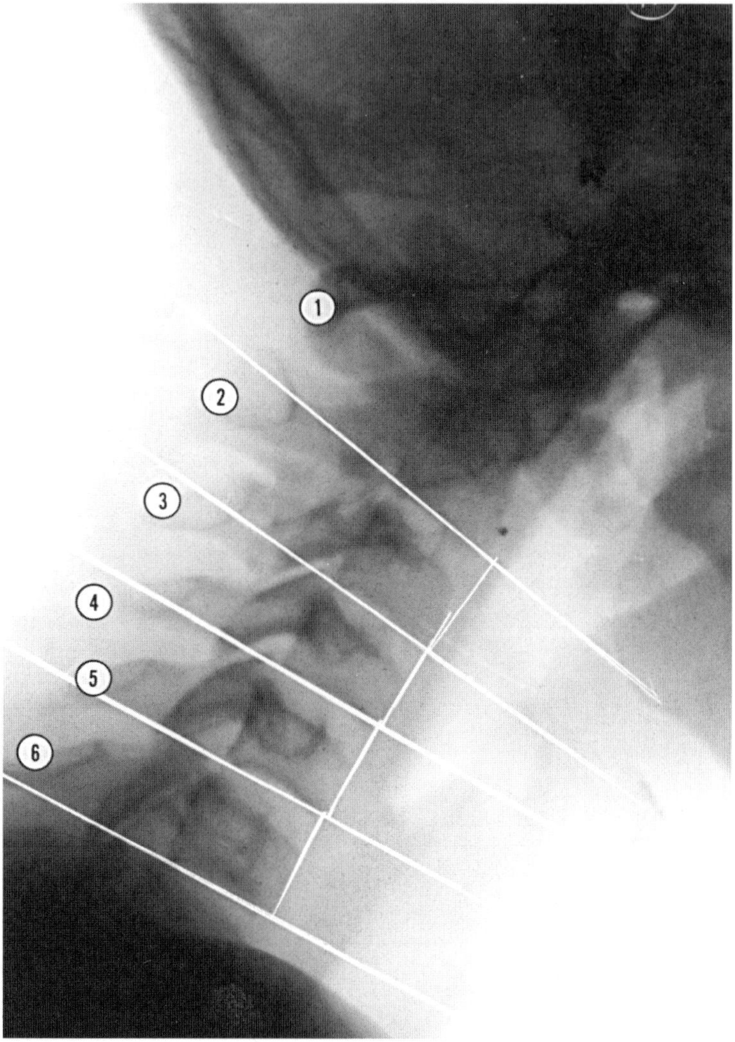

(Ill XI-12) Here on the first lateral x-ray the convergence of the body lines indicates 3rd cervical and Axis are both involved, C 3 was adjusted as the major. Following the analysis given in this text we have a posterior lateral shift of the nucleus between Axis and C 3 and C 3 and C 4. The A.P. x-ray is on page 154.

ANTERIOR LATERAL TORTICOLLIS
After (Eight Days)

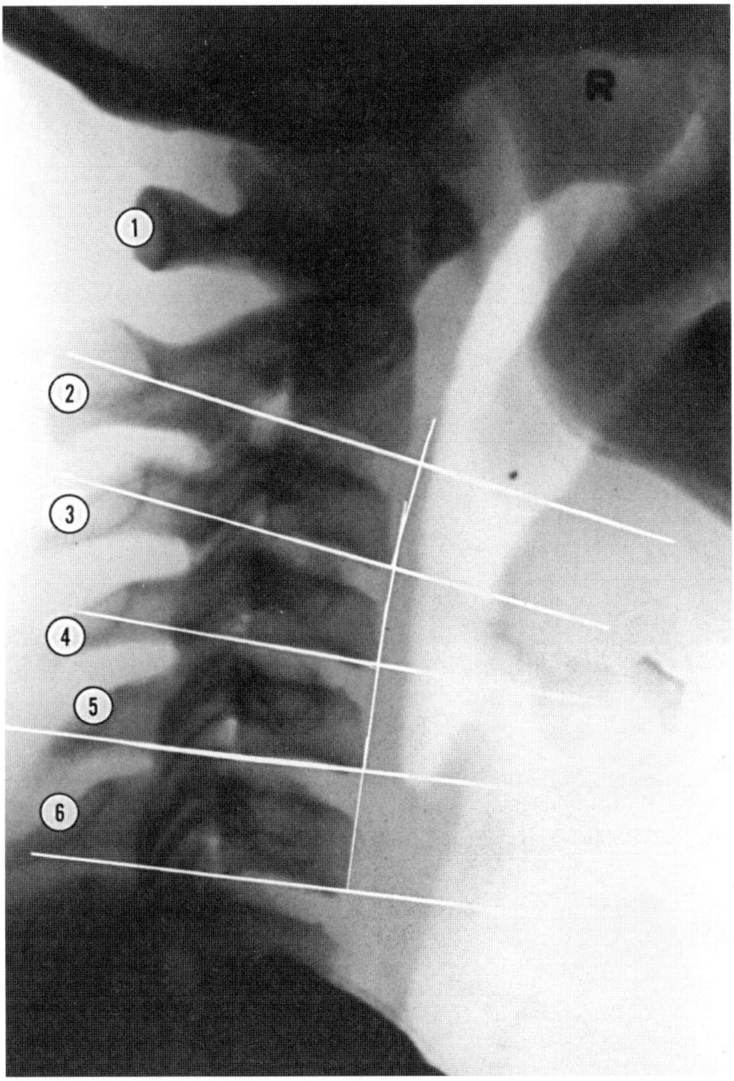

(Ill. XI-13) The x-ray above is the mate to the A.P. on page 155, Ill. XI-11. The acute symptoms are now all but gone. A kyphosis and tendency toward posterior nuclear shift remain. This young man continued to have some problems with his neck and we decided to take a 14x36 A.P. x-ray, see (Ill. XI-14).

FULL SPINE

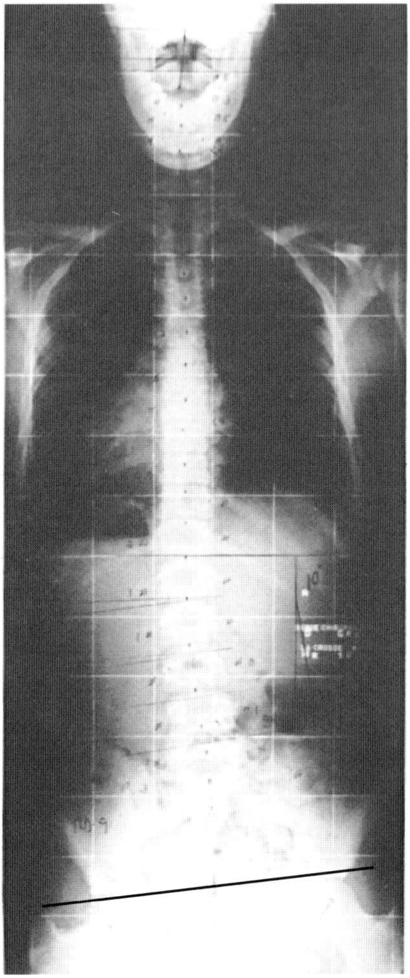

(Ill. XI-14) The x-ray above indicates why I say that many cases of torticollis in youth are caused by a problem somewhere lower down in the spinal column. This torticollis attack was traumatic in origin and the attending doctor took only 8x10 x-rays. When repeated problems occurred he then took the above 14x36 x-ray. There is a 9mm left leg deficiency and resulting compensatory curve. The placement of a left heel lift* has balanced this young man's spine, thus eliminating his reoccurring cervical problems. The x-rays showing this acute problem and its correction are on pages 154 - 157.

* Heel lifts are not placed on the criteria of an anatomically short leg alone. The sacrum must be inferior on the same side and verified by sacral base x-rays! (See page 160.)

ANTERIOR LATERAL TORTICOLLIS
After (Six Months)

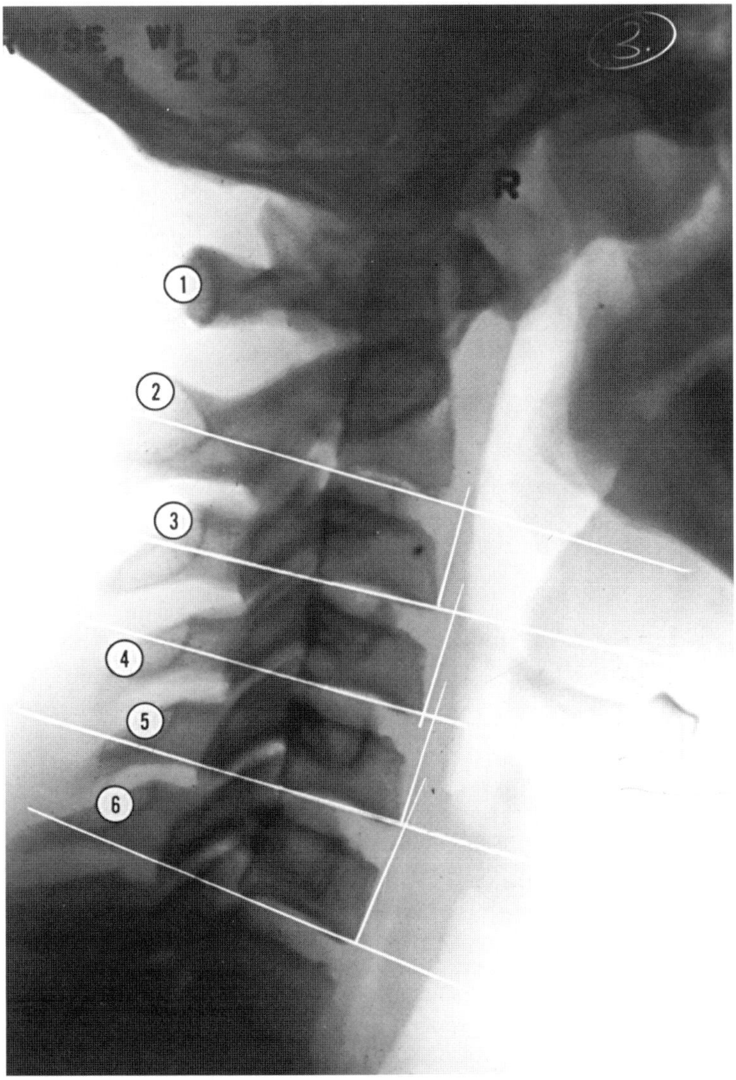

(Ill. XI-15) Six months transpired between this x-ray and x-ray shown on Ills. XI-12 & 13. The lateral x-ray above shows a return of the normal cervical lordosis. Notice that the improved lordotic curve has not been accomplished by a tipping back of the head! The occiput and mandible are at the same angle as Ill. XI-13 page 157.

THE SACRAL BASE

The spine displays a typical distortion on the frontal, or A to P plane. The absolutely straight spine is non-existent and to attempt to achieve orthoganal alignment either segmentally or globally throughout the spine is folly. The spine commonly exhibits a typical distortion, often called today the physiological curve. It has been recorded in anatomy books in the late 19th century and Willard Carver LLD, D.C. referred to it as "Distortion by Compensation."* He entitled this physiological curve, "Carvers Typical Distortion" and described it as the "Typical Complex, Opposed, Rotational Scoliosis," herein I quote his exact wordage. (In this quote ventral refers in its classical sense to the anterior).

"Right innominate headward in its relation to the sacrum; left innominate crest-ventral; sacrum rotated ventral aspect to the right turning the fifth and fourth lumbars with it, but less far in proportion to distortion of intervertebral discs; third lumbar in gravity plane or crossing; second and first lumbars rotated by the ventral aspect to the left as are also the twelfth, eleventh, tenth, and ninth thoracics; eighth and seventh in gravity plane; sixth, fifth, fourth, third and second thoracics rotated by their ventral aspects to the right, forming a right scoliosis; first thoracic and seventh cervical in gravity plane; sixth, fifth, fourth, third and second cervicals rotated by their ventral aspects to the left, which fails to bring the Axis fully to the gravity plane, hence the Atlas is rotated by its ventral aspect to the right, sufficiently to bring its weight-carrying aspects to the gravity plane."

On the facing page I have reproduced Dr. Carver's illustration of this typical distortion, the physiological curve of the human spine. Most scoliotic curves, such as the "Double Major Thoracolumbar Scoliosis," follow this physiological design. It has been related to right handedness and other factors. Those seeking more information on the physiological curve I would refer you to my text SCOLIOSIS. But for now it must be understood that the spine will seek to compensate for sacral inferiorities and in so doing create distortion through compensation. If the sacrum is anatomically low on one side the spine will compensate. In "THE NEURODYNAMICS of the VERTEBRAL SUBLUXATION,"[25] Dr. A. E. Homewood had this to say:

"It is doubtful that there exists a more important area of the vertebral column than the sacrum for the determination of the

* See Carvers texts, Carver Chiropractic Analysis, cira 1920s.[27]

CARVER'S TYPICAL DISTORTION[26]

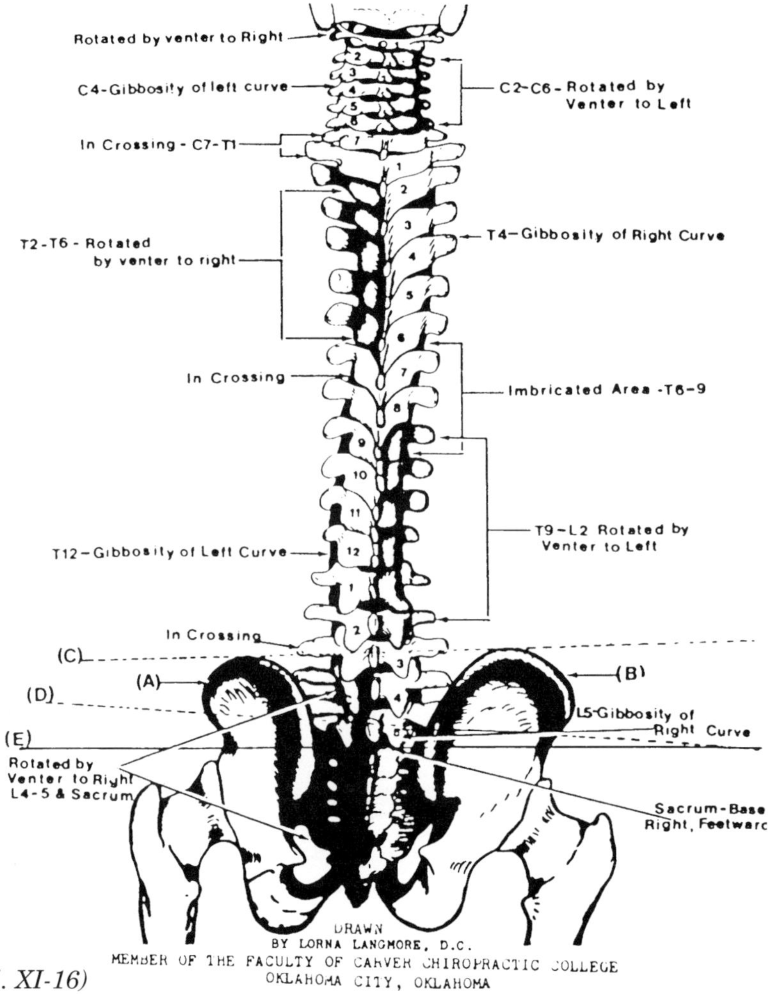

(Ill. XI-16)

true cause of the average patient's health problem. For here is the base and as the base goes, so goes the superimposed spine. The necessity for compensation for basic distortion creates areas of stress within the spine which tend to give way under added stress that would be insufficient to overcome the inherent resistance of a normal spine."

I heartily agree, and stress in the areas of compensation can create acute manifestations and torticollis is one such result.

Dr. H. B. Logan D.C. said it this way:[20]

"We might safely say that distortions throughout other parts of the body are largely or wholly dependent upon distortions of the spinal column. Adjusting locally subluxated vertebrae is valuable, since it is indisputably true that we have obtained results, in some instances outstanding results, therefrom. But if, as we now know, subluxations are dependent upon spinal distortions originating from unequal or uneven base or foundation, then they cannot remain adjusted or corrected until such major distortion is corrected, or until the base or foundation is made level."

As I have said before, and as Dr. Crowder mentioned in his chapter; torticollis can often be a symptom of chronic underlying spinal problems. Thus after the acute attack is resolved it is best to look for such problems. In looking for infragenic causes, the sacral base x-ray is imperative. Due to the angle of the sacrum its base is obscured on the common A.P. Lumbopelvic x-ray. Methods to determine its level on the common A.P. Lumbopelvic x-ray are commonly in error. Therefore in 1962 this author devised a way to x-ray the actual sacral base; the sacral base x-ray. First the sacral angle is determined on the lateral x-ray. (Ill. XI-17)

DETERMINING THE SACRAL ANGLE

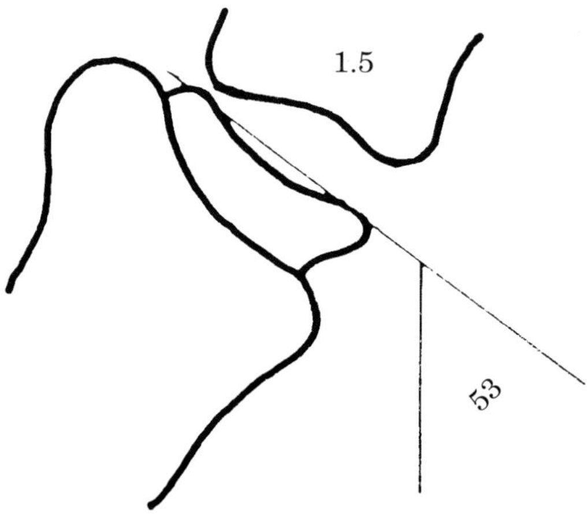

(Ill. XI-17) The Barge sacral angle is determined by drawing a line across the superior aspect of the sacrum and measuring the angle it makes with the vertical edge of the film.

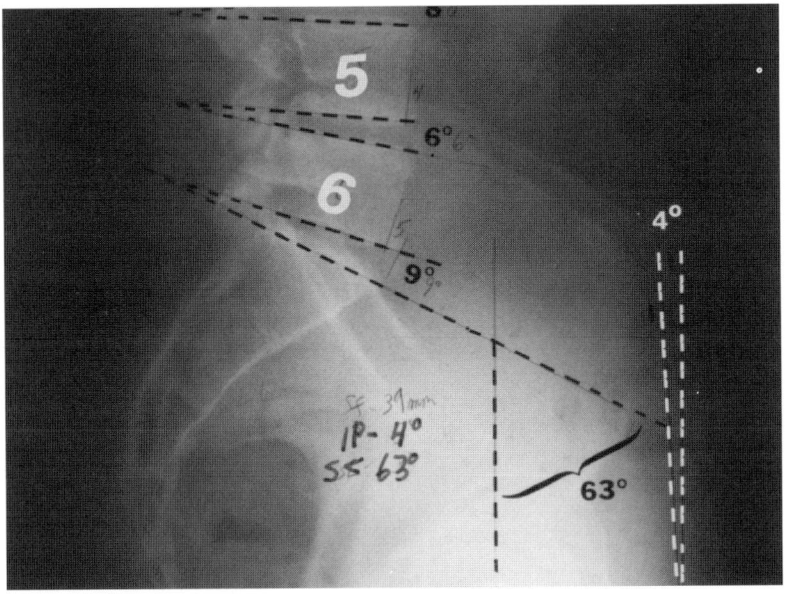

(Ill. XI-18) Determing the Sacral Angle.*

The taking of the sacral base film requires a knowledge of the sacral base angle as determined previously by lateral x-ray. (Ill. XI-18 above). The tube is tilted to correspond to the angle of the sacral base. The patient is positioned before the bucky as in the A. to P. x-ray using a 14x17 film. Take pains to eliminate pelvic rotational distortion. The tube will have to be moved considerably closer to the patient. (Ill. XI-19) Gauge this position using a light device or a string. Because of the central ray angle, the film bucky placement will need to be several inches higher than the horizontal anterior to posterior shot. The KV must be determined with the calipers held at the same angle showing the need for considerably greater penetrating distance. With a bit of trial and error a suitable technic can be worked out to the doctor's satisfaction. When there is an acute sacral angle the patient may have to stand on a platform in order to achieve decent tube distance. (Ill. XI-19 next page)

The sacral base x-ray reveals the true level of the sacral base. It often reveals structural anomalies that will create compensatory distortions. See (Ill. XI-20).

* For the other determinations shown on this x-ray, see VOL. I TORTIPELVIS.[16]

PATIENT — TUBE PLACEMENT

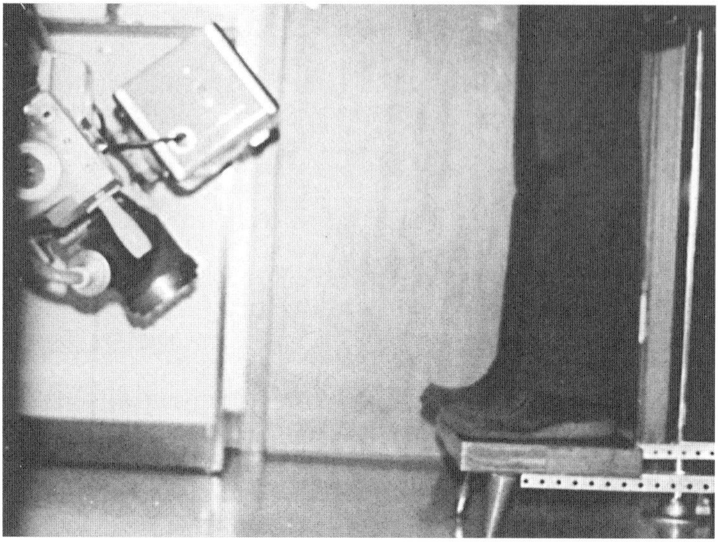

(Ill. XI-19) The platform you see here folds up against the wall (behind the bucky) when not in use.

PLATEAU SACRUM DEFICIENT ON ONE SIDE

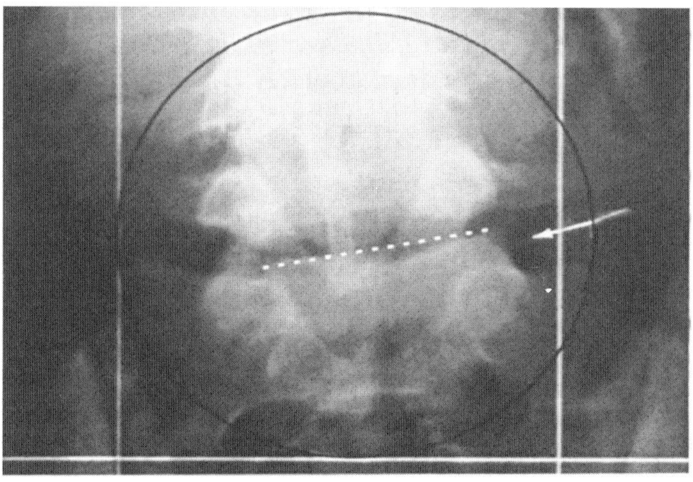

(Ill. XI-20) This congenital anomaly can be familial in origin and produce the so-called hereditary scoliosis.

UNILATERAL SACRAL INFERIORITY

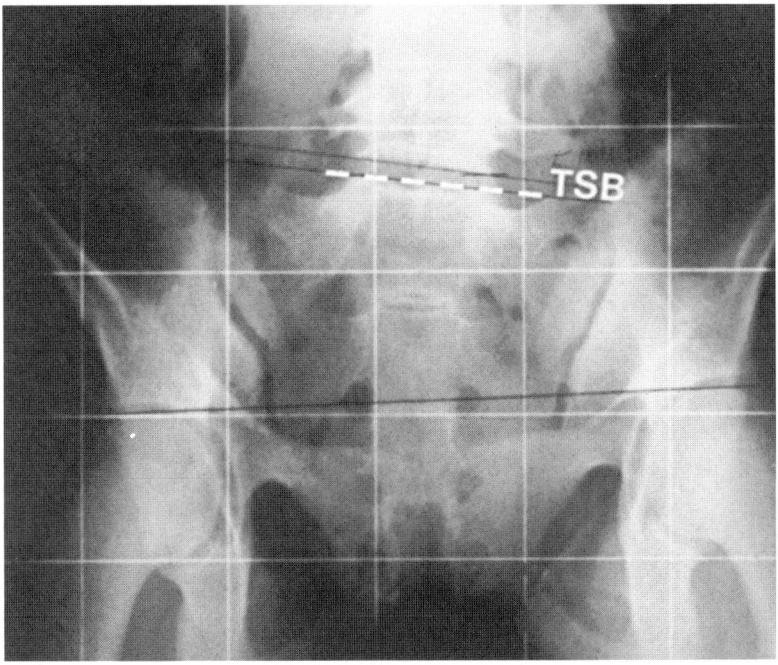

(Ill. XI-21) Sacral base films have revealed to us that as far as the sacrum is concerned, anomaly is more the rule than the exception. Furthermore, sacral inferiority is often opposite the side of leg deficiency. Lifts must not be placed according to leg deficiency alone. The sacral base film is the only way to determine true sacral inferiority.

My own research and the research at the Logan College of Chiropractic are both reported in my text SCOLIOSIS, but the readers of this text should grasp the point intended here. There are problems in the lower spine that set up compensatory curvatures which can lead to acute episodes of torticollis and tortipelvis.

SCOLIOSIS

For the reader who is interested in complete study of this deforming progressive rotatory scoliosis of youth I refer you to my final volume of this triology of books, VOL. III SCOLIOSIS.[21] For the purpose of this text let it be noted here that unilateral sacral inferiority has been found to be a frequent cause of this scoliosis.

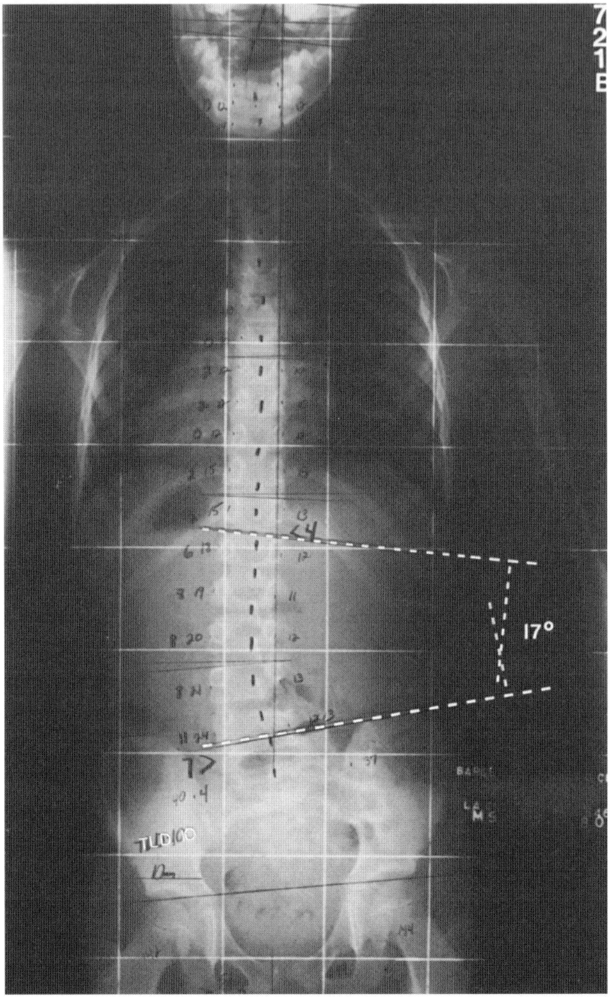

(Ill. XI-22) Standing 14x36 x-ray.

14x36 x-rays reveal the effect that an anatomical short leg has on the spine. On the x-ray above you can see how the cervical spine tips back to plumb endeavoring to achieve balance. Such spines are prone to develop scoliosis and those so afflicted commonly suffer acute attacks of torticollis. Notice also that the odontoid **is not** centered over the sacrum. This balance problem may also involve the "righting reflex" — read on.

THE RIGHTING REFLEX

The spine is a concatenation, a connected series of joints, a tightly linked chain so to speak; the twisting of one end influences the other. It is designed as a vertical pillar in man with three distinct sagittal curves and therefore balance is necessary as gravitational stress can cause distortion. Early chiropractic pioneers, Drs. Carver and Logan, both spoke on these factors. Both of these early writers on spinal structure based their observations on infragenic problems that cause the superimposed spine to accommodate. But, as B. J. Palmer tried to point out, there are factors other than structural that set the stage for spinal distortion. In all spinal distortion **supragenic** and **infragenic** forces play a part. In this chapter I have briefly touched on infragenic problems such as lumbar scoliosis and unilateral sacral inferiority; now let us turn to the supragenic forces, the proprioceptive reflex mechanisms that control spinal balance. These balance mechanisms are located in the brain stem and in the cervical spine. My text, VOL. III SCOLIOSIS[21] goes into this thoroughly and I will now quote from pages XIV and XV from said text. Quoting "SPINE":

"In a paper written by Maquire, Madigan, Wallace, Leppanen and Draper, they mention as 'A possible cause of Scoliosis;'[28]

'Spinal cord reflexes play an integral role in the maintenance of posture. These complex polysynaptic segmental reflexes are regulated by a variety of descending suprasegmental systems, by peripheral afferent impulses and within the spinal cord by a network of interneurons and propriospinal neurons."

Yes, the maintenance of correct posture is controlled by the nervous system. As B. J. Palmer stated, "faulty attitude or habit" seldom creates scoliosis. It does little to berate little Jane or Johnny to "straighten up" when the child in no way can control that which he/she is not in command of.

Ever since Yamada and Yamamoto reported in SPINE[29] in a paper by scoliosis investigators Nachemson and Sahlstrand that equilibrium mechanisms may be involved in the cause of scoliosis, investigators have written on this basic cause of the problem. Nachemson and Sahlstrand[29] stated in the aforementioned paper:

"Considering these facts, it is conceivable that a functional asymmetry or disturbance somewhere in the vestibular-spinal reflex arc might be a contributing mechanism in idiopathic scoliosis. The level of dysfunction might be in the peripheral sensitivity of the labyrinthic reception mechanism, in the junctions centrally located

in the brain stem, or in the spine."

Yes, the disturbance could well be in the "brain stem" and thus, the work of upper cervical chiropractic practitioners that clearly indicates the restoration of spinal balance through upper cervical care becomes clear in the light of the understanding that the Atlas/Axis/Occipital subluxation can interfere with the area in the cord wherein this mechanism is housed. The above quote from Nachemson & Sahlstrand also states, *"or in the spine."* Timothy G. Gerhart, D.C., reported this in his paper, "The Role of Cervical Joint Dysfunction in Balance and Coordination"[30], herein he quotes the work of Cohen and States:

"... the loss of sensory input from cervical joint receptors results in signs and symptoms very similar to those of inner ear dysfunction. Indeed, cervical mechanoreceptor function is as essential as labyrinthine function for normal balance and orientation.

Cohen demonstrated this quite graphically in his work with primates. Following anesthetic block of the first, second and third cervical verve roots with resulting impairment of mechanoreceptor sensation, the animals were released into a specially equipped gymnasium. In each case, severe defects in balance, orientation and motor coordination affecting the entire body were present. The animals displayed in wide-based, unsteady gait, disturbed hand-eye coordination and alterations in skeletal muscle tonus. The resultant locomotion was described as similar to that of a severely intoxicated human with accompanying disorientation and incoordination.

The key to understanding these results lies in the function of the joint mechanoreceptors. Type I, II, and IV sensory receptors reside in the synovial capsules of the cervical facet joints and joints of von Luschka."

So you see, facet subluxations of the cervial spine and the subsequent inflamatory process involved, can influence the proprioceptive reflex mechanisms located in the capsular ligaments of these structures and impair balance.

Author's Note

As reported by Timothy G. Gerhart, D.C., Success Express [30] Vol. 7, No. 1 Spring 1984, *cervical joint dysfunction can impair balance and coordination.* ***Joint mechanoreceptors reside in the synovial capsules of the cervical facet joints and joints of von Luschka.*** *This point is clear, cervical subluxation can impair equilibrium function.*

SPINAL BALANCE CORRECTION

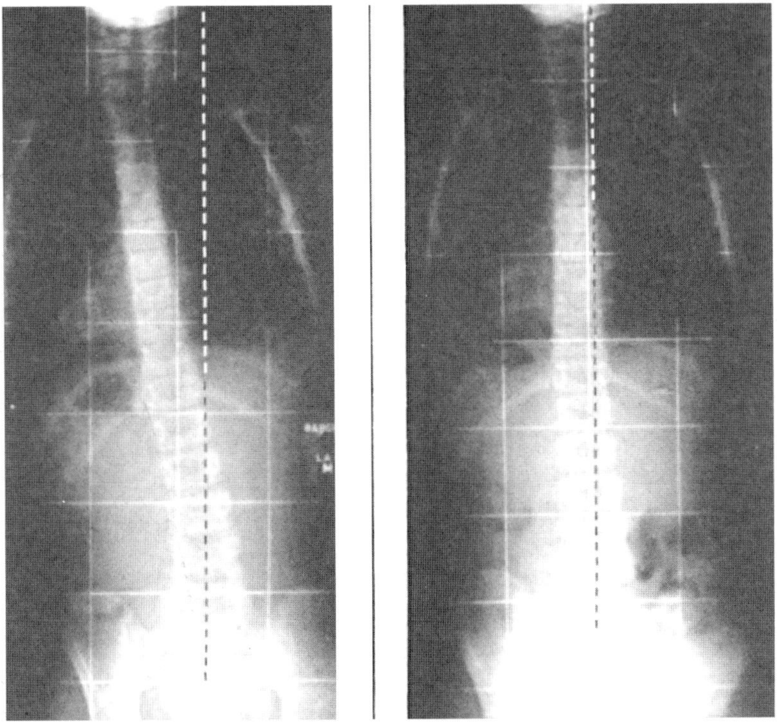

BEFORE AFTER

(Ill. XI-23) The above two x-rays indicate the correction gained through upper cervical adjustment in less than four months time. The spinal balance has been greatly improved (odontoid over sacrum). The child was also an epileptic and this problem too is responding nicely to chiropractic care.

When balance is impaired the spine will throw its weight to one side or the other, forward or backward, or a combination of directions. 14x36 A.P. and lateral x-ray evaluation is an important tool in determining equilibrium malfunction. On the x-ray above (Ill. XI-23) we can clearly see the problem in spinal balance caused by a cervical subluxation. 14x36 **lateral** x-rays are also necessary in determining spinal balance problems. When the body inclines forward due to impairment of balance, all secondary curves of the spine flatten and the thoracic spine becomes hypokyphotic (Ill. XI-24).

SPINAL BALANCE

LATERAL X-RAY Before LATERAL X-RAY After

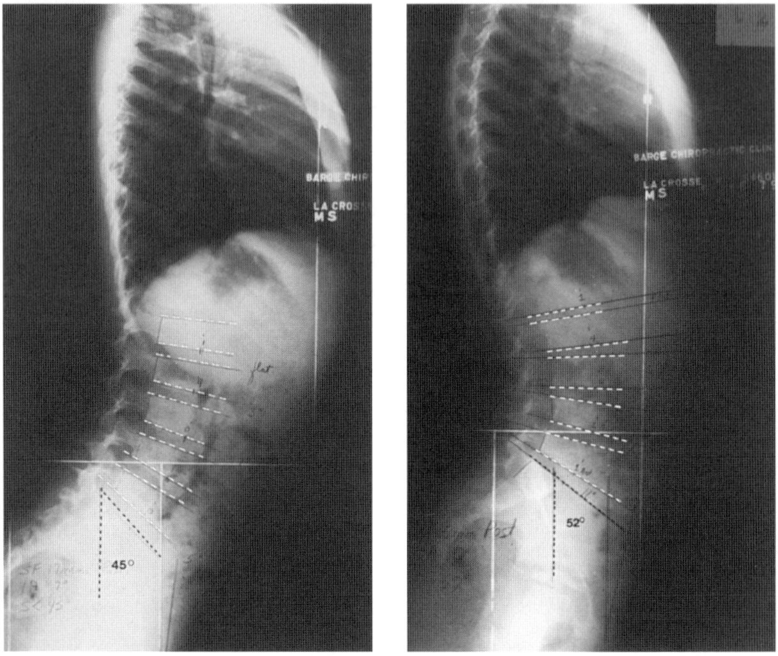

(Ill. XI-24) When the weight is borne forward a flattening of the lumbar and cervical lordoses occur and the thoracic spine becomes hypokyphotic. Chiropractic adjustments allowed the child's spine to assume its normal sigmoid contours in 3 1/2 months. Cervical 8x10 x-rays showed first a cervical kyphosis and then a return of the normal cervical lordotic curve.

Other than 14x36 x-rays, bilateral scales and plumb line devices (Ill. XI-26) can help monitor the improvement in spinal balance as adjustic correction of subluxations correct the cause.

Pes cavus (Ill. XI-25), in my opinion, is a righting reflex problem. When a child bears their weight forward they tend to be "pigeon toed" on **both** sides and exhibit pes cavus; they carry their weight forward on the "balls" of their feet and thus raise the arch. Now this is expressing a rather bold opinion by the author but research seems to indicate impaired balance is implicated in pes cavus. In SPINE, Vol. 19 #11, 1994, in a paper entitled "The Relationship Between Pes Cavus and Idiopathic Scoliosis,"[31] the authors state:

"In conclusion, a statistically significant correlation was observed between the incidence of pes cavus and scoliosis. Spina Bifida occulta was ruled out as an etiologic factor. Therefore, it is believed that in certain patients with idiopathic scoliosis who have other disorders, such as pes cavus, the deformity may be due to a malfunction of the system of balance at some level of the nervous system."

It has also been my observation that when the spine towers to one side the pelvis on the same side rotates to the anterior (Logan P.A., Gonstead EX). Thus the foot on the same side toes in. Adjustic correction of the pelvic rotation eliminates the toeing in problem but it quickly returns if the balance mechanism continues to cast the spine's balance to one side. The adjustment of the cervical subluxation solves the problem.

So in the ending of this chapter, let us reflect on the technics developed through the years chiropractically. A comprehensive study of both B.J. Palmer's upper cervical technic and H. B. Logan's concepts of unilateral sacral inferiority can bring forth a thorough understanding of the supragenic and infragenic forces that can combine to cause acute episodes of spinal dysfunction such as tortipelvis and torticollis. In youth both of these acute spinal problems should be considered harbingers of scoliosis and 14x36 x-ray studies should be taken after the acute episode subsides. A heel lift may be necessary to prevent scoliotic progression, this is clearly the need on (Ill. XI-22). The placement of a heel lift solved the problem in this case. VOL. III SCOLIOSIS[21] has a complete chapter on the appropriate use of heel lifts for those interested in the placement of this most useful tool in scoliotic spinal correction.

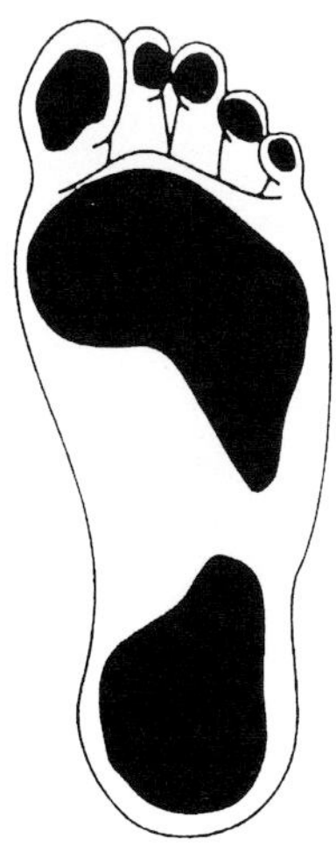

(Ill. XI-25) Pes cavus first is indicated by a reduction of the outside edge of the footprint. In grade #2, we see a disappearance of the outside edge, in grade #3, the outside edge disappears altogether.

PORTABLE MASTERS SPINALYZER

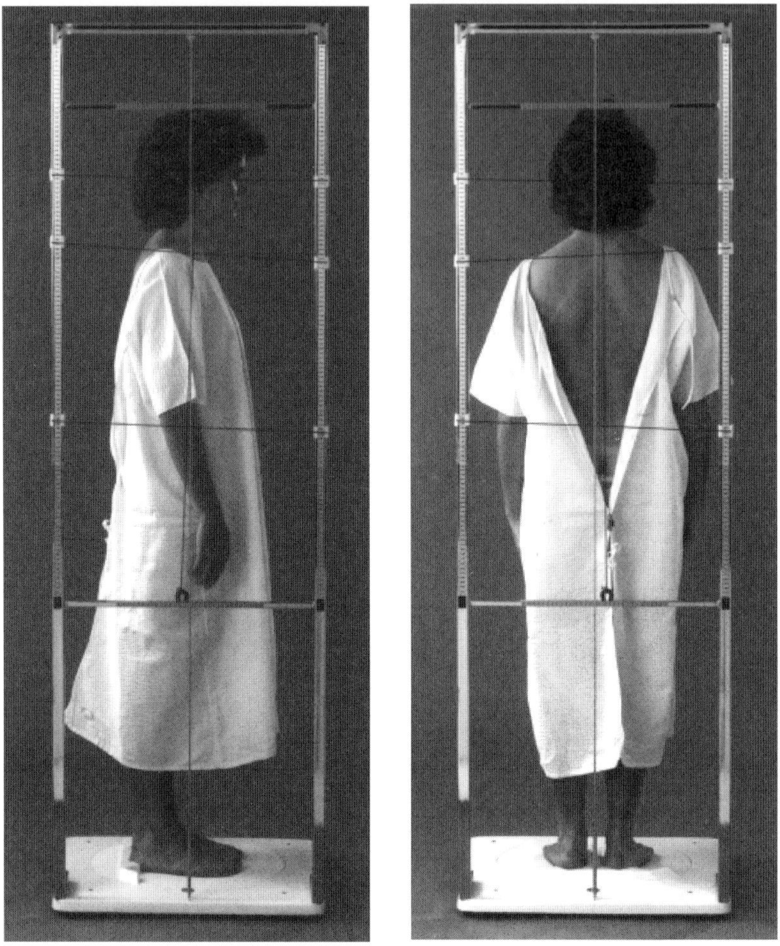

(Ill. XI-26) The Masters Spinalyzer is available with interchangeable turntable "T" footplate and bilateral scale.

Lloyd's Spinalyzer is a chrome posture standard that visually analyzes and measures spinal scoliosis in a matter of seconds. A turntable "T" footplate provides analysis from posterior, lateral and face-on views. It includes dual position foot notches for Dr. DeJarnette's sacrooccipital procedures. The Spinalyzer sets up quickly anywhere. Lloyd Table Co., Lisbon, Iowa.

CHAPTER XII
THE CHRONIC TORTICOLLIS SUBLUXATION

The chronic torticollis subluxation manifests itself upon x-ray by revealing an uncorrected disc block subluxation in the cervical spine. The subluxation is apparent on x-ray, but the patient may exhibit no objective or subjective symptoms of the old acute problem. The condition may be completely asymptomatic; or the patient will complain of symptoms as they relate to the neurological level of the subluxation. Brachialgia syndromes are particularly common in many of these cases. Numbness of the arms and hands, loss of strength in the upper extremities, tendinitis, myocytis, bursitis and carpal tunnel syndrome are common symptoms related by patients with this chronic spinal distortion.

Then too, systemic problems may be involved in the symptomatic picture; frequent sore throats and earaches are common in children who have chronic cervical subluxations. In the adult, facial neuralgias, laryngitis, sinusitis and the like, all can be related to the nerve root impairment caused by cervical subluxations; the disc block subluxation, in its chronic state, is often the culprit.

It is not the purpose of this text to discuss chronic spinal conditions, however, we feel that the reader should be cognizant of this subluxation in its chronic state so to better prognosticate recovery time. Chronic disc block subluxations are slow to respond to spinal adjustment, thus the doctor may want to indicate guarded prognosis and extend the recovery time when discussing results with patients.

We shall briefly discuss this subluxation in three categories:

1. **Chronic Lateral Torticollis Subluxation**
2. **Chronic Anterior Torticollis Subluxation**
3. **Chronic Anterior Lateral Torticollis Subluxation**

1. The Chronic Lateral Torticollis Subluxation

Upon A.P. full spine (14x36) x-ray analysis one can be suspicious of chronic lateral torticollis when analysis reveals a normal spine except for a cervical rotatory scoliosis. If analysis indicates a disc wedge with its wide (open) side on the concavity of the scoliotic curve it is commonly the chronic disc block subluxation of torticollis. The tipping of this vertebra creates an inferiority and the vertebrae above then create the adaptive rotatory scoliosis. In an acute torticollis this adaptive curve is not present, but the vertebrae above the subluxation tip laterally to one side in a leaning tower type scoliosis.

If a torticollis subluxation remains uncorrected in the juvenile spine, it will not only create a cervical scoliosis, but will also reflect a scoliosis down into the thoracic spine.

Chronic lateral torticollis type subluxations are often found in the full spine x-ray examination of scoliosis. These chronic disc block subluxations are usually the problem causing subluxations. They are commonly found at the base of the curves and in the transitional areas between the curves. (Ills. XII-4 & 5)

2. The Chronic Anterior Torticollis Subluxation

This subluxation, in its early stages (without outstanding pathology), can often be seen in the lower cervicals. (Ill. XII-2) Above the chronic disc block subluxation the spine attempts to again form the normal lordotic curve. As time goes on the chronic subluxation will exhibit degenerative change. Thinning of the disc, exostotic spurring, ebernation and Schmorl's Nodes will be evident. When we see a kyphosis in the cervical spine and yet a normal lateral is exhibited in the dorsals and lumbars we must suspect trauma or an uncorrected torticollis subluxation. Carefully question the patient on incidences of neck pain or a stiff neck that may have occurred in years past. I hold that these chronic subluxations are often the result of uncared-for, uncorrected anterior torticollis subluxations. Remember the public and the medical doctors often regard such acute events as trivial, take an aspirin is the common advise given. As I say in my lectures, "When nature (Innate) sends us a message in the form of pain we should make sense out of it not numb our senses to it." Time will prove the folly of today's penchant for pain killing drugs.

3. The Chronic Anterior Lateral Torticollis Subluxation

Upon A. P. and lateral film analysis you will find the combination of a lateral disc block subluxation and a posterior nuclear shift (reverse disc wedge). In this chronic distortion much pathology becomes evident as time goes on (Ill. XII-1); there can even be an anterior slippage of a vertebra due to the articular laxity that is produced by the stretched facital capsular ligaments. Ebernation, Schmorl's Nodes, exotosis, vertebral body wedging all become apparent in chronic torticollis as the vertebral malposition stresses the dynamics of the intervertebral joints. So look for the disc block subluxations in all chronic curvatures of the spine. Be especially aware of these subluxations in the lumbar and cervical spine as the causation of the youthful idiopathic rotary scoliosis.

It is becoming increasingly apparent to me that the activities of youth, especially sports-related trauma, set the stage for the majority of destructive pathological deteriorative vertebral and disc changes in later life. Early detection and chiropractic correction could truly bring B. J. Palmer's prophetic statement into full light, "Chiropractic adds life to years and years to life."

On the next four pages I have illustrated x-rays with chronic torticollis type subluxations (chronic disc block subluxations). Such chronic subluxations have trauma or episodes of torticollis in their etiology.

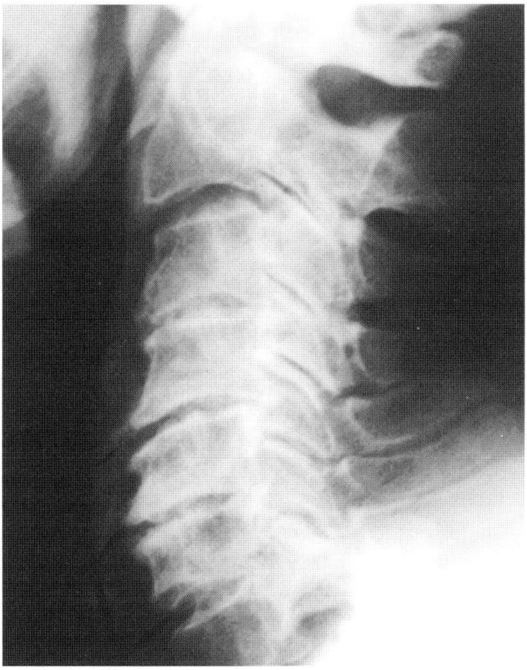

(Ill. XII-1) It is the author's opinion that chronic vertebral subluxations are the major cause of the deteriorative pathology so evident in our adult and senior citizen population. Ignoring symptomatology by simply taking pain relieving drugs, rather than remedial action, sets the stage for deteriorative/degenerative change as seen on the x-ray above.*

* X-ray courtesy Dr. E. L. Crowder.

CHRONIC ANTERIOR TORTICOLLIS SUBLUXATION

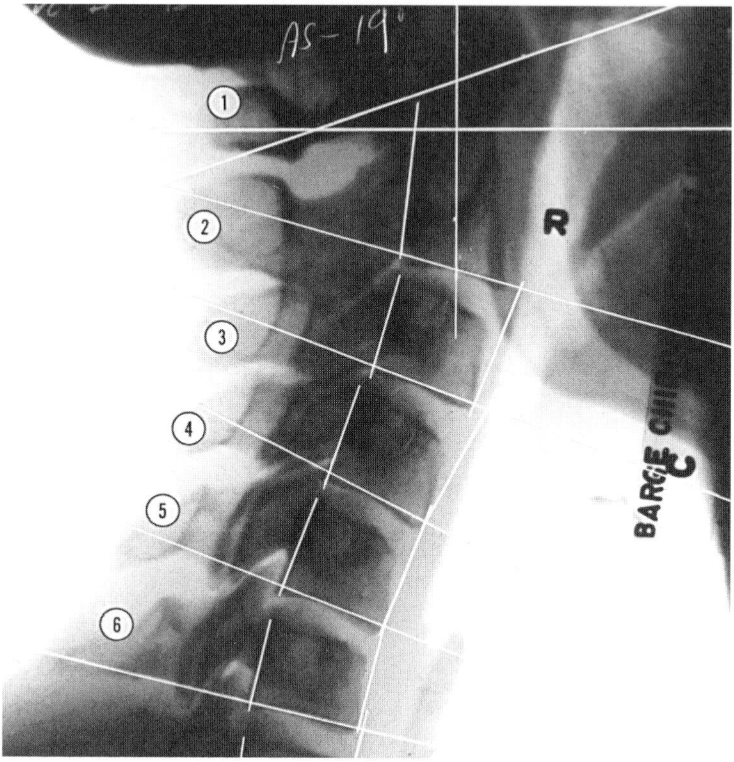

(Ill. XII-2) Converging plane lines indicate the chronic disc block subluxation of anterior torticollis exists between C 4 and C 5 … C 5 and C 6. *Notice how the cervical spine again tries to create a lordotic curve above these chronic subluxations.* This problem is not long standing as no deterioration is evident as yet. A spinal condition such as this can be reduced through proper chiropractic adjustment. In long standing chronic conditions one can suspect chronic anterior torticollis when there is a flat disc space with ebernation and Schmorl's Nodes in the posterior aspect of the vertebrae above and below. Exostosis and calcareous deposits are usually evident around the old lesion. The posteriorally shifted nucleus erodes into the vertebral bodies and creates the aforementioned pathological manifestations. When the full spine lateral x-ray displays normal contours and only the cervical is kyphotic, either chronic anterior torticollis or trauma, or both, is commonly the cause of the kyphotic change.

CHRONIC ANTERIOR TORTICOLLIS SUBLUXATION

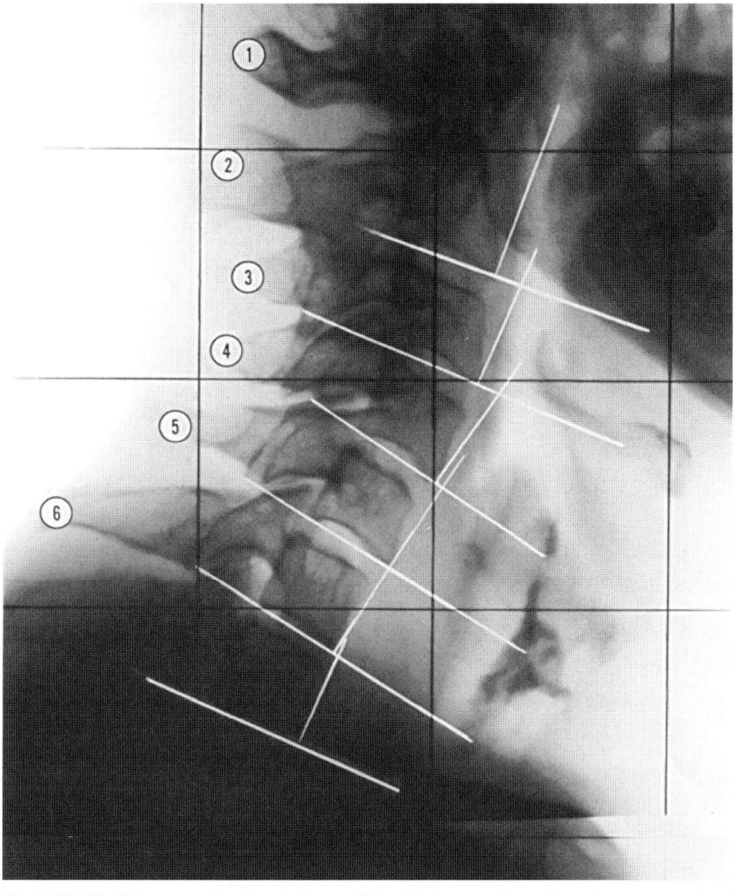

(Ill. XII-3) 6th cervical along with C 4 are involved segments in the x-ray above. Note the body plane lines converge to the anterior ... the perpendicular lines intersect. The disc between 6th and 7th cervical is thinning and showing signs of deterioration. Again, this is not an advanced state of deterioration and, in my opinion, reduction of the subluxation will prevent further degenerative change. Case histories reveal that most patients that exhibit such problems on x-ray relate incidences of neck pain or stiffness. Mild cases of torticollis are often ignored or assumed to be a strain or sprain. People today commonly take analgesics or muscle relaxers rather than seek care and thus nature's warnings go unheeded.

CHRONIC LATERAL TORTICOLLIS SUBLUXATION

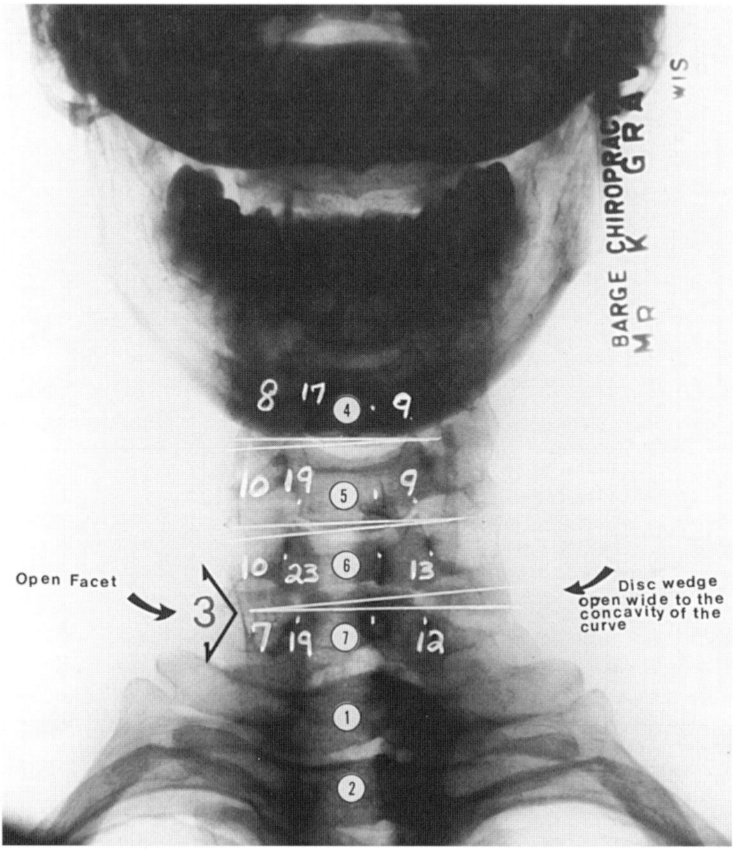

(Ill. XII-4) This degree of a chronic disc block subluxation is often missed in routine x-ray analysis. Notice the disc wedge open wide to the right (concavity of the curve) between the 6th and 7th cervical. The 6th cervical vertebra is rotated 10mm body left away from the wide side of the disc wedge, the 7th cervical 7mm. Thus C 6 is rotated 3mm away from the wide side of the disc wedge compared to C 7. The facet is "open" on the left! Neurological problems would occur on this side and the facet would be palpably swollen and elicit pain upon palpation. Notice the adaptive rotatory change above this subluxation, **all other disc wedges are open to the convexity of the curve. The disc block subluxation reveals itself by showing a disc wedge open to the side to the concavity of the curve.**

CHRONIC LATERAL TORTICOLLIS SCOLIOSIS

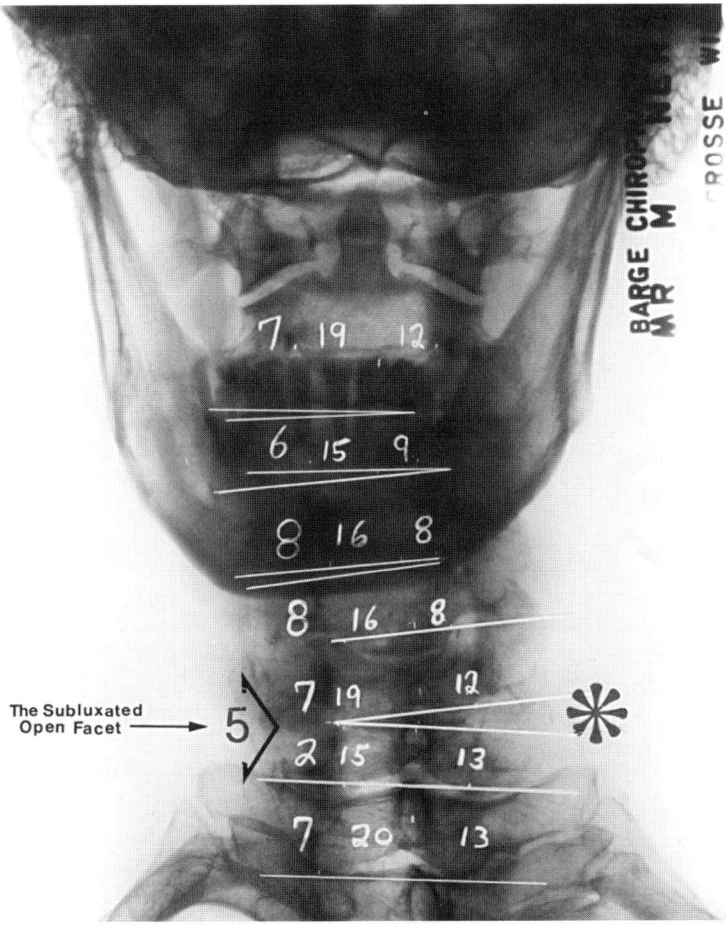

(Ill. XII-5) This is a classic example of a chronic lateral torticollis subluxation. When you see a disc wedge on the concavity of a cervical rotatory scoliosis suspect a chronic disc block subluxation. Here the 6th cervical is (body) rotated 5mm away from the wide side of the disc wedge in relation to the 7th cervical. The nucleus of the disc between C 6 and C 7 has shifted to the right creating an inferiority on the left and thus the compensatory left rotatory scoliosis above this point. Again either trauma or torticollis created this disc block subluxation. Now compare this x-ray to the one on the next page (Ill. XII-6).

COMMON ROTATORY SCOLIOSIS

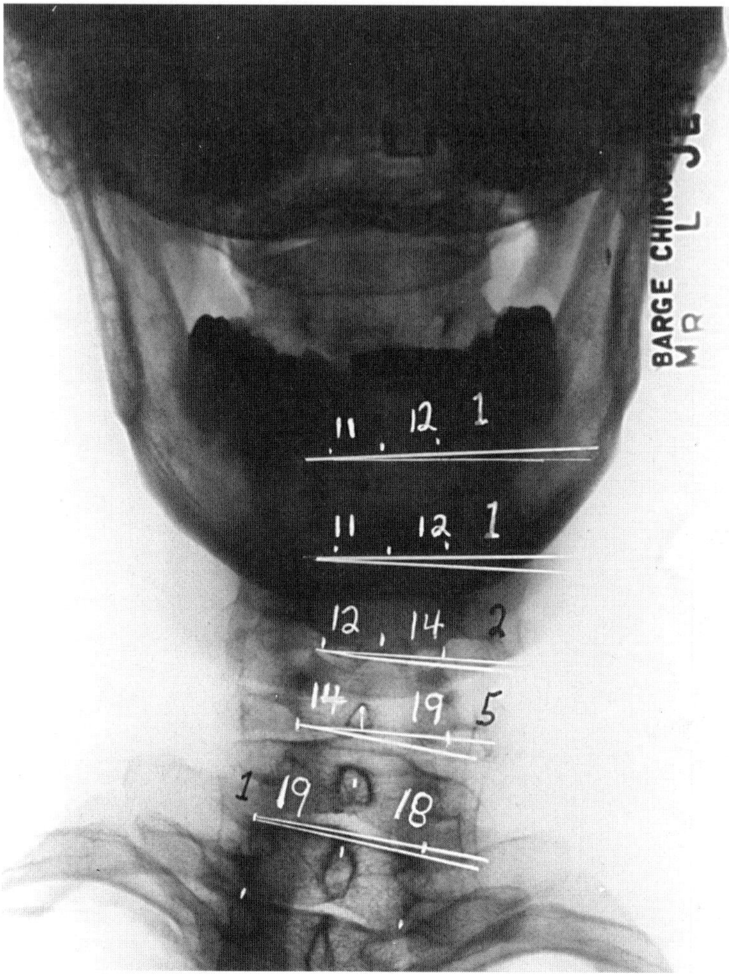

(Ill. XII-6) This x-ray illustrates a common right rotatory cervical scoliosis. All disc wedges are open wide to the convexity of the curve, all body rotations are toward the convexity. There is no disc wedge "open" to the concavity of the curve. Look closely at this x-ray and the one on the last page, compare one to the other and when you analyze x-ray films the existence of the chronic lateral torticollis (tortipelvis in the lumbars, Ill. XII-8) subluxation will become evident to you. Such subluxations are chronic disc block subluxations. There will be a disc wedge open wide to the concavity of the curve, (Ill. XII-4) page 179.

SUMMARY

Chapters I – XII

At this point in this text I want to summarize some significant aspects of this treatise on torticollis. First I would like to emphasize once more the importance of the disc block subluxations of torticollis and tortipelvis. If not corrected in youth, they can lead to the destructive adaptive curves of scoliosis! In the adult these subluxations are found commonly in the cervical and lumbar spine and are involved in severe neurological disturbances such as sciatica and brachialgia. The x-ray on page 183 is a classic example of a tortipelvis subluxation of the 4th lumbar creating a scoliosis. This subluxation could have easily been corrected in youth.

This young adult female, age 29, had received no help from the usual medical approach, and was finally told to see a psychiatrist. She suffered headache and low back pain, which responded excellently to chiropractic care. Notice the 4th lumbar disc block subluxation on her x-ray, such subluxations neglected in youth cause scoliotic adaptation. The injury is often summarily dismissed medically as a sprain, strain, or muscle spasm and when the subluxation becomes chronic, the spinal adaptation creates scoliosis. I repeat, as I have said in VOL. I TORTIPELVIS, "I am convinced there is no simple backache." There are very few purely muscular backaches. Backache and neck pain are caused by vertebral subluxations, neglect of which can raise havoc with the growing spine. To simply numb ones senses to pain through the use of pain killing drugs makes as much sense as putting cotton on the clapper of a burglar alarm and allowing the burglar to go to work. But I speak of this in my philosophy texts so let me carry on with torticollis.

Chiropractic vertebral adjustment facilitates the body's effort to restore subluxated vertebra to their normal position, thus preventing scoliotic adaptation. The adjustment and reduction of the malposition of such subluxations, in their chronic state, can reduce abnormal spinal contours and prevent further spinal degradation.

We must look carefully as to how we handle our infants. Normal spinal contours must be allowed to develop before the child assumes the upright posture. Spinal exercises (pages 184 and 185) used in our school systems should be tailored to provide maintenance and development of the normal secondary curves of the spine. Chiropractic examinations should be routinely given to all school children. The screening for scoliotic problems should begin in the first year of school, even kindergarten, as the prevention of scoliosis is dependent upon the early detection and correction of inferiorities and spinal balance mechanisms.

The cervical spine holds the key to correcting disturbances in the body's proprioceptive balance mechanisms which are located in the brain stem and the capsular ligaments of the facet joints and the joints of Luschka. Cervical subluxations cause disturbances in spinal balance which can lead to the development of faulty spinal postures, curvatures and scoliosis. For a treatise on the five basic causes of scoliosis I refer the reader to my third text in this chiropractic trilogy, SCOLIOSIS. First published in June of 1981, the text is now available in its second expanded edition which was published in 1996.

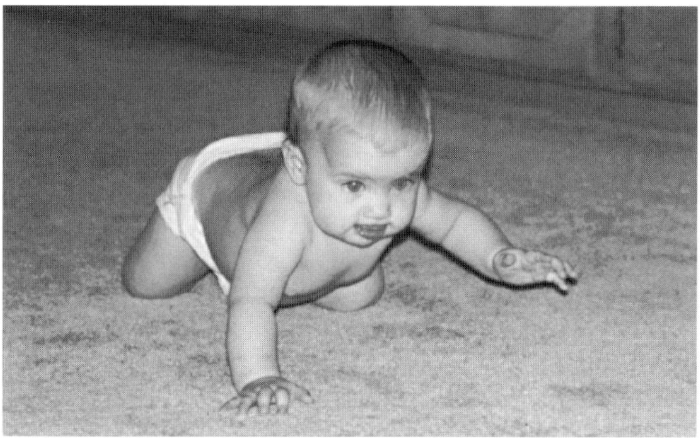

(Ill. XII-7) As explained in Chapter IV, to properly develop the sigmoid curve, the normal sagittal contours of the human spine, a baby should be allowed to creep. Creeping maintains the thoracic kyphosis, nurtures the cervical lordosis, and initiates the development of the lumbar lordosis. A baby will walk when it is ready to do so, early walking should not be encouraged too greatly by the parents. The baby above is the daughter of Dr. & Mrs. David Ragland, baby Brittini.

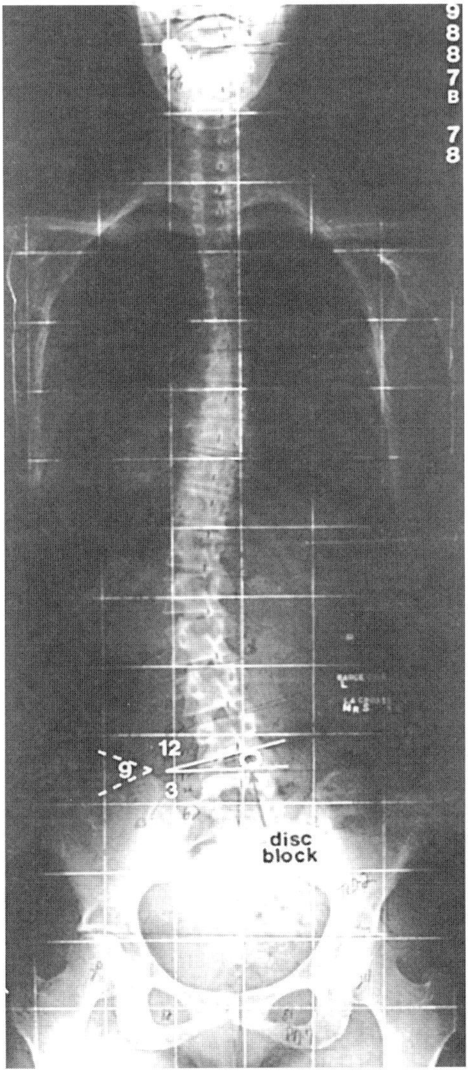

(Ill. XII-8) Notice the classic disc block subluxation between 4th and 5th lumbar. The 4th lumbar is rotated 9mm away from the wide side of the disc wedge in relation to L 5. The author contends that this scoliosis could have been prevented by early chiropractic correction of this disc block subluxation. The disc wedge is "open" to the side of the **concavity** of the scoliotic curve. The lateral view of this case is shown on page 144.

SPINAL EXERCISES

Man should observe nature. Often through such observations we can learn of our mistakes.

Ever watch an animal stretch in the morning? They arch their neck, back and lower back down in. Only man bends over forward upon rising, puts on his shoes and slippers and thus strains the lower back and discs.

Nature's way to stretch observed in the dog.

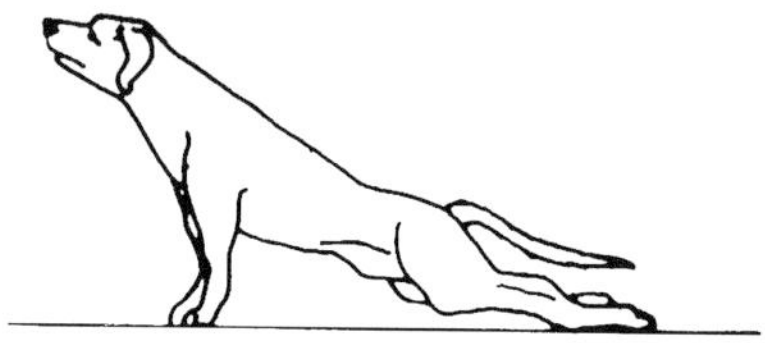

Man, too, can stretch this way with the use of the X.R. wheel:

Exercises with the X.R. wheel

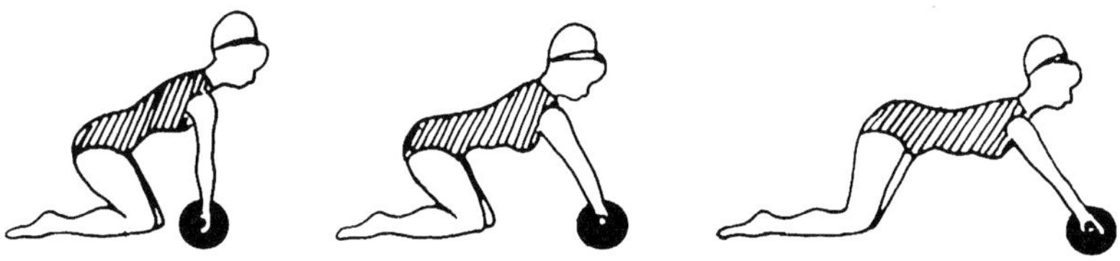

Exercises without X.R. wheel

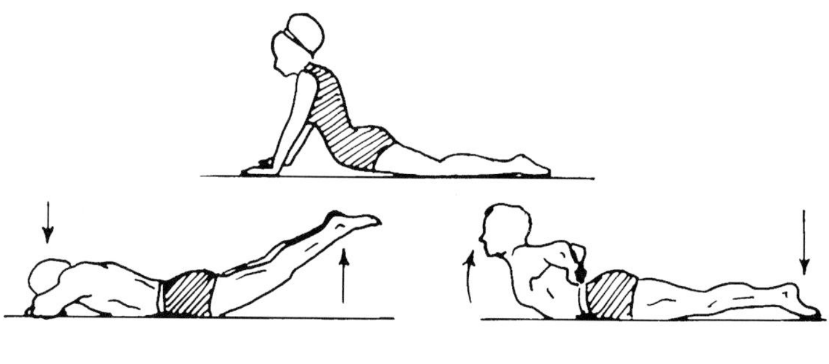

(Ill. XII-9)

CERVICAL SPINAL EXERCISES

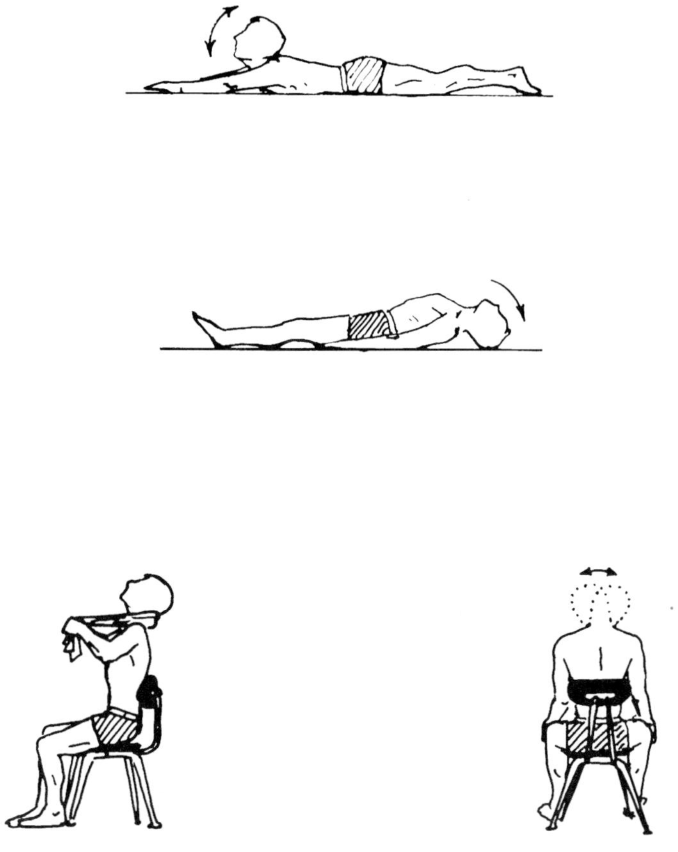

(Ill. XII-10) Exercises: After the correction of an acute torticollis subluxation, x-ray evaluation very commonly indicates a cervical kyphosis. As stated earlier in this text, the kyphosis is the predisposing factor in most disc block subluxations. The exercises shown are those used by the author to promote the formation and preservation of good lordotic curves in the cervical spine. **Such exercises should be done in moderation**. "No pain, no gain," is nonsense. We should not try to **force** change in the spine. Remember a cervical kyphosis is often an adaptation to a thoracic hypokyphosis. Our body's innate intelligence (nature) will decide the curve that it finds best to accommodate the sagittal spinal contours that best balance the spine. These exercises simply are intended to **encourage** an improved lordotic contour.

INFANT TOGGLE "DROP" HEADPIECE

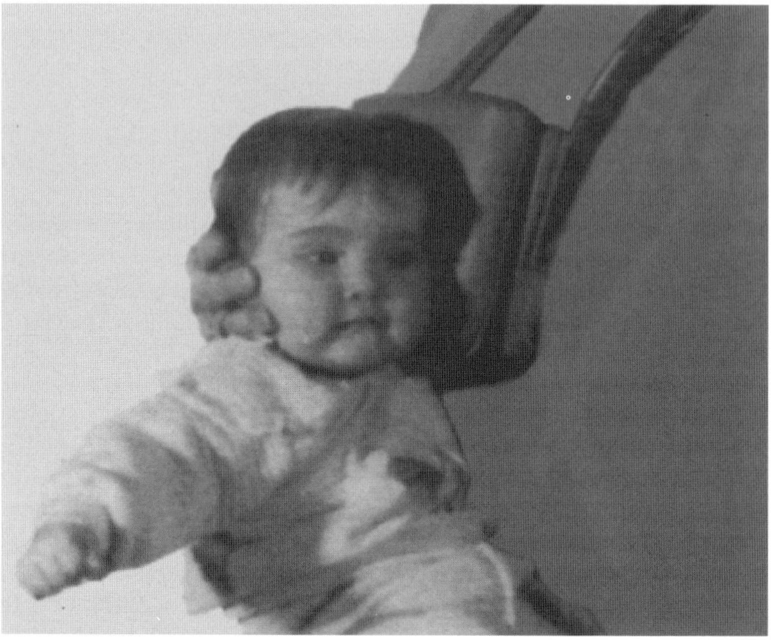

(Ill. XIII-1) The method of suspending a portable drop headpiece mechanism from the parent's or the doctor's neck, in the adjustments of infants, was developed by the late Dr. Larry Webster, D.C., chiropractic educator and research clinician who focused on the care of children. The author was a friend of Dr. Webster and taught in his pediatric programs. This method allows the infant to be adjusted while cradled in the doctor's or parent's arms. Such headpieces feature adjustable tension in respect to the drop mechanism and an adjustable neck strap. The strap suspends the headpiece from the doctor's or the parent's neck and the child is held against the headpeice as illustrated above.

Once a comfortable position is achieved, a contact on the vertebra to be adjusted is made and the thrust delivered towards the headpiece. The headpiece "drops," facilitating the adjustic correction of the subluxation. Adjusting the tension on the headpiece allows the doctor to vary the force needed to apply the thrust. The headpiece used by the author is shown on (Ill. XIII-4), page 191.

CHAPTER XIII
INFANTILE TORTICOLLIS

Dorland's medical dictionary's (26th Edition) definition of "congenital" states - - "existing at, and usually before, birth ... "Existing at," yes but "usually before birth"? To this I would have to render my opinion that torticollis before birth would be rare indeed. I contend that it is **usually** due to the rigors of birth, or the mishandling of the infant during delivery (or soon thereafter). Birth trauma is the chief cause of infantile torticollis.

Often the condition is summarily dismissed by the attending physician as a customary consequence of a difficult birth and the parents are advised that it will disappear within a few months; such was the case of baby A. W. whose case report is given on page 211. In this day of medical enlightenment in respect to chiropractic care, such medical neglect and lack of referral is appalling. Especially to a chiropractor like myself who has practiced over four decades and has often seen the unfortunate consequences of such medical neglect. Asymmetry is not common at birth, but it certainly **will** occur from torticollis as the infant grows into the tortuous position dictated by the bend of its cervical spine; and I remind you, that growth in the first six months of life is rapid indeed! Unusual pressures on the facial structures create apparent asymmetry within the first six months.*

As oft stated in this text, "Torticollis is a subluxation" and infants thus afflicted are no exception. The x-raying of infants for the critical analysis of the vertebral subluxation can be essential in some cases, but the tortuous position of the infant's neck, combined with adept palpation, is often all that is needed to determine the vertebra involved and the listing of the vertebral subluxation. To be purposely redundant let me repeat again, if the head is bent to the right the disc wedge is open (wide) to the left, the vertebral body rotation of the subluxated vertebra will be to the right and thus the facet is **open** on the right, the side of vertebral incline. The spinous process of the subluxated vertebra is left and becomes a convenient lever for the adjustic correction. The chiropractor has only to ascertain the vertebral segment involved to give the adjustment and this can commonly be accomplished through palpation. Careful case history, of course, must rule out the possibility of trauma that might have caused facet dislocation. Torticollis, in the author's opinion, is a disc lesion

* On page 239, I have reprinted a paper by Dr. Gutmann on infant adjusting that mentions the facial asymmetry in torticollis.

subluxation and can occur from a subluxation of any cervical vertebra that rests upon a disc, and that leaves only one cervical vertebra out, the Atlas. But the Atlas too, may have to be adjusted, to completely resolve a case of torticollis.

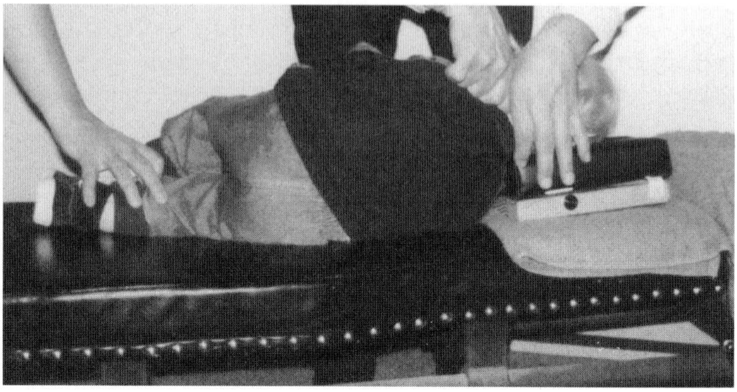

(Ill. XIII-2) While mother helps stabilize the child, Dr. LeRoy Otto delivers a thumb contact toggle recoil adjustment to the spinous process of the Axis vertebra on the drop headpiece mechanism.

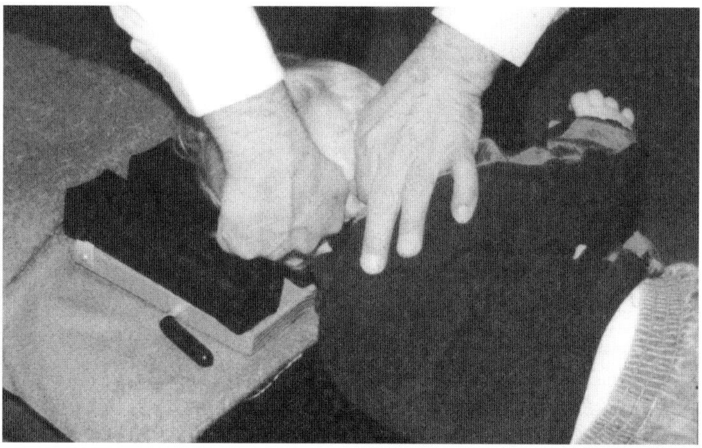

(Ill. XIII-3) With the thumb of one hand on top of the other, the thrust is delivered to the laterally deviated spinous process of Axis. The toggle recoil adjustment is a high velocity low amplitude adjustic thrust developed by Dr. B. J. Palmer. The drop mechanism was invented by Dr. J. Clay Thompson. Upon the thrust, the headpiece drops a fraction of an inch and stops abruptly thus facilitating the adjustment. Instantaneously the adjustor's hands recoil, allowing the patient's own innate mechanisms to accomplish the complete adjustment.

THE TOGGLE RECOIL ADJUSTMENT

For the chiropractor who has specialized in the upper cervical specific toggle recoil adjustment this technic is excellent for the correction of Axis and even 3rd cervical. In infants I have often found the subluxated vertebra is Axis. The toggle recoil thrust is appropriately delivered to the spinous process of Axis and this is the author's preference when toggle recoil is used. (Ills. XIII-2 & 3) Many are the baby toggle headpiece adjusting apparatuses available in the chiropractic profession today. This technic, the drop headpiece technic, was developed by my good friend and teacher, the late Dr. J. Clay Thompson and it has become a leading method for the correction of the cervical subluxation in the infant. (Ills. XIII-4 & 5) The late Dr. Larry Webster's technic involves a unique way of placing the infant on the drop headpiece for the adjustment as described on the next page and on (Ill. XIII-1.)

In using the drop headpiece technic, the patient can be placed on the headpiece in the most comfortable position, this is commonly the convexity of the curve up. The spinous process of the subluxated vertebra rotates towards the convexity of the curve and thus the toggle recoil of the spinous process is easily accomplished. The headpiece is preset by the doctor to the desired tension to accommodate the weight of the baby's head and yet allow for a low force, low depth, high velocity thrust to be given downward upon the deviated spinous process. The headpiece drops, the doctor recoils and the vertebra is directionally impelled to reduce and correct the subluxation. Care should be taken to be positive of the exact spinous process contacted.

If it becomes impossible to lay the baby on the side of the lateral head tilt, (convexity up) the baby may be placed upon the opposite side. The transverse process of the subluxated vertebra is then the contact point as the transverse would be listed as posterior on the side opposite the spinous process deviation. This, however, **is not** the preferred positioning. When the child is laid convexity up, the open side of the disc wedge would be **up** and thus the thrust down on the spinous process would not only close the facet on the contralateral side but also this directional force would favor the closing of the lateral disc wedge.

Thus the usual and prefered side posture patient positioning for this thrust would be:

1. Concavity of the curve down, convexity up.
2. Open facet down.
3. Open disc wedge up.
4. Deviated spinous up.

Now this same adjustment may be given with the headpiece suspended from the adjusting doctor's neck, the baby held against the doctor's chest and abdomen in a sitting position and the spinous simply pulled towards the doctor's chest. This thrust was developed by the late Dr. Larry Webster D.C. (Ill. XIII-1)

The doctor may choose to use or not use the drop mechanism, the headpiece serves as a contralateral support to the occiput as the force of the adjustment is specifically applied to the subluxated vertebra.

Contralateral support of the occiput can be achieved through the use of a paperback book with a blanket or diaper as a cushion. The occiput is supported, the vertebra is impelled to move by the directional thrust of the adjustment.

This author personally likes to use the drop mechanism of the headpiece as its abrupt stop at the end of the adjustic thrust, facilitates the adjustic correction.

Fortunate, indeed, is the female chiropractor with her small and dexterous hands in the adjustment of infants. If the practitioner's hands are small, the rotatory lift move or the transverse thrust adjustment as described for the adult in Chapter IX may be used. This can be accomplished with the baby held in its mother's arms or the doctor can elect to use a supine cervical on the adjusting table. (see page 213) Other technics are employed throughout the chiropractic profession for the correction of this subluxation. The important thing, of course, is to determine the exact malposition and the vertebra involved. Simply slipping your hand under the baby's neck, baby lying supine, with the chiropractic index finger contacting the spinous and the other hand rotating the skull a wee bit, is a move that I have used effectively in adjusting infants in torticollis. Again, once the subluxation is thoroughly understood, its adjustic correction can accommodate almost any situation and pain syndrome presented.

LLOYD INFANT TOGGLE HEADPIECE

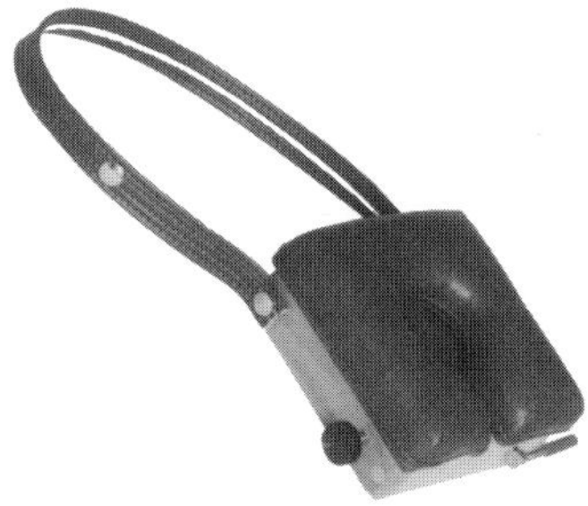

(Ill. XIII-4) This specially designed portable adjusting tool allows precision low force adjustment while the infant is in the doctor's or parent's arms. It features adjustable tension and adjustable straps, and is available in a choice of colors, Lloyd Table Co., Lisbon, Iowa, 52253-0899.

PORTABLE "DROP" ADJUSTING MECHANISMS

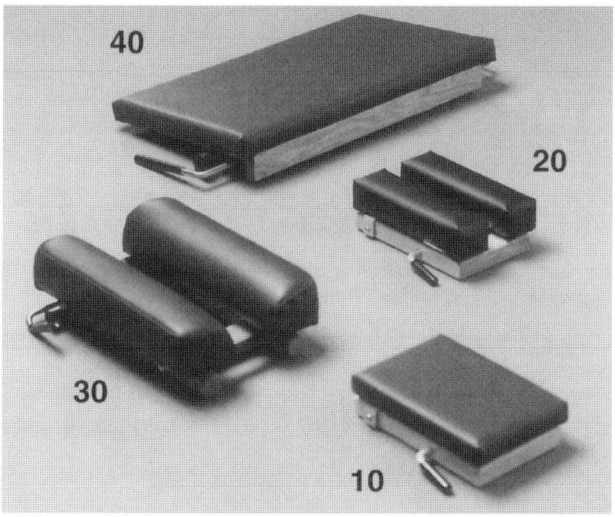

10–SINGLE CUSHION DROP PIECE (8½" x 6" x 2½")
20–DOUBLE CUSHION DROP PIECE (8½" x 6" x 3½")
30–PORTABLE HEADPIECE (12½" x 10" x 4")
40–THORACO-PELVIC DROP PIECE (12" x 20" x 3½")

(Ill. XIII-5) Drop mechanisms available through THULI TABLES INC., 4160 Rohowitz Road, Dodgeville, WI 53533.

ADJUSTING INFANTS AND CHILDREN IN TORTICOLLIS

Chiropractors have always adjusted children and infants. Some of the most dramatic responses to chiropractic care have been in the wee ones. There is nothing unusual about this, they have spines just like adults and they too become subluxated. Subluxation pathology has had little time to develop in young children and thus their responses to care are often dramatic.

In my early years of practice I built strongly upon my first case, who was an epileptic juvenile. From the success in this case I came to see many epileptic children plus a myriad of other childhood disorders such as constipation, asthma, bronchitis, otitis media, intraventricular septal defects, pyloric spasm, colic, scoliosis, heart arrhythmias, heart murmurs, Baker's cysts, Osgood Schlatter's syndrome, tonsillitis, sinusitis, chronic sore throats, upper respiratory infections and more. The gratifying results gained, led me to focus strongly on children in my practice.

It is important to understand that the chiropractic profession holds forth **no cure** for the diseases of children, nor for those conditions I have listed in the last paragraph. Chiropractors simply adjust subluxations of the spine paying particular attention to the neurogenic levels of vertebral involvement that coincides with the disease syndrome of the patient involved. Chiropractors also address the upper cervical spine as we hold that subluxation in this area can result in impaired function throughout the entire human body. Through the reduction and correction of vertebral subluxations the neuroforaminal occlusion, inherent in all vertebral subluxations, is reduced and the resultant improvement of neurological communication within the human system restores normal tissue function, tone, and homeostasis. This restoration of normal body function creates a return to wellness in the patient involved.

It is important for those uninformed on such matters to understand that chiropractors have a different outlook in respect to the cause of disease. Chiropractors hold that disease starts out first as body malfunction. Then in consequence the body exhibits the symptoms that today we name as diseases. In infectious diseases the germ must first find a fertile soil to establish itself in, and thus the body's malfunction sets the stage for the germ, which is an agent of disease, to wreak its havoc.

Chiropractic science holds that the major cause of body malfunction is the lack of normal nerve supply caused by vertebral subluxations and thus the chiropractor's approach is to adjust the subluxations rather than treat the disease.

I apologize to my chiropractic readers for this rudimentary, freshman discussion on chiropractic philosophy, but I want to firmly establish to the uninformed reader that chiropractors focus on adjusting the cause of malfunction rather than treating the symptoms of the problem.

For instance, torticollis is the symptom of the disc block subluxation. The subluxation initiates the painful reflex muscular tensions exhibited by the patient. Medicine seeks to treat the symptoms of discomfort, the muscular contracturing, the pain, etc. Chiropractors simply adjust the cause, the vertebral subluxation.

In my practice I have adjusted a host of juveniles and infants in torticollis. The results were always gratifying and as a young practitioner I considered this just to be the way it was, nothing unusual here. After all, I watched my father, aunts, uncles and cousins, my instructors and professors; all adjust people and many cases of torticollis were cared for. On weekends when Dad made house calls I would often accompany him and observe his adjusting. As number nine in my family to pursue a chiropractic career, I, too, was adjusted from infant on up - adjusting children has always been the realm of chiropractic care.

I do wish I had taken the time to document all of the cases of infantile torticollis I have adjusted. As a recognized authority on this problem, many chiropractors have referred infant patients to me for care. But then a practitioner is seldom a research clinician and it wasn't until the medical profession began to focus on scoliosis that I decided to document the chiropractic results achieved. In this text I have described the adjustment of the infant in torticollis. The infantile years are from birth to age three and infants present unique considerations in respect to vertebral adjustment. When a child has assumed full ambulation of the upright posture, adjusting technics are essentially the same for the child as for the adult.

SYMPTOMATOLOGY OF THE INFANT IN TORTICOLLIS

The infant in torticollis is seldom in evident pain from the tortuous position he/she is locked in. In severe cases the distortion is easily recognized (Ill. XIII-6 A, page 213) but in mild cases the baby may just be more comfortable with his/her head slightly bent to, or facing to one side. In the mild case the baby's head may be manually turned or bent to the other direction without much discomfort; but the baby almost immediately resumes its more comfortable positioning. In severe cases you cannot force the baby's head out of the position it is in without the child crying out in pain. In these cases when one waits for six or more weeks before correction, facial asymmetry and cervical scoliosis become an apparent complication of the problem.

As stated before, torticollis in infants is commonly due to birth trauma. Difficult delivery, the use of suction (such as bell jar delivery), forceps and manual traction extension and rotation imposed upon the infant's head and cervical spine create the subluxation. I have never seen an infant that I would hold to be an intrauterine victim of torticollis. I hasten to add, I am not saying this cannot exist, but I do believe that it would be rare indeed. What we see in the infant is usually a traumatically caused disc block subluxation.

Any vertebra with a disc can be the culprit in this disc lesion subluxation. From Axis on down throughout the cervicals, the subluxation can exist. I personally have found it most frequently at the Axis and 3rd cervical level. When Axis is involved the Atlas rotates in the opposite direction endeavoring to face the head forward. In the author's opinion, this contra-rotation is an antalgic positioning and should not be assumed to be a subluxation; see pages 41-43, 78 and 79.

THE STERNOCLEIDOMASTOID TUMOR

Throughout the history of the description of torticollis in medical texts the "sternomastoid" or more correctly the sternocleidomastoid tumor is frequently mentioned. Under the heading of Congenital Torticollis, Boyd's Pathology,[32] 1970 Edition, made this interesting observation.

"This is a condition due not to ischemia, but rather to excessive congestion of muscle. The wryneck usually develops about the age of four years. In these cases the history goes back to the so-called "sternomastoid tumor of infancy," which generally appears about ten days after birth. A spindle-shaped swelling develops in the sternocleidomastoid; this is peculiarly hard and feels like cartilage. The swelling persists for two or three months and is then gradually absorbed, disappearing entirely in four to six months after birth. If the muscle is now exercised it is found

to consist entirely of fibrous tissue with complete replacement of the muscle fibers. The neck lengthens rapidly in the fourth year, and as the fibrosed muscle is unable to grow, the head is pulled over to that side - a condition of congenital wryneck. The sterno-cleidomastoid tumor is produced as the result of acute venous obstruction due to pressure on the veins during labor, rendered permanent by thromobsis of the veins. When the artery to a muscle is tied experimentally or the artery and vein together, the result is simple atrophy. But when the vein above is tied, the arterial supply being left intact, the muscle becomes acutely swollen, hard and tender, and very cyanosed. The fibers disintegrate and the muscle is densely infiltrated with round cells. In the course of a few months such a muscle is completely replaced by fibrous tissue. When the vein alone is obstructed the autolytic products from the breaking down muscle fibers are not carried away from the part and appear to stimulate proliferation of fibroblasts. The marked edema of the muscle also favors the formation of fibrous tissue."

Dr. William Boyd's theory on veinous obstruction may have merit and at least casts some light on the fibrous mass that can develop from an unattended lesion. However, the injury is traumatic, the torn tissues could block veinous drainage and the infant is invariably in some degree of torticollis at this time, the time of birth. Torticollis in infants is not always dramatically apparent, only a slight malposition of the head and neck may at first be the only sign; or the baby may constantly favor one position for its head. It is in such incidences that neglect, medically speaking, is often the case. The problem being summarily brushed off with some comment such as "Oh, this often occurs in a difficult birth, it will solve itself in a few weeks." Nor necessarily true, chiropractic examination should be sought forthwith in any case of suspected torticollis. Chronic spinal distortion, facial asymmetry and a lifetime of disfigurement have evolved from such neglect.

In her fine book, "CHIROPRACTIC AND PREGNANCY"[33], noted chiropractic author, clinician and educator Dr. Joan Fallon D.C. illustrates the tumor's location, see page 200.

In a paper written by Drs. Fallon and Peter N. Fysh, (contained in this chapter), they discuss this so-called "tumor."

Quoting with permission from her aforementioned book, and from correspondence with Dr. Fallon, I now include some of her comments. As to the SCM Tumor, Dr. Fallon states;

"A painless lump in the SCM which appears after the first week of life due to trauma at birth. It is seen very frequently after a breech birth, and is almost always accompanied by torticollis. Chiropractic care of this condition can usually bring about a resolution to this problem in 2-3 weeks. Soft tissue work on the actual lump, which is no more than a muscular "knot," can aid in the resolution of the torticollis along with the adjustments."

Dr. Fallon's opinion and mine concur in that we both state that when this so-called "tumor" is present the child invariably is in a state of torticollis; **and it is due to birth trauma!** Another quote from Dr. Fallon states;

"Torticollis is one of the most common pediatric conditions seen in the chiropractor's office. Congenital torticollis is seen often after a difficult birth or as the sequelae of birth-related trauma. Frequently the torticollis is accompanied by a large nodule located in the belly of the sternocleidomastoid (SMC) muscle of the child's neck on the concave side of the torticollis. This nodule is most often referred to as a sternocleidomastoid "tumor." Many times this "tumor" is seen after the following types of birth scenarios: 1) breech presentation, 2) posterior presentation, 3) forceps delivery, 4) vacuum extraction.

The tumor consists of taut and contracted fibers which are allowed to persist as a result of the torticollis. These fibers will cluster in the belly of the SCM muscle. The "tumor" needs to be differentially diagnosed from a contusion which would present within the first 48 - 72 hours with discoloration and also the "tumor" can easily be distinguished from primary lymph swelling which would not be present directly in the muscle belly as is the "tumor."

The SCM "tumor" will develop as a result of traction to the cervical spine which includes flexion, extension and unequal lateral flexion. The SCM muscle which receives the most stretch with these cervical traction movements will ultimately develop the "tumor."

Very often the child is brought into the chiropractor's office with the suggestion of surgery confronting the parents. Surgery is very often prescribed especially when the "tumor" is not responding to the medical treatment which consists most commonly of a "wait and see" program. This "tumor" however ***does respond very well and very quickly to chiropractic adjustments, and soft tissue treatment.*** (emphasis added)

When approaching the problem of an SCM "tumor" in the

chiropractor's office, it is most important to examine the duration of the existing tumor, and the measure of firmness of the nodule. The longer the nodule has been present the more resistant to treatment it will become. The first mode of treatment will be to assess the subluxation. Often times if the child is a newborn when presenting in the office, a very simple and efficacious way of determining subluxation of the upper cervical region would be to use the McMullen Reverse Fencer Reflex. Among other things, the MRF reflex relies on the child's ability to turn its head with the appropriate proprioceptive stimulus. Even with the presence of the SCM "tumor" the child will be able to turn its head albeit restricted in its range of motion. Once the child's subluxation is established an adjustment should be rendered. Since the SCM "tumor" is located on the side of the concavity of the torticollis, it will be difficult as in some techniques to adjust into the concavity, ***and this situation will call for an adjustment into the convexity of the torticollis."*** (emphasis added)

Again I concur with Dr. Fallon, this time in respect to the adjustic correction of this subluxation, Illustrations XIII-2 and 3 on page 188 show Dr. LeRoy Otto adjusting into the **convexity of the curve**, the contact is the deviated spinous process of the subluxated Axis. Dr. Crowder illustrates the Axis spinous toggle thrust on (Ill. X-12) page 135.

Dr. Fallon goes on to describe the soft tissue work she applies to the SCM "tumor."

"Soft tissue treatment most commonly used for the 'tumor' is the process often referred to as 'milking the muscle.' This technique in its various forms has been used by chiropractors such as Dr. Nimmo for years in removing muscular restriction such as that found with the 'tumor.'

"The chiropractor will run his/her hand along the SCM muscle which has the 'tumor' in the belly from superior to inferior beginning at the base of the occiput and completing the traverse to the clavicle. In doing this maneuver, the SCM on the concave side is stretched from its contracted state and this enables the child to more readily 'hold' his/her adjustment.

"Chiropractic adjustments are very important to the resolution of this condition. Without chiropractic adjustments the 'tumor' will very often persist for months, ***and may cause significant problems for the child which range from eating difficulties through the full range of subluxation induced conditions."*** (emphasis added)

As to my emphasis in the last paragraph, I refer you to the paper by Dr. Gutmann reprinted from "Manuelle Medizin," page 239. The permission to reproduce this paper was gained by the I.C.A. I originally had the paper translated for my own information, the I.C.A. received permission to print the translated version from "Manuelle Medizin." The grave consequences of "untreated torticollis" are thoroughly elucidated by Dr. Gutmann.

And now with the kind permission of Dr. Fallon and Dr. Fysh; Dr. Maxine McMullen and the International Chiropractor's Association, I present their fine paper, "Chiropractic Care of the Newborn With Congenital Torticollis." J.C.C.P., Vol. 2, No. 1, January 1997.

Author's Note

Joan Fallon, D.C., F.I.C.C.P. continues on in her research and writing on chiropractic pediatrics. In the October 1997 issue of J.C.C.P. she has published another paper entitled, "The Role of the Chiropractic Adjustment in the Care and Treatment of 322 Children with Otitis Media."[34] *She states in the Abstract, quote:*

"To our knowledge this is the first time that tympanography has been used as an objectifying tool with respect to the efficacy of the chiropractic adjustment in the treatment of children with otitis media. As tympanography has been used extensively in the medical assessment of children with otitis media, it also serves as a bridge from which the chiropractic field and the medical field can begin to communicate with respect to otitis media. The results indicate that there is a strong correlation between the chiropractic adjustment and the resolution of otitis media for the children in this study."

Yes, many infectious conditions of youth respond beautifully to the subluxation correction care of the Doctor of Chiropractic.. I recommend the reading of this paper.

Chiropractic Care of the Newborn with Congenital Torticollis*[35]

Joan M. Fallon, D.C., F.I.C.C.P.
Peter N. Fysh, D.C.,B.APP.Sc(CHIRO), F.I.C.C.P.

Abstract

Objective: To discuss the various causes of congenital torticollis in the newborn infant and to present an approach to the chiropractic management of torticollis based on the authors' experiences.

Method: Congenital torticollis has been estimated to affect approximately two percent of newborn infants. The frank breech birthing position has been reportedly associated with the highest incidence of torticollis, with up to 34 percent of infants born in this position being affected. It has been suggested that a fetal posture with both the knees and the cervical spine extended is responsible for much of the high incidence of congenital torticollis resulting in stretching of the sternocleidomastoid muscle during the delivery process. The most common type of congenital torticollis is that associated with subluxation of the upper-cervical spine. Chiropractic management of congenital torticollis is primarily directed at reducing cervical spine subluxations which have been identified as commonly present with this condition. Chiropractic evaluation and management techniques appropriate for this condition are described.

Conclusion: Chiropractic management of congenital torticollis, using a combination of spinal adjustments, cranial re-alignment and soft tissue therapies can produce rapid resolution in many cases of congenital torticollis and plagiocephaly in the newborn infant. Spinal adjustments have been demonstrated to be efficacious to the resolution of the congenital torticollis. Before commencing a course of conservative spinal care however, accurate identification of the cause of the torticollis must be made to rule out complicating conditions which may result in high morbidity or mortality. The typical course of spinal adjustments for torticollis is usually of short duration requiring just a few treatments. Early correction of congenital torticollis should be the goal since prolonged contraction of the SCM can be the cause of cranial and facial anomalies as well as scoliosis.

The medical approach to a protracted torticollis is surgical

*Reprinted with permission from the "Journal of Clinical Chiropractic Pediatrics," Vol. 2, No. 1, Jan. 1997, published by The I.C.A. Council on Chiropractic Pediatrics.

intervention. While surgical intervention is typically a solution of last resort, it is frequently the only solution considered by the medical community. Chiropractic care is considered essential to the health and maintenance of the child's spine and nervous system. It is therefore important that the doctor of chiropractic become part of the multi-disciplinary team and that medical doctors become aware of chiropractic management as a solution to the most common causes of congenital torticollis.

Key Words: congenital torticollis, chiropractic, spinal adjustments.

INTRODUCTION

Torticollis is a condition of the newborn infant which has been reported to respond to spinal adjusting.[1] Defined as a unilateral contracture of the sternocleidomastoid muscle (SCM), torticollis has numerous causes. This paper discusses the most common etiologies of this condition in the neonate and provides recommendations for management. Clinically, torticollis presents with the head tilted (laterally flexed) toward the side of the contracted SCM and with the chin rotated to the contralateral side[2,3] (Figure 1). This position of the head is produced by the action of the SCM which will be found to be in a significantly contracted state. Torticollis which is present at birth or which develops during the first few weeks of life is appropriately described as congenital torticollis. In addition to the head tilt characteristic of torticollis, often the face and head will be distorted with a condition known as plagiocephaly.

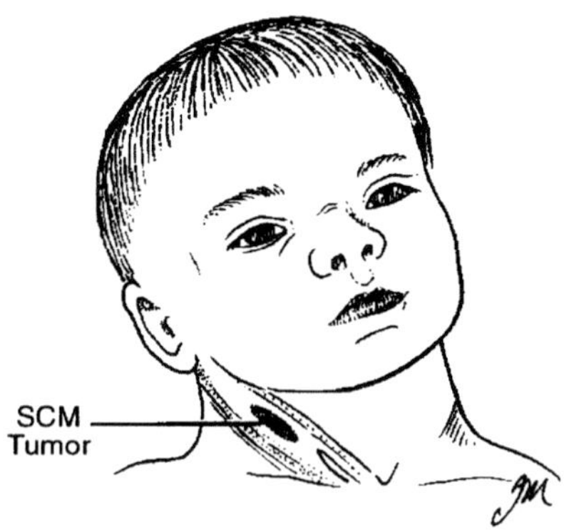

(Figure 1). Neonatal torticollis with SCM "tumor." *(From Fallon J. Textbook of Chiropractic & Pregnancy. 1st ed. ICA, 1994.)*

ETIOLOGY

The etiology of torticollis in the neonate may include stretching of the SCM during delivery resulting in development of a pseudotumor, subluxation of the upper cervical vertebrae from in-utero positioning or a difficult birth, or due to pressure on the spinal cord caused by a spinal tumor. Of these etiologies, pseudotumor and upper cervical subluxation are the most common, with spinal tumor being a relatively uncommon cause of neonatal torticollis. Spinal cord tumor however is an important consideration in the differential diagnosis of neonatal torticollis and one which requires accurate early diagnosis and treatment. Malposition such as posterior presentation *(Figure 2)* and

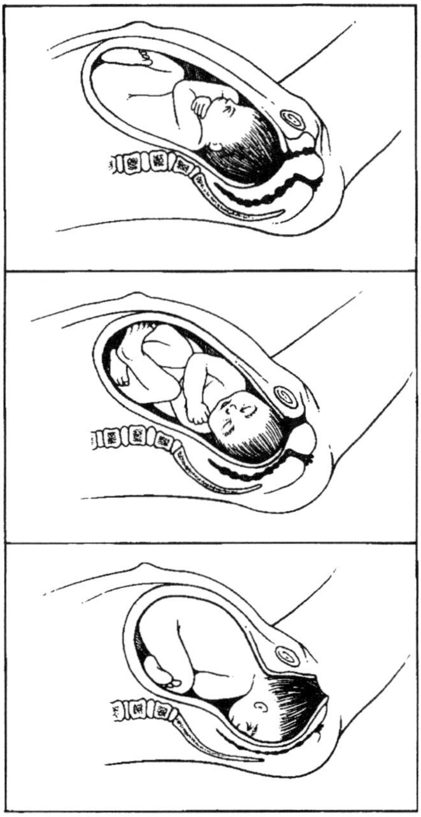

(Figure 2.) Occiput posterior presentation with 135 degree correction. *(From Fallon J. Textbook of Chiropractic & Pregnancy. 1st ed. ICA, 1994.)*

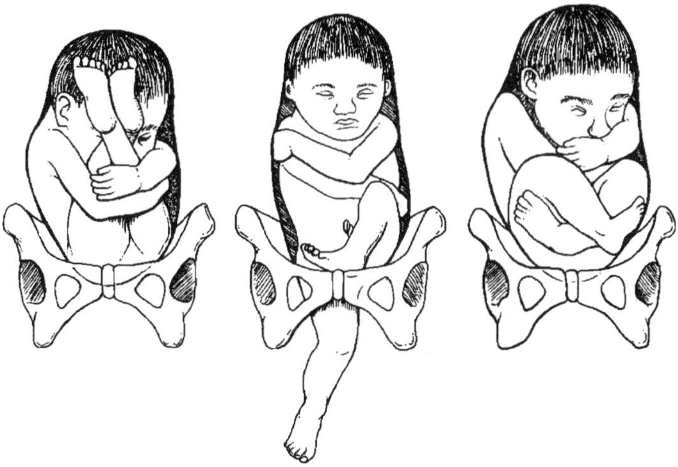

Frank Breech | Incomplete (Footing) Breech | Complete (Full) Breech

(Figure 3.) Breech presentation. *(From Fallon J. Textbook of Chiropractic & Pregnancy. 1st ed. ICA, 1994.)*

breech presentation *(Figure 3)* account for the majority of cases of torticollis found in the neonate.[4,5,6] These two malpresentations, in particular, can cause excessive flexion, extension and lateral flexion of the cervical spine resulting in subluxation of the atlanto-occipital and/or atlanto-axial motor units.[3,5,6,7,8,9] The overall incidence of torticollis has been estimated to be 1.9 percent of which 1.2 percent were cephalic presentations, 6.5 percent double breech presentations, 4.2 percent footing presentations and 34.0 percent were single (frank) breech presentations.[10] The use of forceps *(Figure 4)* and vacuum extraction *(Figure 5)*, as aids in the delivery process, also have been implicated in the development of torticollis in the neonate.[5,6,9]

PSEUDOTUMOR

Congenital torticollis is frequently accompanied by a fibrous nodule known as a pseudotumor in the muscle belly of the SCM[2,3] *(Figure 1)*. The occurrence of pseudotumor has been reported in 10 to 20 percent of the cases of newborn torticollis.[11] Pseudotumor is the result of abnormal stretch on the SCM during the birth delivery process producing an aggregate of torn and contracted muscle fibers and eventually, at about 2 to 3 weeks of age, fibrosis and contracture of the damaged section of muscle.[2,3] Pseudotumor is reported to occur most commonly as a sequelae of birth malposition and presentation with associated delivery trauma.[2,3,4,5,6,7,9] The primary medical intervention for this condition involves massage and stretching of the sternocleidomastoid muscle while waiting for the condition to resolve. In the absence of an appropriate resolution, surgery is then the treatment of choice to release the contracted muscle.

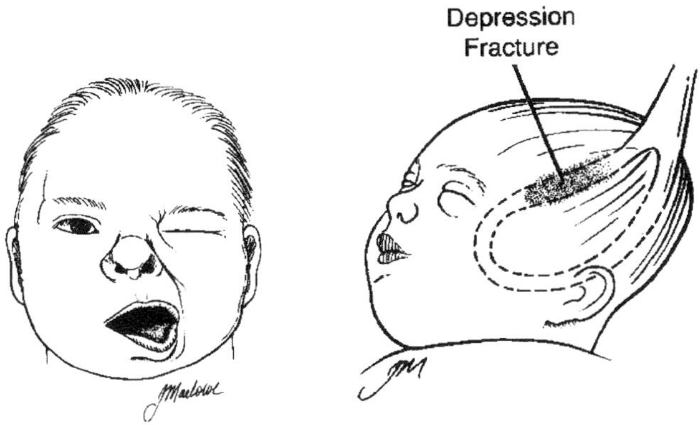

(Figure 4.) Use of forceps during delivery. *(From Fallon J. Textbook of Chiropractic & Pregnancy. 1st ed. ICA, 1994.)*

UPPER CERVICAL SUBLUXATION

Congenital torticollis has been described as a function of the subluxation of the spinal vertebrae, most commonly of the atlanto-occipital and/or atlanto-axial motor units.[4,8,12,13] Studies have demonstrated cervical spine involvement to be present in up to 50 percent of cases of congenital torticollis.[13,14] The most common area of subluxation has been identified as being at the C 1-C 2 level, with the majority (92 percent) having anterior rotation of C 1 on the side opposite the side of SCM contracture.[13] Subluxation of the lower cervical vertebra and/or the upper thoracic vertebrae, to a lesser extent, has been implicated in the etiology of torticollis.[8,12] According to Slate, et al, recognition of cervical subluxation in patients with congenital muscular torticollis may help to explain residual head/neck posturing problems even after successful neck muscle therapy.[13]

SPINAL CORD TUMOR

Spinal cord tumors, which are present at birth, may demonstrate torticollis as one of the clinical manifestations. Spinal cord tumor is an idiopathic lesion yet one which can have serious consequences for the infant. The fact that these tumors can sometimes be missed at birth and not identified until several months later as has been reported in the literature.[15] It is imperative to differentiate congenital torticollis due to spinal tumor from other less invasive causes. Cervical radiographs can be helpful in identifying the presence of a spinal cord tumor. Expansion of the spinal canal can be identified on plain film radiography in many cases of spinal cord tumors. If the outlines of the spinal canal are abnormal, magnetic resonance imaging scans should be obtained to rule-out the possibility of a tumor.

CONGENITAL ANOMALIES

Anomalous development of the vertebral structures may manifest as congenital torticollis. Hemivertebra at any level of the cervical spine or of the upper thoracic spine may manifest as torticollis in the newborn infant. Hemi-segmentation of the C 1 vertebra is a rare congenital anomaly which may cause a rather severe and progressive torticollis. Despite this deformity, when a child is young and the neck quite flexible, the torticollis can be passively corrected. However, in some patients it can become increasingly severe and fixed and may require surgical correction.[16]

ASSOCIATED CLINICAL FINDINGS

Congenital torticollis can also be associated with asymmetry of the cranial and facial bones (plagiocephaly), scoliosis and congenital hip dysplasia.[11,14,17] Plagiocephaly is an asymmetrical and twisted condition of the head and face due to irregular closure of the cranial sutures. Plagiocephaly frequently occurs in conjunction with congenital torticollis.[3,4,7,13] In one study, it was demonstrated that 26 of 30 subjects had consistent flattening of both the contralateral occipital-parietal region and the ipsilateral fronto-orbital region relative to the side of the torticollis.[13] Congenital hip dysplasia is reported by various authors to occur in from 10 to 20 percent of cases of newborn torticollis.[11,14,17]

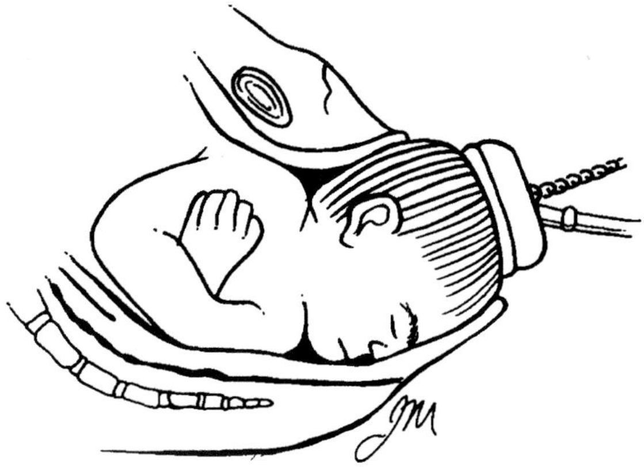

(Figure 5.) Vacuum extraction during delivery. *(From Fallon J. Textbook of Chiropractic & Pregnancy. 1st ed. ICA, 1994.)*

DIFFERENTIAL DIAGNOSIS

Differential diagnosis is an important step in the evaluation of any newborn infant. This is particularly so for the infant presenting with torticollis, since it may be caused by conditions with high morbidity such as spinal cord tumors. Differential diagnoses should include the following etiologies: subluxation of the upper-cervical complex, congenital anomalies such as hemivertebra, cervical lymphadenopathy, localized hematoma, retropharyngeal edema or tumor, spinal cord tumor, reflux esophagitis (Sandifer's syndrome), abducens nerve palsy, child abuse and injury.[3,6,7,8,9]

Differential diagnosis of cervical lymphadenopathy can be made based on the presence of swollen and edematous lymph nodes being located alongside the SCM muscle. Retropharyngeal edema and tumor as well as reflux esophagitis both will present with difficulty in swallowing, vomiting, and occasionally a persistent cough.[3,7] Torticollis with pseudotumor may present with a localized hematoma of the SCM which can be identified by discoloration of the overlying tissue due to aggregate pooling of blood in the injured tissues. Spinal cord tumors and other CNS disorders can usually be ruled out by performing a detailed neurological examination, including neonatal reflexes such as Babinski and Chaddock.[3,7,12] Hermivertebra and other congenital bony anomalies can be identified or ruled-out by obtaining cervical radiographs.

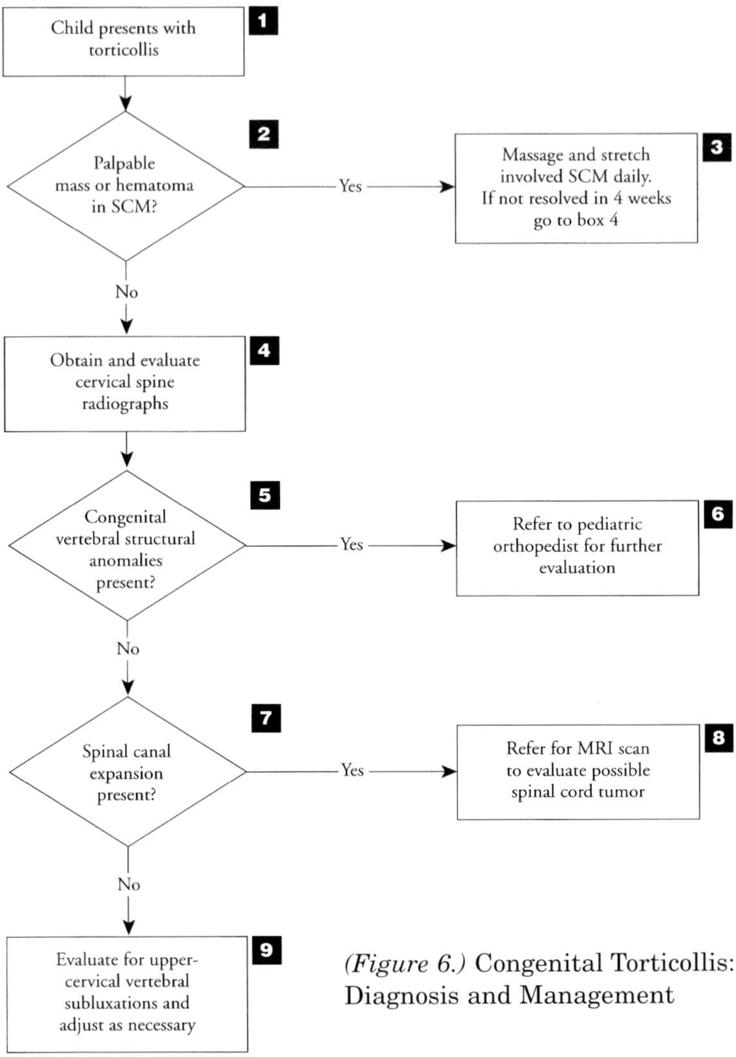

(Figure 6.) Congenital Torticollis: Diagnosis and Management

Abducens nerve palsy can produce a head tilt similar to torticollis but will also present with aberrant unilateral ocular movements, i.e. one eye fixed in lateral gaze.[3,12] Torticollis associated with abducens nerve palsy is rarely seen in the neonate but is seen more commonly in the infant and toddler.[12] Child abuse and other traumatic injuries may also be a cause of torticollis. In such cases, contusions and abrasions or evidence of "shaken baby syndrome" often will present where trauma has occurred.[3,7,12]

The newborn infant with torticollis should be evaluated for the presence of a pseudotumor, manifesting as fibrotic contractures or a hematoma in the involved SCM. If fibrotic contractures or a hematoma is the cause, then a mass, usually 1 to 3 cms in diameter, can be palpated in the involved SCM. If no such mass is palpable then cervical radiographs should be obtained to rule out other possible causes.

EXAMINATION AND TREATMENT

Spinal adjustments have been demonstrated to be efficacious in the resolution of congenital torticollis. In one study, 78 of 79 infants with torticollis responded favorably to a short course of conservative spinal care.[1] Once an accurate diagnosis has been established, and the cause of the infant's torticollis has been identified as being associated with spinal subluxation, a course of conservative chiropractic spinal adjustments should be administered.

Treatment of the child with congenital torticollis should be commenced promptly for best results. The "watch and wait approach" adopted by some physcians would appear to be inappropriate since studies have indicated that congenital muscular torticollis which persists beyond one year of age is unlikely to respond spontaneously.[18] For the infant with torticollis caused by upper-cervical subluxation, determination of the direction of subluxation can be performed by palpation, radiography or with the McMullen reverse fencer reflex.[19] This reflex has been suggested to determine with some accuracy the level of subluxation in the neonate, using a variation of the infantile automatism known as the tonic neck reflex.[19]

Management of an infant with upper-cervical subluxation as the cause of a torticollis requires accurate determination of the position of the upper-cervical vertebrae prior to the administration of any adjustment. If cervical radiographs have previously been obtained, then an accurate determination of misalignment can be obtained visually. In the absence of radiographic evidence, palpatory findings are frequently used as the basis for applying a light adjustive thrust to the fixed segment(s).

Normal spinal biomechanics dictate that with lateral flexion of the neck a concomitant ipsilateral vertebral rotation will occur. As a result of this positioning, the spinous processes of the upper cervical vertebrae will be palpated prominently on the side opposite to the head tilt. Because of the lateral flexion of the neck and its associated coupled motion, the area of fixation will be difficult to determine by motion palpation. Since the most common area of fixation of the vertebral motor units has previously been described as being at the C1-2 motion segment, we will describe an appropriate adjustment at this level.[13] The goal of the adjustment is to restore proper alignment and motion while reducing and eventually eliminating the neurofacilitation responsible for the spasm of the SCM.

The adjustment is performed typically with the patient in the supine position, while laterally flexing the head slightly to the contralateral side a light adjustive thrust is applied with the medial tip of the index finger to the prominent spinous process of the C 2 vertebra.* Light tissue pull should be taken from inferior to superior to remove any tissue slack and the direction of thrust should be lateral to medial and posterior to anterior. If it is determined that the motion segment to be adjusted is at C 0-C 1, then the same set-up is performed except that the segmental contact point is shifted to the transverse process of Atlas on the contralateral side of SCM contracture.

After making appropriate correction of associated vertebral subluxations, the second tier of work can be performed which includes stretching and bending exercises for the SCM. While supporting the child's head with the doctor's hand on the convex side of the torticollis, the doctor will run his/her thumb from the origin of the contracted SCM on the mastoid process to its insertion on the clavicle, while at the same time rotating the child's head toward the concave side of the torticollis. This maneuver should be performed by the doctor three times prior to and after the administration of the adjustment. This will insure that the adjustment can be maintained by the body, and will encourage the SCM to elongate. As an adjunct to spinal adjustments, soft tissue therapy to the involved SCM should enable the child to attain maximum improvement.

CONCLUSION

Chiropractic management of congenital torticollis, using a combination of spinal adjustments, cranial realignment and soft tissue therapies can produce rapid resolution in many cases of congenital torticollis and plagiocephaly in the newborn infant. Spinal adjustments have been demonstrated to be efficacious to the resolution of the congenital torticollis. Before recommending a course of conservative spinal care, however, accurate identifica-

* See page 214.

tion of the cause of the torticollis must be made to rule out complicating conditions which may result in high morbidity or mortality. The typical course of spinal adjustments for torticollis is usually a short duration requiring just a few treatments. Early correction of congenital torticollis should be the goal since prolonged contraction of the SCM can be the cause of cranial and facial anomalies as well as scoliosis. Figure 6 represents a flow chart for the evaluation and management of congenital torticollis as it is presented in the chiropractor's office.

The medical approach to a protracted torticollis is surgical intervention.[5,8,10] While surgical intervention is typically a solution of last resort, it frequently is the only solution considered by the medical community. Chiropractic care is considered essential to the health and maintenance of the child's spine and nervous system, it is therefore considered important that the doctor of chiropractic become part of the multi-disciplinary approach and that medical doctors become aware of chiropractic management as a solution to the most common causes of congenital torticollis.

REFERENCES

1. Biedermann H. Kinematic imbalances due to suboccipital strain in newborns. *J Manual Med.* 1992; 6:151-6.
2. Fallon JM. Textbook of Chiropractic & Pregnancy. Arlington: 1st ed. ICA,1994:126.
3. Stacy M, Jankovic J. Childhood dystonia. *Pediatr Ann.* 1993; 22:157.
4. Cruilshank DP, White CA. Obstetric malpresentations: Twenty years experience. *Am J Obstet Gynecol.* 1973;116:1097.
5. Levine MG, Holroyde J, Woods JR, et al. Birth Trauma: Incidence and predisposing factors. *Obstet Gyneol.* 1987; 156:928.
6. Collea JV, Rabin SC, Weghorst GR et al. The randomized management of frank breech presentations: vaginal delivery vs cesarean section. *Am J Obstet Gynecol.* 1978;131:186.
7. Tredwell SJ, et al. Instability of the upper spine in Downs Syndrome. *J. Pediatr Orthop.* 1990;10:602.
8. Cox D. The condyle subluxation in infants. Articles on Pediatrics. *Int Rev Chiro.* 1994;2: 56-59.
9. Bird CG. The use of the vacuum extractor. *Clin Obstet Gynecol.* 1982; 9:641.
10. Suzuki S, Yamamuro T, Fujita A. The aetiological relationship between congenital torticollis and obstetrical paralysis. *Int Orthop* 1984;8(3):175-81.
11. Porter SB, Blount BW. Pseudotumor of infancy and congenital muscular torticollis. *Am Fam Physician.* 1995;52(6):1731-6.
12. Bradord DS, Hensinger RN. In: The pediatric spine, New York: Thieme. 1985:88.

13. Slate RK, Posnick JC, Armstrong DC, Buncie JR. Cervical spine subluxation associated with congenital muscular torticollis and craniofacial asymmetry. *Plast. Reconstr Surg.* 1993;91(7):1187-95.
14. Binder H, En GD, Gainer JF, Koch B. Congenital muscular torticollis: results of conservative management with long-term follow-up in 85 cases. *Arch Phys Med Rehab.* 1987;68(4):222-5.
15. Shafrir Y, Kaufman BA. Quadriplegia after chiropractic manipulation in an infant with congenital torticollis caused by a spinal cord astrocytoma. *J Peds.* 1992;(26):266.
16. Eubousset J. Torticollis in children caused by congenital anomalies of the atlas. *J Bone Joint Surg.* (AM) 1986;68(2):178-88.
17. Morrison DL, Macewen GD. Congenital muscular torticollis: observations regarding clinical findings, associated conditions, and results of treatment. *J Pediatr Orthop.* 1982; 2(5):500-5.
18. Canale ST, Griffin DW, Hubbard CN. Congenital muscular tortiollis. A long-term follow-up. *J Bone Joint Surg.* (AM) 1982; 64(6):810-6.
19. McMullen M. Assessing cervical subluxations in infants under six months of age. Articles on pediatrics. *Int Review Chiro.* 1994;1:5-8.
20. Grover G. Disorders of the Spine.In: Berkowitz CD,ed. Pediatrics: A Primary Care Approach. Philadelphia: WB Saunders. 1996:324-9.

The astute reader will realize that I do not agree with the rotational listing of the Atlas vertebra "anterior on the side opposite the side of SCM contraction" found by Slate, Posnick, Armstrong and Buncie, as quoted on page 199 in the foregoing paper. However, I do agree with the conclusion of Drs. Fallon and Fysh that the **deviated spinous process** of the subluxated vertebra (usually Axis) is on the side opposite the contracture and that it is the preferred contact for the adjustic thrust. Opinions differ on the subluxation listing of the Atlas in respect to torticollis and more research is needed to shed light on this matter.

This author has not used any therapeutical approach to the care of torticollis in the infant or adult. However, I pass no judgement as to the use of soft tissue therapies. Ancillary procedures used pre and post to chiropractic adjustic care are based on the judgement and the experience of the practitioner.

Let us now turn to a case study of patient A. W., an infant with, so-called, "Congenital Torticollis."

CASE STUDY

This case study is presented by my former associate Dr. LeRoy Otto, D.C. Dr. Otto owns chiropractic clinics in Lake City and Redwing, Minnesota. As a young lad he was my protégé and today he remains my confidant and assistant in my lecturing. A 1976 graduate of The Palmer College of Chiropractic, Dr. Otto is active in practice and research, he is a member of the Minnesota State Board of Chiropractic Examiners.

• • • •

A CASE STUDY, ALEX W.

LeRoy Otto, D.C.
127 South High Street
Lake City, Minnesota 55041

Many parents today, awaiting their first child, are well prepared. They have attended most of the suggested prenatal classes and they have received the usual indoctrination into the medical world of childbirth. They have also been convinced on the necessity of a medically acceptable delivery so just in case something goes awry, the doctors will be able to intervene and help them make what they feel is the right decision.

Sometimes, however, medical **procedures** go awry. Personally, I feel these procedures are more dangerous when new parents choose to utilize their hometown general practitioner who they have always seen for colds and flu, adenoids and hemorrhoids; rather than an obstetrician who just may be a bit more adept when utilizing manual methods of delivery and hopefully less reliant on invasive procedures. Today, when asked well in advance, some obstetricians will avoid the use of invasive procedures as best they can.

For whatever reason, in July of 1989, during his delivery, Alex became the victim of one or more of these circumstances. The G.P. delivering him used a vacuum procedure to assist his delivery. Alex would spend the next three months in some degree of torticollis and suffer reoccurring infections of the ears, U-R-Is, and inconsistencies of the bowels. I became privy to the records of the medical physician after the parents contacted an attorney regarding the matter. Technically, Alex suffered from what is medically termed "acquired acute torticollis."

The birth trauma evidently subluxated the baby and the repeated infections Alex suffered obviously complicated and perpetuated the condition. In 21 years of practice, Alex is the only child I have seen in such a severe state of torticollis. It is interesting to note that despite the problems suffered by Alex, in February of 1992, Alex's sister was born and suffered even more extensive trauma at the hands of the same G.P.; utilizing the same procedure resulting in a seizure and significant hair loss at the crown of the head. To date, the mother reports both children have had learning disabilities and both suffer from numerous infections. The hair loss on the crown of the child's head is now permanent. (Ill. XIII-7)

The following case history focuses on Alex's traumatic torticollis. On August 2, 1989, Alex's mother brought him to my Lake City Clinic with severe right lateral torticollis and moderate anterior distortion, and the symptoms of colic; the usual gassy inconsistent bowel and crankiness. As his mother put it, "He screams all day." I've often felt the diagnosis of colic is easily made in the waiting room. One look at the mother's fatigued eyes, even if the baby is momentarily quiet, is all it takes to confirm the diagnosis.

In Alex's case, as the photos illustrate, (Ill.XIII-6A) the diagnosis was easily made. Examination revealed the usual orthopedic findings for right lateral, anterior torticollis, i.e., absolutely no left lateral flexion, no possible right rotation, extension foraminal compression to the right elicited no response from the infant. All other range of motions were impossible. Neurological examination was unremarkable. The infant's grip was substantial and equal bilaterally. Ophthalmological examination was normal. All reflexes were intact. Palpatory findings yielded all the usual suspects; extreme tautness evident in the right SCM. Flaccidity on the left and involvement of the Atlas/Axis. Alex's Axis vertebra palpated spinous left and superior on the left; it was fixated, however the Atlas seemed somewhat mobile during what limited palpation I could accomplish.

I utilized a supine adjustment initially, contacting the body of the Axis on the right. After the second visit, the anterior torticollis began to resolve. For the next six visits, the Axis held, but so did the right lateral torticollis. Throughout his initial visits, I also adjusted secondary subluxations when necessary, and symptomatically, the colic resolved. The rotatory and lateral

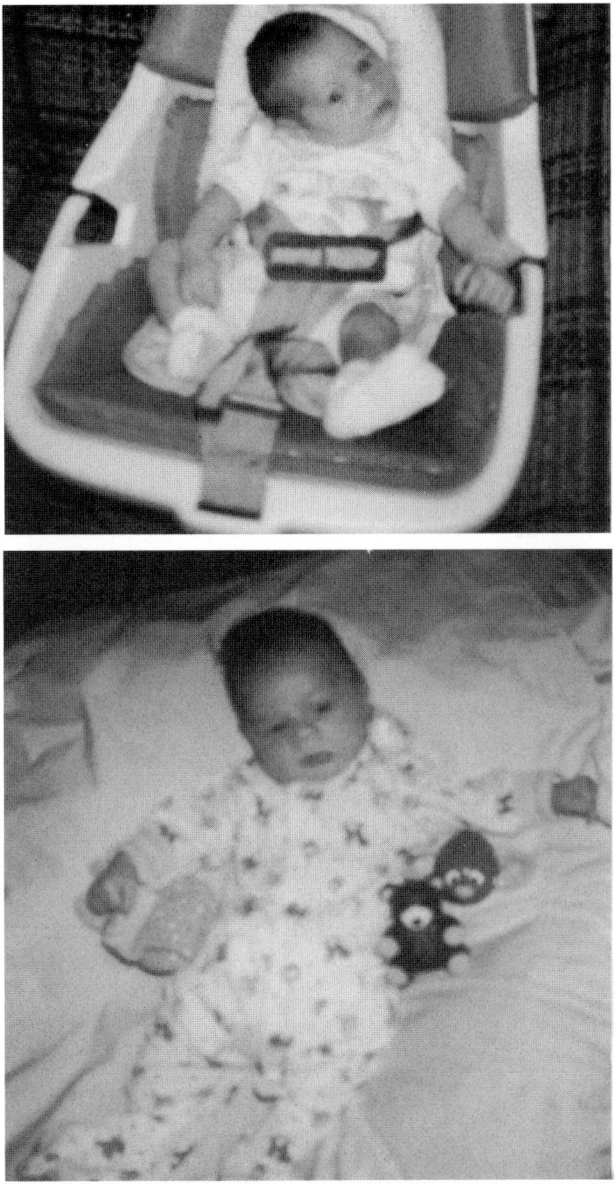

A.

B.

(Ill. XIII-6 A & B) The before and after pictures of baby A. W., (A) shows the baby on his initial visit. (B) shows the improvement after two visits using the toggle adjustment of Atlas and the "spinous pull and lift adjustment" of Axis as mentioned on the next page.

aspect of the torticollis did not. I knew that Dr. Fred would be traveling to a Minneapolis lecture in a few weeks, so I made the necessary arrangements to have Alex examined by him.

On August 30, Dr. Fred utilizing the baby toggle, set the Atlas (ASL) and utilized a spinous pull and lift (spinous left) on the Axis. Within seven days, and after two visits utilizing the toggle, (see page 188) Alex began lifting his head upright. Fatigue would again return the condition. Within three more visits, Alex would have successive days without much "tippage" at all. After eight more visits, the torticollis was resolved.

On Alex's last visit to me on January 13, 1994, he still had not suffered a reoccurrence of torticollis. Soon after he and his family moved about an hour and a half away from my office and I was unable to follow the case further. The photos of the illustrations on page 188 and (Ill. XIII-8) on the next page demonstrate the methods utilized in this case. The condition as it presented initially and upon follow-up are seen on (Ills. XIII-6A & B).

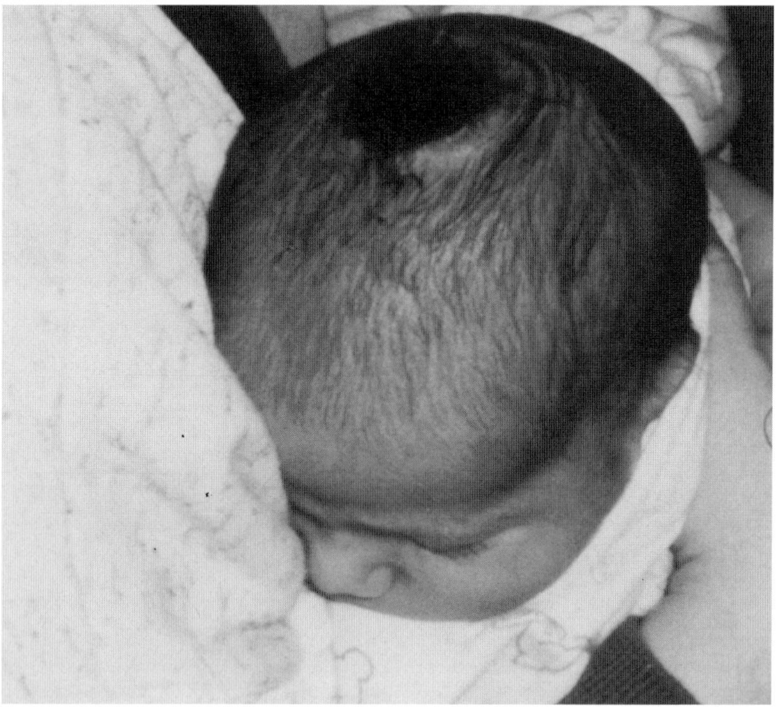

(Ill. XIII- 7) The suction lesion on the crown of the head of patient A.W.'s sister. Such occurrences are quite common after "vacuum extraction" delivery.

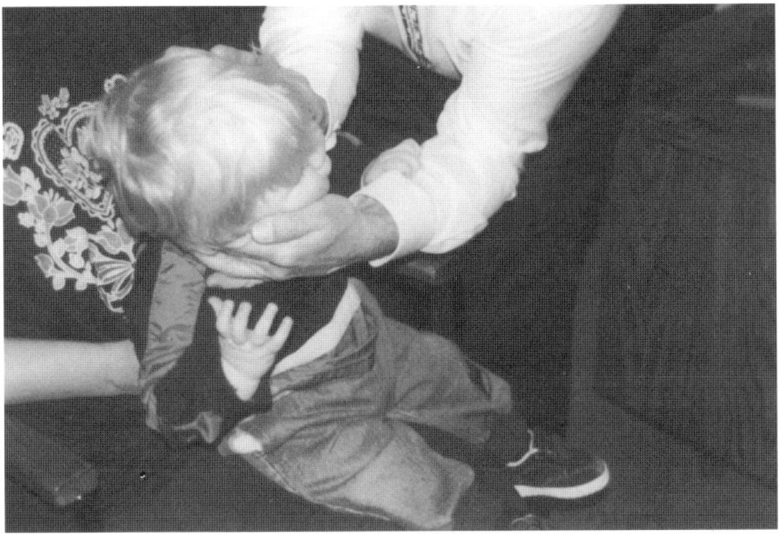

(Ill. XIII - 8) Dr. Otto delivering the spinous pull and lift move on a young lad sitting on his mother's lap. This adjustment is very effective in torticollis, regardless of the patient's age. In the juvenile, adolescent and adult it is the author's preferred adjustment. (See Chapter IX)

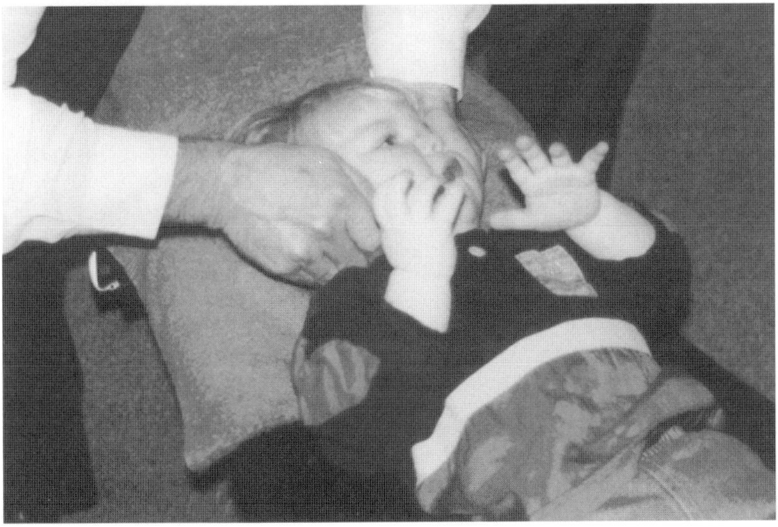

(Ill. XIII - 9) The deviated spinous process can also be adjusted using nail point 6, the lateral tip of the pointer finger. This is a traditional supine cervical thrust commonly taught in chiropractic adjustic technics. See Dr. Fallon's description on page 208.

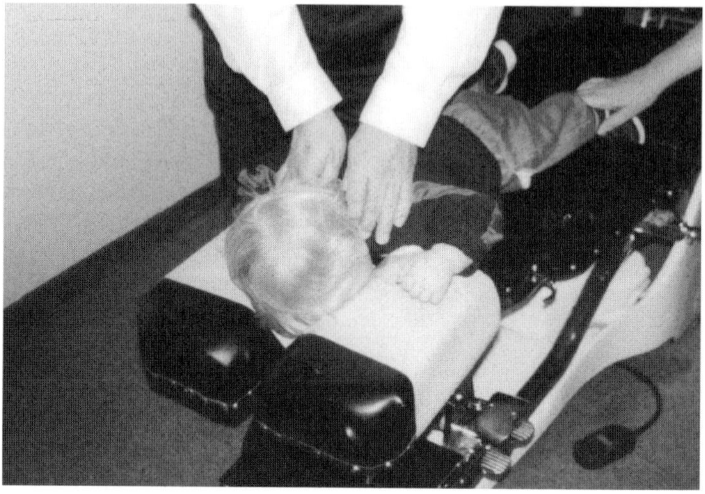

(Ill. XIII-10) Closing the headpiece opening as tight as it can be made to close, the posterior cervical thrust as described in Chapter IX pages 101-105 can also be an effective thrust in accomplishing full correction of the torticollis subluxation in children. This thrust, however, should not be used until after the major correction of the acute subluxation is addressed as before described.

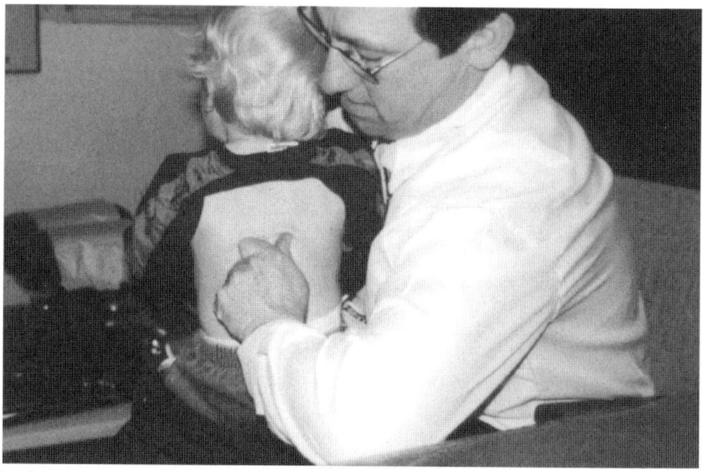

(Ill. XIII-11) At times a thoracic adjustment is called for in torticollis. Using the tip of the thumb (nail point 9) and the knuckle of the index finger, is the author's favorite method of adjusting the dorsal spine in children. The child may sit on your lap or the mother's for this adjustment, Dr. Otto has this child sitting on his knee.

CHAPTER XIV
THE CHIROPRACTIC CARE OF CHILDREN

In 1987 I was elected to serve as president of The International Chiropractors Association. During my three year tenure of office it was my pleasure to initiate and call for the first National Conference on Chiropractic Pediatrics. Since that time the movement has grown into an annual conference sponsoring lecturers on the chiropractic care of children. Through the efforts of the I.C.A., a diplomate program is available to the profession, co-sponsored by the Palmer College of Chiropractic, graduating diplomates annually.

You see, chiropractors have always cared for children and the remarkable recoveries from a host of childhood maladies are legend within the profession. In early years testimonials were widely used by chiropractors, the testimonials detailed the case histories and often depicted photographs of the unfortunate children. One such case was reported in 1913 with an "affidavit" available from the parents. It was contained in a patient brochure on chiropractic published by Dr. R. E. McNamara D.C., B.Sc of Quincy Illinois. (Ill. XIV-1 A & B)

B. J. Palmer published a monthly periodical called The Chiropractor. The inside cover page of Vol. 13, Feb. 1916, is reproduced on (Ill. XIV-2), notice the child on the adjusting table of Dr. Lyons, an early Palmer graduate.

Yes, the chiropractic adjustment of children is nothing new. The recent focus on chiropractic pediatric care has, however, caught the attention of the medical profession and the usual vitriolic criticism has spewed forth from organized medicines political forces. However, today medical doctors are indeed referring to chiropractors and the referrals of children are no exception. Dr. Joan Fallon's rapport with medical physicians in New York is a typical example and in my work in scoliosis I see much improved communication between the two professions. Later in this book I will present the paper by Dr. Gutmann that demonstrates the adjustments efficacy in the care of infectious conditions of infants. Dr. Fallon recently presented a study on the care of over 300 cases of Otitis Media chiropractically. It was recently published in the

"Journal of Clinical Chiropractic Pediatrics," Vol. 2, No. 2, Oct. 1997

All of these studies again point to host factors in regards to infectious conditions. Claude Bernard's famous quote comes to mind. (See page 220).

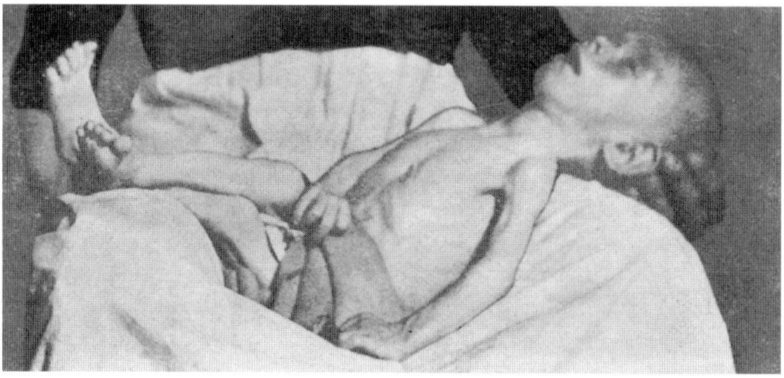

A From this condition

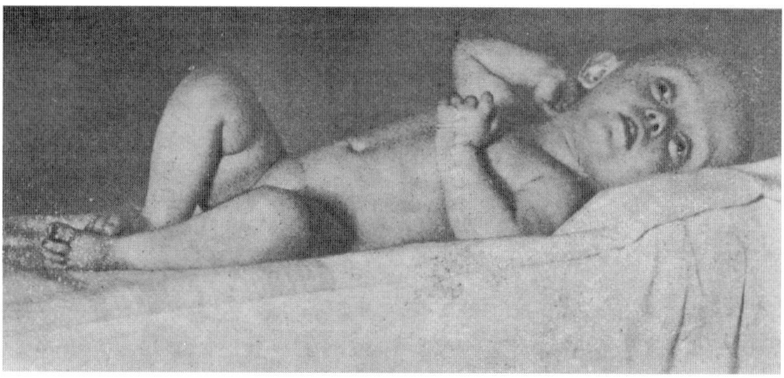

B to this.

(Ill. XIV-1A & B)

The Chiropractor

(Reg. U. S. Pat. Off.)

FOR PEOPLE WHO BELIEVE IN FREE THOT, FREE SPEECH AND GOOD HEALTH

PUBLISHED MONTHLY BY

THE CHIROPRACTOR PUBLISHING CO.

(Copyright 1915 by B. J. Palmer)

F. P. MYERS, Managing Editor

OFFICIAL ORGAN OF THE UNIVERSAL CHIROPRACTORS' ASSOCIATION

OFFICIAL ORGAN OF THE PALMER SCHOOL OF CHIROPRACTIC

Entered at the Postoffice in Davenport, Iowa, as second-class matter

Subscription price, United States, $1.00; Canada, $1.25. Advertising rates on application.

Vol. 13 FEBRUARY, 1916 No. 2

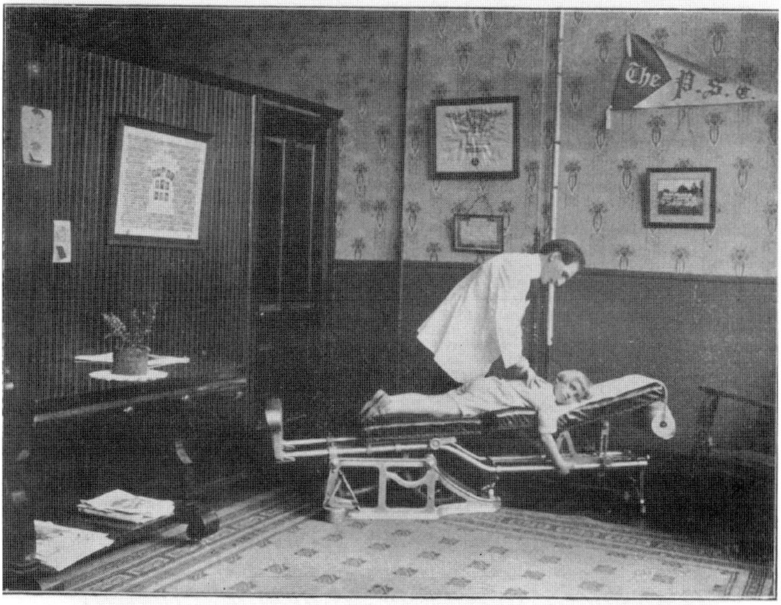

View of Adjusting Room of H. L. Lyons (P. S. C.), Glenwood, Iowa.

(Ill. XIV-2)

"Illnesses hover constantly above us, there seeds are blown by the wind, but they do not set in the terrain unless the terrain is ready to receive them."

Yes, I agree but not only are they "blown by the wind," they are found **within**, and when the host is weak they proliferate. Chiropractic care has never claimed to cure any disease. We give the credit to the doctor within each and every one of us to perform this task. Chiropractors simply adjust the cause of the nerve interference that disturbs the coordinate body function that is necessary to produce health.

Today much emphasis is being put upon genetics by the medical fraternity. Host factors are gaining strong recognition but, certainly, it is not all genetics, systemic malfunction still remains the imminent cause of most of the common maladies suffered by we humans and all vertebrata. In all body function, the control of the nervous system, even over the immune system, reigns imminent.

Nowhere can this be more clearly seen than in the case of cojoined twins. In the annals of Palmer chiropractic history, cases of cojoined twins have often been recorded. Though I have not been able to find case histories on the twins pictured herein, modern case history reports indicate that cojoined twins **do get ill separately**!

Cojoined twins are always identical, the product of a single egg; they are identical genetically. For some unknown reason the egg failed to divide completely during the first few weeks of gestation. On (Ill. XIV-3)* we see B. J. Palmer with a set of cojoined twins and two other unidentified males in the Palmer Clinic gardens.

Violet and Daisy Hilton are shown on (Ill. XIV-4)* with Dr. Mabel Palmer. The twins shown on (Ill. XIV-5)* were also pictured on the cover of the June 1927 issue of "The Chiropractic Educator, Vol. II, Number 6." This periodical was produced by The Palmer School of Chiropractic, for use in chiropractors' offices.

The twins are "The Gibb Sisters," Margaret and Mary. They were cared for by Nestor Alzarez, D.C. who stated they appeared on vaudeville stage. The illustration contained herein shows them in the good doctor's office examining skeletal specimens.

* Photographs courtesy Palmer College of Chiropractic Archives.

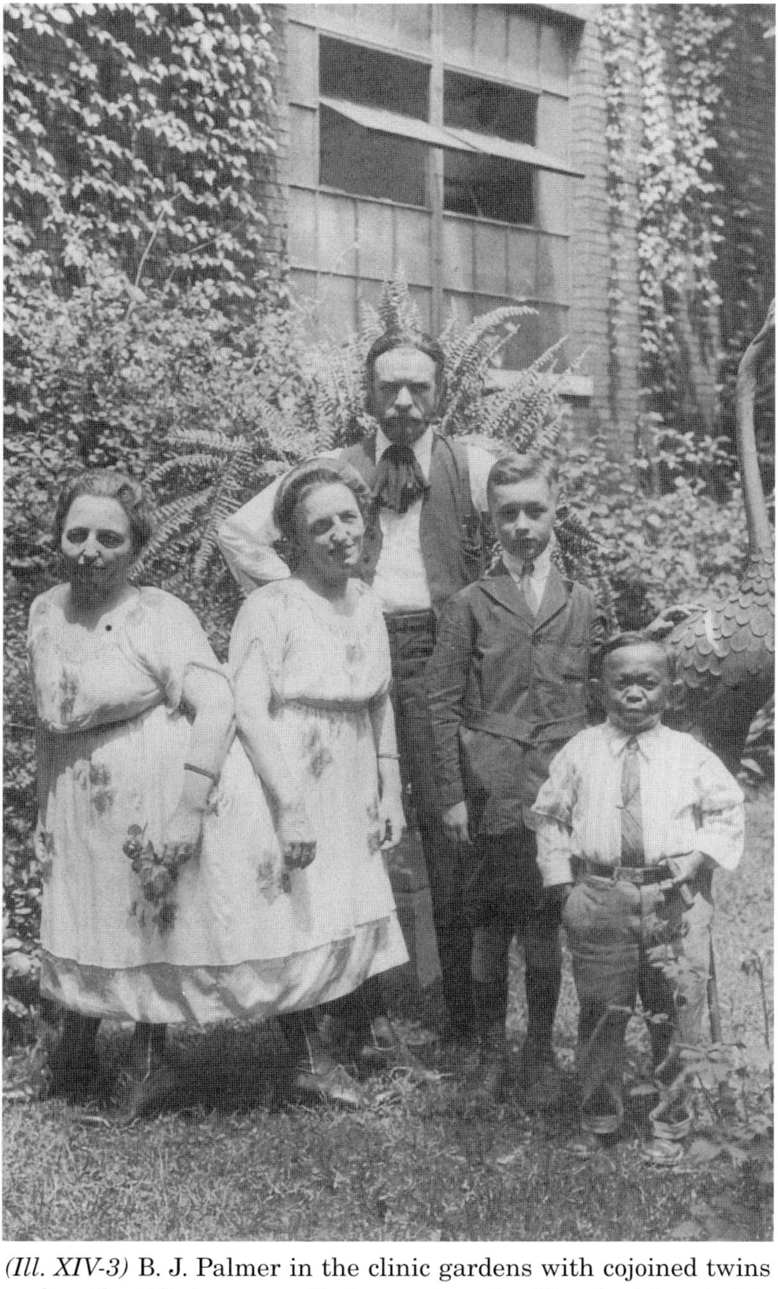

(Ill. XIV-3) B. J. Palmer in the clinic gardens with cojoined twins and unidentified persons. B. J. mentions the Blazak sisters in his writings, possibly it is they who are pictured above.

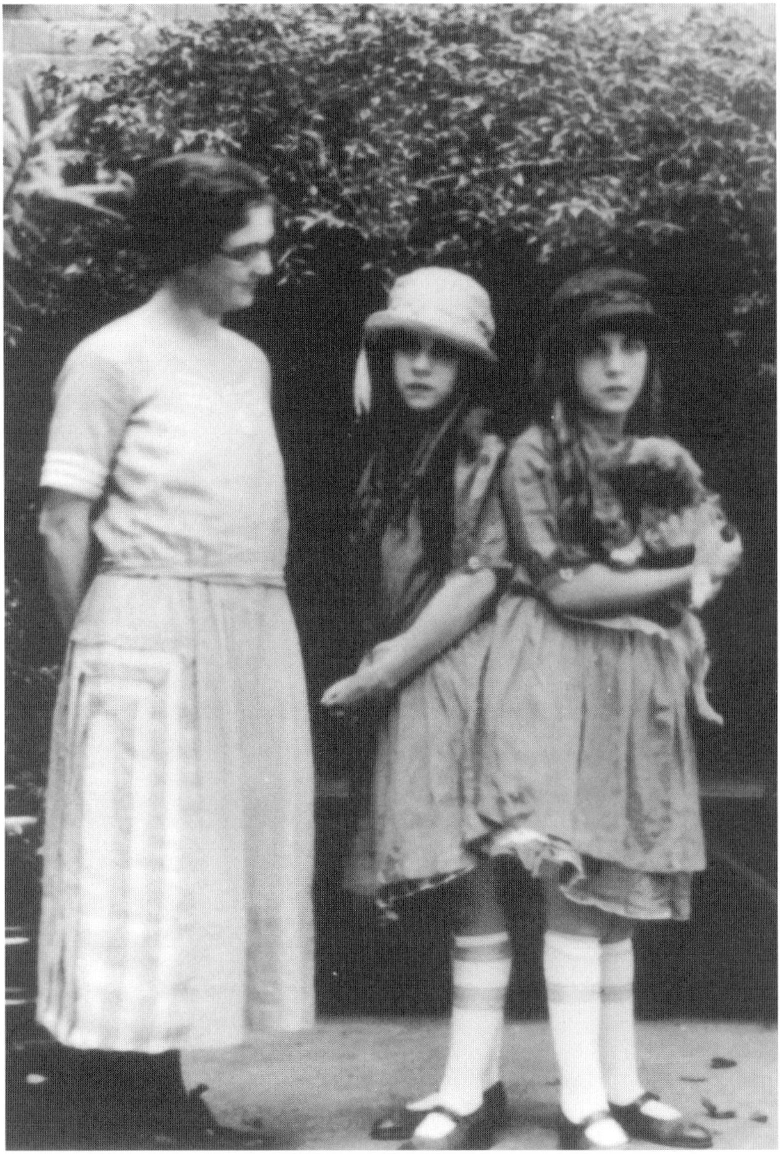

(Ill. XIV-4) Dr. Mabel Palmer with the Hilton twins, Violet and Daisy.

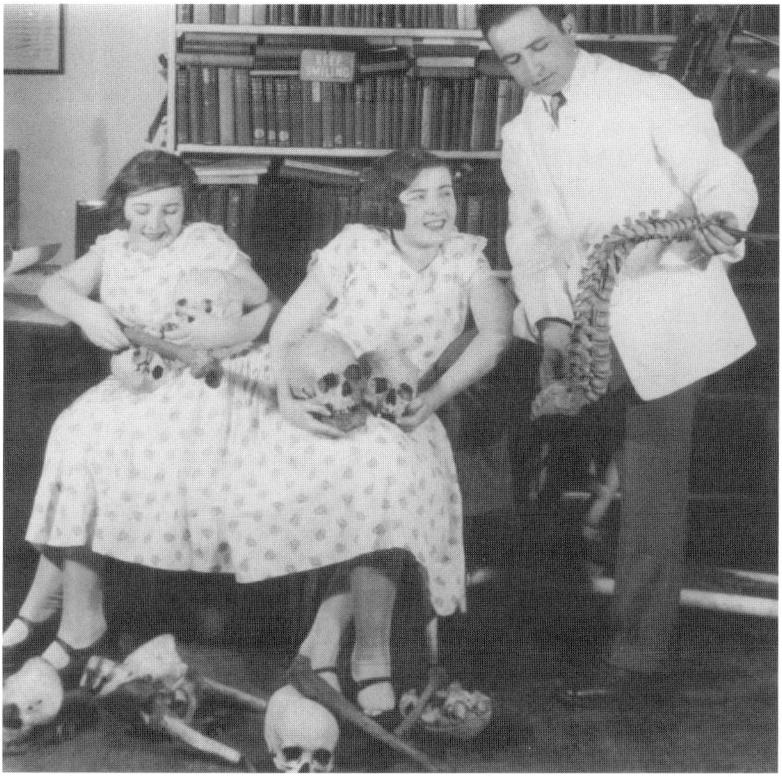

(Ill. XIV-5) Margaret and Mary Gibb and Dr. Alzarez, notice the early Hilo table behind the doctor. 1927

The cases of cojoined twins clearly indicate that factors more than genetic are involved in health. In the April 1966 *Life Magazine*[36], there appeared an article entitled, "Rare Study of Siamese Twins in Soviet - MASHA and DASHA." This set of cojoined twins were born on January 4, 1950. To my understanding their parents were told they were stillborn but they were actually well-cared for in Moscow medical clinic and studied under the supervision of eminent Soviet Physiologist, Pyotr Anokhin. The girls were five years old before they learned to walk as they shared two legs between them and the left leg was controlled by Dasha and the right leg by Masha. Their pelvic bones were joined and their spines met at the coccyx. Their circulatory systems were inter-connected, the article stated, "if one were bit by a poisonous snake the venom would quickly spread to both. Although their spines connect their spinal cords did not. Hence their nervous systems, e.g. sense of touch, are totally distinct, they become ill separately ..." The article goes on to state that their intestines are connected at the level of the lower intestine, they have four kidneys but only one bladder and they have a common reproductive system. With everything so interconnected except their nervous systems, the germ theory and genetic theory of disease certainly reveal their fallibility; **these children become ill separately.** I thank the good Dr. Carl S. Cleveland Jr. for bringing the case of Masha and Dasha to the attention of the entire chiropractic profession, in his lectures he mentioned them often.

Most recently another set of cojoined twins were brought to light in the March 25, 1996, issue of TIME.[37] In an article entitled, "The Most Intimate BOND," Abigail and Brittany Hensel are discussed and pictured. They have much in common with Masha and Dasha as they share two legs and each controls one side of their connected body, their sensations such as urination and the need to sleep and eat are separate. Again, **their nervous systems are distinct** but their circulation and many organic functions are shared. If one child takes a medicine it will treat both, the same is true for vitamins; yet these two twins do get ill separately. For instance one may have a cold when the other does not, one may get an ear infection yet the other may be free of the malady. The mother stated the twins need only one set of vaccinations. While we as chiropractors may question the validity and need for vaccinations, this certainly proves the interconnection of their circulatory systems.

Yet, their spines are separate and join only at the pelvic level, their nervous systems are separate and distinct. And **yes**, they can subluxate separately and thus suffer the consequences of ill health separately.

B. J. Palmer studied the cases I have illustrated in this text and it was his belief that a subluxation in the mother caused the problem. For historical purposes and to end this chapter on "The Chiropractic Care of Children," allow me to quote from page 403 of "The Bigness of the Fellow Within." Written in 1949, Vol. XXII of B. J. Palmer's, "Green Books,"[38] states this:

"Due to subluxations, possible in the mother pre-natally, we often have pre-natal monstrosities such as the Hilton Sisters, Gibb Sisters, Blazak Sisters, Eng and Cheng Siamese twins as they are known. We have known all first three personally. So far as we know we were the first and only people to radiograph the Hilton Sisters and know exactly how they were united. So far as we also know, we were first to make a physical examination of the Blazak Sisters and know how and where they were united.

"Here are cases of where twins were in the making. Instead of two blastoderms being independent and separate from each other, they became mixed and grew united to each other and developed that way for 280 days. Their fusion was abnormal, pathologically premised, even though their tissue cell expansion process was otherwise comparatively normal which was almost so with the Hilton Sisters. This was not true of the Blazak Sisters. Their blastodermic fusion and tissue cellular expansion were both abnormal and pathological. They had two separate upper bodies, one middle body with one lower backbone, sacrum and rectum between them, and two separate lower pairs of legs. Certain parts of the blastoderms of one or the other did not develop, therefore, they had to divide what they had.

"In each of these cases there was a vertebral subluxation in the mother which hindered normal reproduction function from carrying through normally. Function being abnormal, product followed suit."

Yes, B. J., you made your viewpoints well known and time has proven you correct in many points you have made.

But the fact remains cojoined twins do become ill separately and so we see again the imminence of the nervous system in the coordinate functioning so necessary to produce health. And the subluxation, the primary cause of incoordinate functionating can be corrected through chiropractic vertebral adjustment.

As we look at the correction of vertebral subluxations in infants, children, and adults, one outstanding technic developed by the chiropractic profession became known through the efforts of its founder, Dr. C. S. Gonstead of Mount Horeb, Wisconsin. He was a 1923 graduate of the "Crusader Class" at the then Palmer School of Chiropractic in Davenport, Iowa. He was a classmate and seat partner of my father, Dr. H. A. Barge who practiced, as do I, in LaCrosse, Wisconsin. Dr. Gonstead and my father were friends throughout life and it was at the insistence of my father that I interned with Dr. Gonstead after I returned home from my graduation from Palmer and a nine month postgraduate course at The Logan Basic College of Chiropractic. I wanted to begin practice at once with my father and I did so, I simply traveled to Mount Horeb on weekends and Dr. Gonstead graciously allowed me to observe his patient care; he practiced every day of the week.

Today the Gonstead Clinic carries on and the Doctors Cox teach his work worldwide. In 1995, working on the preparation of this text, I wrote my friend, Dr. Doulgas B. Cox of the Gonstead Clinic, and asked for any input he might have in respect to the adjustment of an infant in torticollis. He stated that he did not have any specific adjustment to offer except that they often found a "Condyle Subluxation" in infants, he then gave me his kind permission to quote, in whole or in part, from his paper which was published in the March/April 1991, I.C.A. Review.[39]

With the kind permission of the publisher, The I.C.A. Review, and Dr. Cox, I reproduce his paper herein.

The Condyle Subluxation in Infants[39]
by Douglas B. Cox, DC

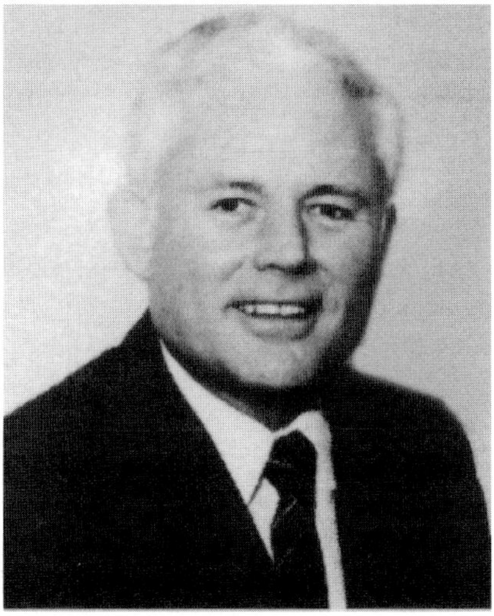

Douglas B. Cox, DC, is in private practice in Mt. Horeb, Wisconsin. A graduate of Palmer College of Chiropractic, he taught for four years at the college as an associate professor. A member of the teaching staff of the Gonstead Seminars, Dr. Cox has conducted over 428 seminars in Europe, Australia, and North America.

Throughout the history of chiropractic, many men and women have made an important contribution to their profession beyond caring for their patients.

Such is the case of the late Dr. C. S. Gonstead of Mt. Horeb, Wisconsin. He developed and perfected a system of carefully analyzing and correcting the subluxation. To my knowledge Dr. Gonstead was the first in the discovery and correction of the anterior superior condyle which occurs especially in infants. It is believed that this is often caused by an injury during the birth process.

This article will deal with the detection, analysis and correction of the occipital condyle subluxation in infants.

Following are some examples of the condyle subluxation and how they are corrected.

Occipital Condyle Misalignment

The occiput and Atlas are optimally aligned when there is maximum patency through the portion of the spinal canal formed by the vertebral foramen of the Atlas, and the foramen magnum of the occiput. This condition can exist only when the plane of the foramen magnum and the AP Atlas plane are parallel. In Figure 1, two dots have been placed on the external, inferior surface of the occiput. The dots are put on the flat, straight surface of the occiput that lies immediately behind the condyles on the lateral film. The anterior dot should be placed at the point where the flat surface and the posterior portion of the condyles are joined. The posterior dot is placed where the flat surface meets the curved external surface of the squama. The line through these dots represents the AP plane of the foramen magnum, and is designated the "foramen magnum line." When the foramen magnum line and the AP Atlas plane line are parallel, there is optimal alignment between the occiput and Atlas.

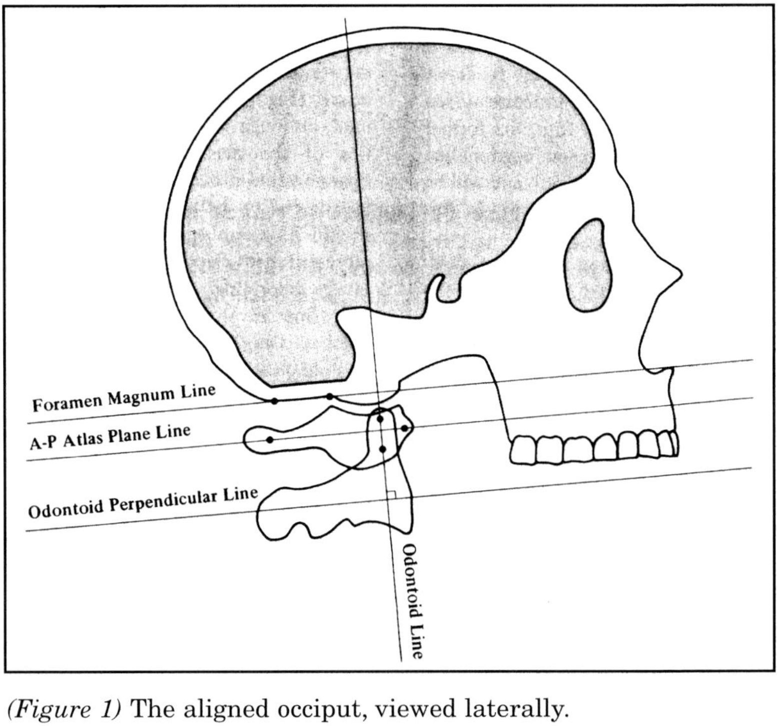

(Figure 1) The aligned occiput, viewed laterally.

"AS" or "PS" Misalignment

When the occiput misaligns with the Atlas, it will first misalign in one of two possible directions. It can either slip anterior and superior, in relation to the Atlas, in which case it will be listed as an "AS" occiput; or, it can misalign posterior and superior in relation to the Atlas which will qualify it as a "PS" (Fig. 3) occiput.

When the occiput slips anterior and superior (AS), the foramen magnum line and the AP Atlas plane line will converge posteriorward (Fig. 2). "AS" misalignment diminishes the space between the posterior arch of the Atlas and the occiput, so that the two structures become approximated (Fig. 2, arrow). Because the occiput and Atlas are fixed in this position, the space will remain closed even when the cervical spine is in flexion.

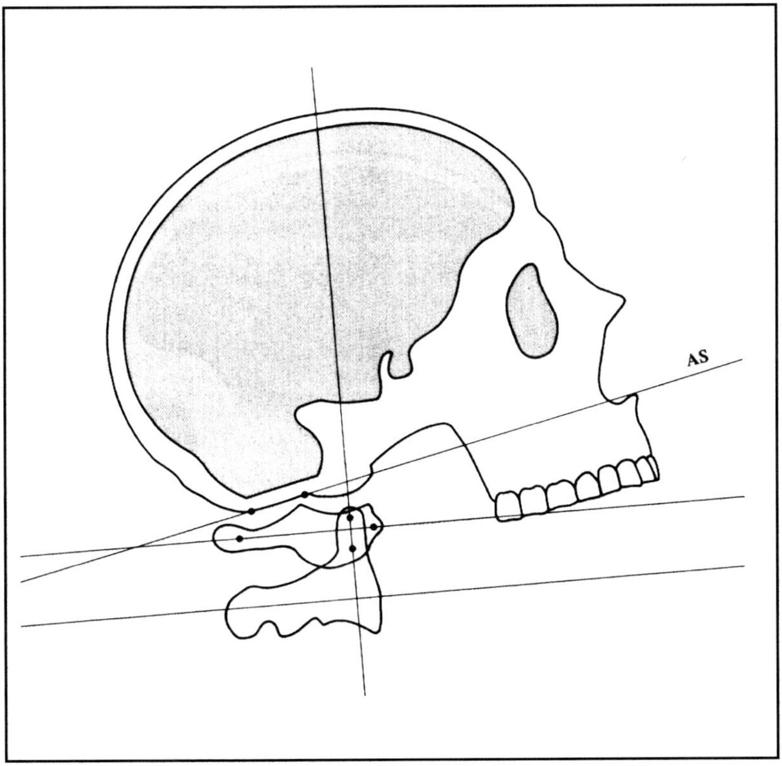

(Figure 2) The "AS" occiput.

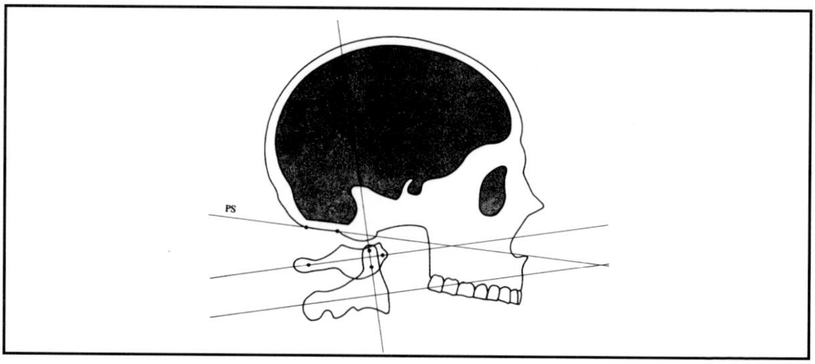

(Figure 3) The "PS" occiput.

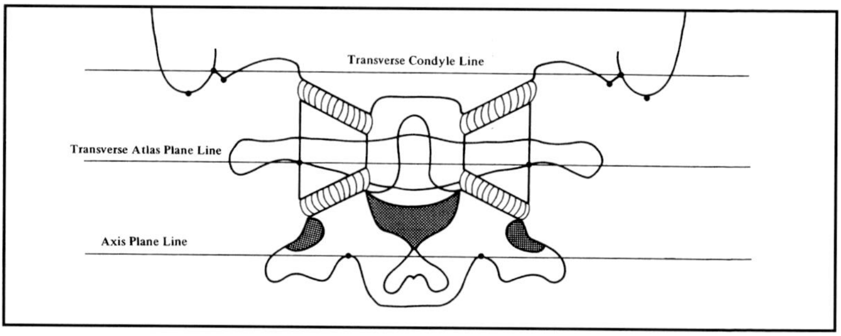

(Figure 4) Optimal occiput-atlas alignment in the reversed anteroposterior view.

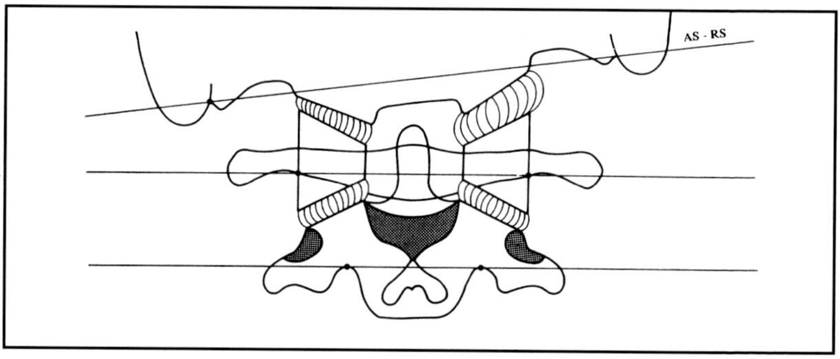

(Figure 5) Occiput misaligned AS-RS.

When the occiput misaligns posteriorward and superiorward (PS), the foramen magnum line and AP Atlas plane line will diverge posteriorward (Fig. 4). This misalignment will cause the space between the posterior arch of Atlas and the occiput to be enlarged (Fig. 4). Even when the cervical spine is in extension, this space will remain relatively wide.

Author's Note - On the AP x-ray viewed from the posterior, the lateral subluxation of the occiput can be determined, (Fig. 5). Optimal alignment (Fig. 4).

Repositioning the Occiput

All "posterior" occipital subluxations, that is, those which begin with a "PS" listing, are corrected with a thrust that drives the occiput anteriorward and inferiorward (Fig. 6). Anterior occiputs are corrected by a thrust which repositions the occiput in the posterior and inferior directions, to correct the "AS" component of the misalignment (Fig. 6).

The same thrust that corrects the "PS" or "AS" factors also reduces the occipital laterality and rotation. In Figure 7, the arrows indicate the direction of thrust, as well as the area of contact for correcting occipital subluxations with right laterality. For "posterior" occiputs, the point of contact is on the temporal bone behind the ear. "Anterior" occiputs are contacted on the glabella of the frontal bone.

All condyle adjustments, both PS and AS moves, should include rotation of the head when rotational misalignment is a part of the listing. (Fig. 5).

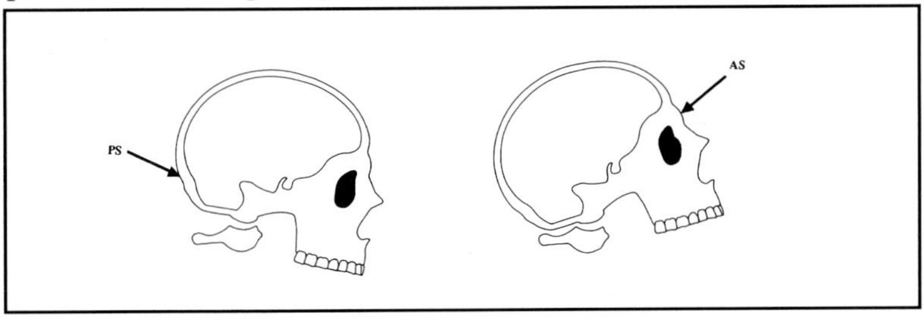

(Figure 6) Direction of thrust for correcting "AS" and "PS" occipital misalignments.

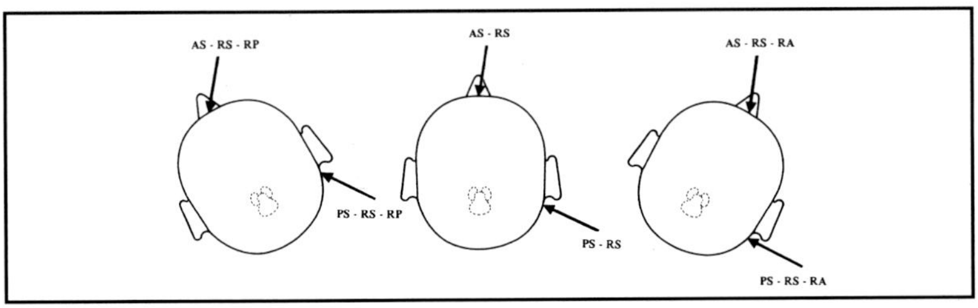

(Figure 7) Direction of thrust for correcting the occipital misalignments with right laterality.

The AS occipital condyle moves are performed with the patient in the supine position. The baby's head should rest on a firm surface to stabilize the occiput. With the doctor standing on the side of contact, the metacarpal heads are placed on the forehead, over the supra-orbital margin, on the side of laterality. The back of the occiput is lifted so that the condyle and Atlas are separated, allowing movement to occur. The thrust is give posteriorward, inferiorward, and medialward. Figure 8 illustrates the setup for an AS-LS occipital condyle adjustment.

An anterior condyle adjustment may also be performed with the child lying supine on the parent's lap. The doctor stands on the side of laterality, and places the pisiform of the contact hand over the glabella. He supports the baby's occiput with his stabilization hand. The setup for an AS-RS occipital condyle adjustment is shown in Figure 9. The thrust is given through the glabella in a posteriorward, inferiorward, and medialward direction. This position may also be used to adjust a straight anterior occipital condyle subluxation. This listing assumes no lateral misalignment or rotation. The doctor may stand on either side, and contact the glabella with either hand. The direction of thrust is posteriorward and inferior.

An optional method for adjusting straight anterior condyle subluxation is with the patient placed supine on the pelvic table. The doctor uses both hands, and places the thenar eminences on the forehead above the supra-orbital margins, as shown in Figure 15. He lifts the back of the occiput to the appropriate angle, and thrusts posteriorward and inferiorward with both thenars.

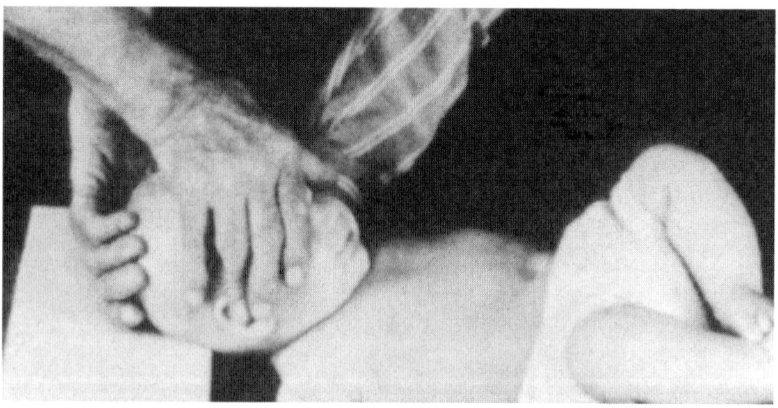

(Figure 8) Adjusting an anterior condyle with an AS-LS listing.

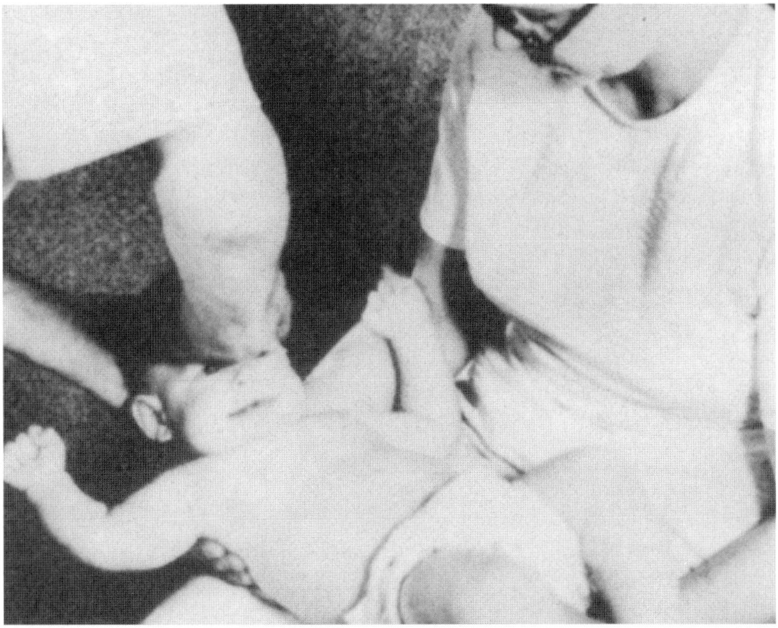

(Figure 9) An AS-RS condyle adjustment while in the mother's lap.

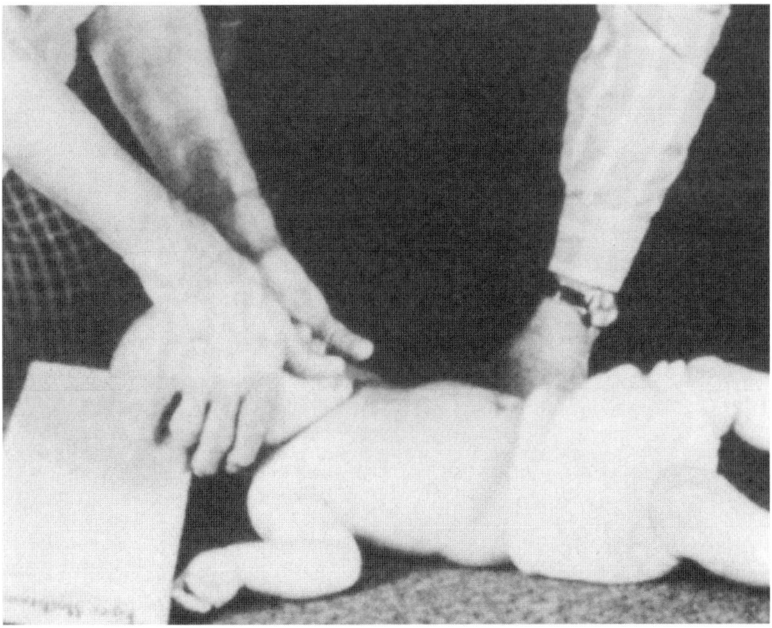

(Figure 10) Adjusting the straight anterior condyle.

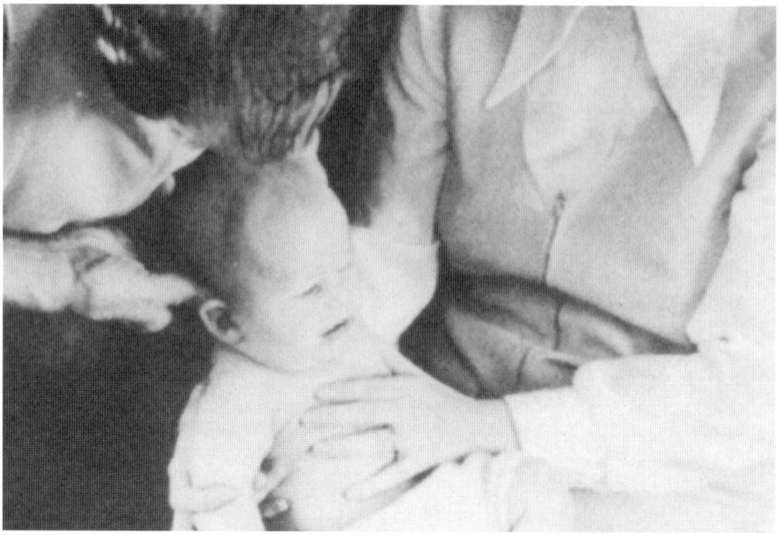

(Figure 11) Adjusting a PS-RS condyle listing.

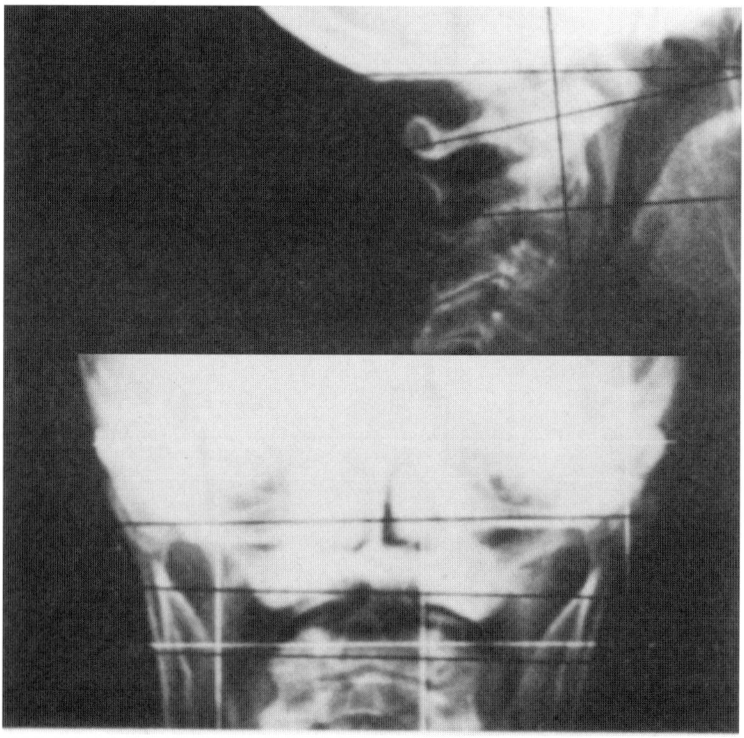

(Figure 12) Occiput listing, PS-RS. (Adult)

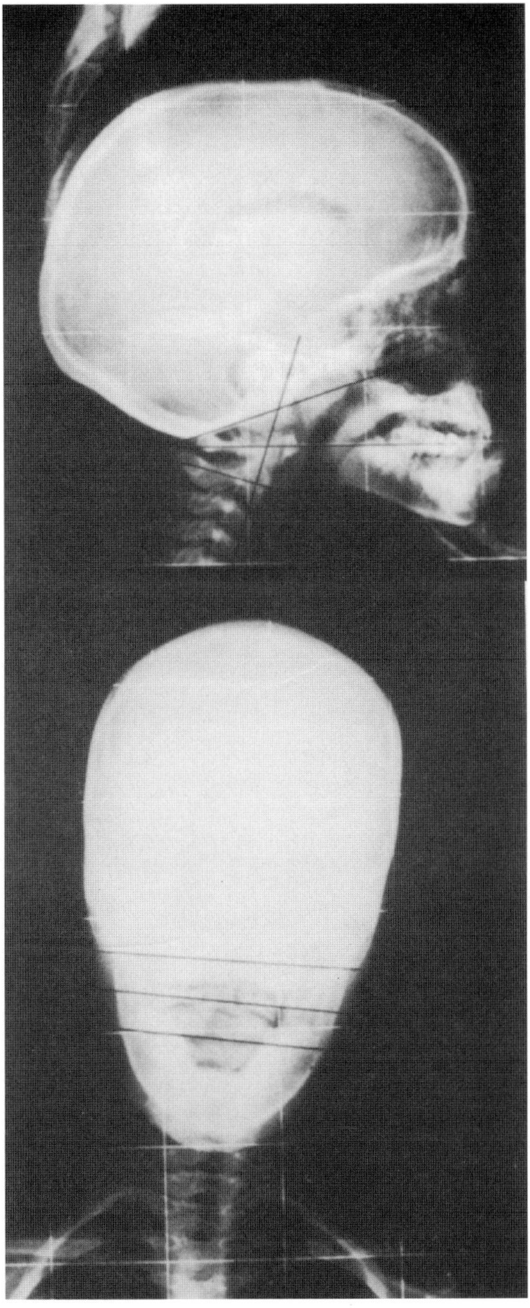

(Figure 13) "Anterior" occiput of a child, listed AS-RS-RA.

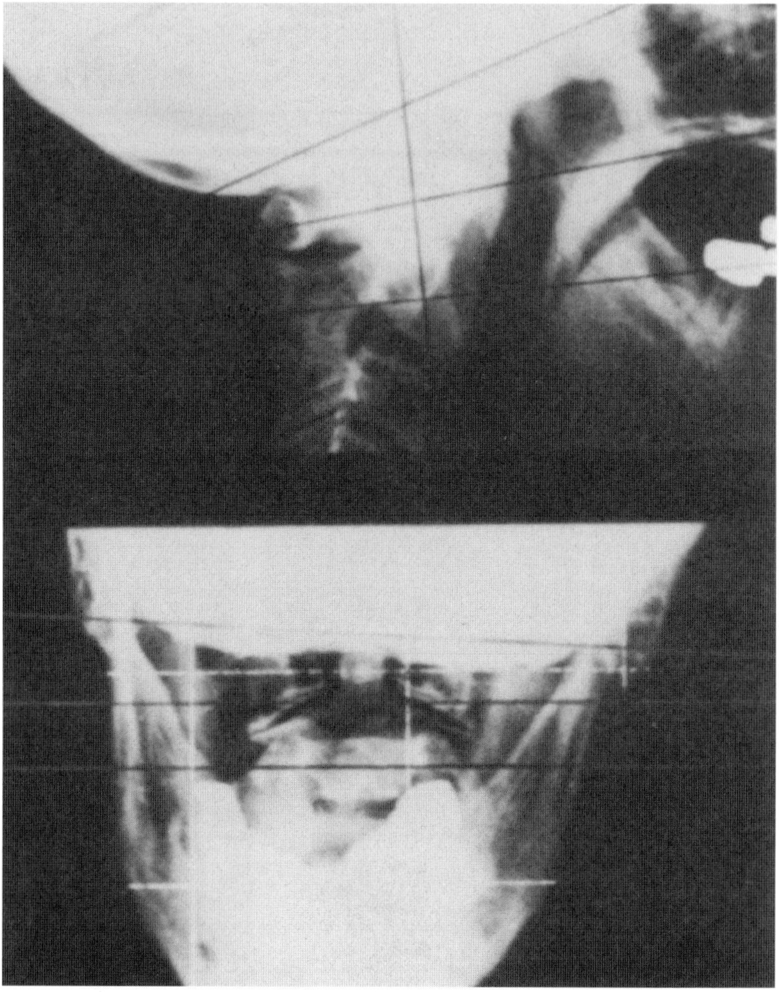

(Figure 14) Occiput listing, AS-LS. (Adult)

Author's Note

There has been some minor editing of Dr. Cox's original paper and the illustration numbers have been changed for the purposes of this text. For questions or information on The Gonstead Technic of Chiropractic contact GONSTEAD, P.O. Box 46, Mt. Horeb, WI 53572.

Throughout this text I have continually emphasized that underlying spinal problems and subluxations can lead to the acute manifestation of the torticollis subluxation. Infragenic problems, such as scoliosis, force the cervical spine to accommodate and create disc wedges that often lead to torticollis. Supragenic problems such as the proprioceptive reflex mechanisms found in the brain stem can also cause faulty spinal balance that in turn can initiate attacks of torticollis and tortipelvis. The Atlas subluxation is often the culprit in such problems. In his chapter on Upper Cervical Specific, Dr. Crowder drives this point home. The Atlas subluxation can create the incoordination that sets the stage for the acute attack of tortipelvis and torticollis. The occipital subluxation too, may be the culprit involved as a predisposing factor in torticollis.

Again, once the acute attack is corrected through adjustment, predisposing factors should be sought out. You may well have to adjust other subluxations, **plus** the torticollis subluxation to fully resolve the problem. In this light let us not forget the occipital subluxation as identified by the late Clarence Gonstead D.C. The chiropractor should always heed the words of Dr. Gonstead when he said:

"Remember, chiropractic always works; when it does not seem to, examine your application do not question the principle."

It is the hope of the author that the adjustic procedures explained in this text, by myself and the other authors, will lead the chiropractor to understand that it is more often the chiroprac**tor** that fails and not chiroprac**tic**.

I believe it was in 1988 that I first read an article in VOICE[40], the periodical published by the "Kentucky Association of Chiropractors." The article was an abstract taken from a paper written in German in Manuelle Medizin (1987), the respected European Periodical. It was reviewed in the "Journal of The Australian Chiropractors Association." Dr. Marcia Segura D.C. brought it to the attention of VOICE and the abstract was printed therein. It stated:

"A most interesting paper by Gutmann was published in German in *Manuelle Medizin* in 1987 and has been reviewed in the September 1988 issue of the *Journal of the Australian Chiropractors' Association.*

"In the abstract to his paper, Gutmann, a prominent specialist in manual medicine from Bad Sassendo, West Germany, concludes:

- Blocked nerve impulses at the Atlas cause many clinical features from central motor impairment to lower resistance to infections— especially ear, nose and throat infections.
- Chiropractic and radiological examinations are "of decisive importance" for diagnosis of the syndrome.
- "Chiropractic can often bring about amazingly successful results, because the therapy is a causal one."

"Gutmann reports examination and adjustment of more than 1,000 infants with Atlas blockage or subluxation. Three case reports are given. One describes a boy of 18 months with early relapsing tonsillitis, frequent enteritis, therapy resistive conjunctivitis, frequent colds and earache, and increasing sleeping problems (fear of lying down or sleeping, falling from exhaustion, screaming during the night). After the first specific adjustment of the Atlas, the child demanded to be put to bed and slept peacefully until morning. The conjunctivitis cleared completely, and previously disturbed appetite returned to normal.

"From his and other German medical studies, Gutmann concludes that approximately 80 percent of all children are not in autonomic balance and that many have Atlas blockage or subluxation. He has been 'constantly amazed how, even with the lightest adjustment with the index finger, the clinical picture normalizes, sometimes gradually, but often immediately.'

"His colleague Frymann, he reports, examined a random group of 1,250 babies five days from post partum. 211 suffered from vomiting, hyperactivity and sleeplessness. Manual examination revealed cervical strain in 95 percent of this group. Release of this strain by specific manipulation 'frequently resulted in immediate quieting, cessation of crying, muscular relaxation and sleepiness.'

"Gutmann's highly significant conclusions are:

I) 'Observations of motor development and manual control of the occipito-atlanto-axial joint complex should be obligatory after every difficult birth'; and

II) 'With any developmental impairment the joint complex should be examined and, if required, specifically adjusted...the success of adjustment overshadows every other type of treatment.'"

For your information, I now present the entire papers.

Blocked Atlantal Nerve Syndrome
In Infants and Small Children[41]

By G. Gutmann

(Published in "Manuelle Medizin" © Springer-Verlag 1987. The "ICA Review" thanks the Barge Chiropractic Clinic of La Crosse, Wisconsin, for having the original paper translated into English by Ronald M. Mazur, PhD, Winona State University, Minnesota. Translation published with permission of "Manuelle Medizen" publishers.)

ICA International Review of Chiropractic July/August 1990 Reprinted with the permission of The ICA, 1997, Barge Chiropractic Publishing, Inc.

Summary: Three case reports are reviewed to illustrate a syndrome that has so far received far too little attention, which is caused and perpetuated in infants and small children by blocked nerve impulses at the Atlas. The clinical picture ranges from central motor impairment and development through idencephalic impairments of vegetative regulatory systems to lowered resistance to infections, especially to ear-, nose- and throat-infections. The theoretical background to this syndrome is indicated. The main factor in the causation concerns the neurophysiological connections between the area of the atlanto-occipital joint and centers in the brain stem. In addition to the case history (birth trauma, etc.) and the pediatrician's diagnosis, chiropractical and radiological examinations are of decisive importance for the diagnosis of this syndrome. If the indications are correctly observed, chiropractic can often bring about amazingly successful results, because the therapy is a causal one.

Key Words: Babies, infants, Atlas, blocked nerves, dysregulation, motor, vegetative, impaired development, resistance lowered to infections, diagnosis and therapy, chiropractical.

We described this syndrome for the first time in 1953, and then again in 1968, with the complex designation, cervical-diencephalic-static syndrome (C.D.S.). In 1984 we described it as cervical-diencephalic-kinesiological syndrome in small children.

Even though it is among the most satisfying indications of the effectiveness of manual therapy, evidently even experts in our own ranks have hardly gained access to this occurrence at all. Only the pediatrician Mohr (30) has checked our reports and confirmed them in full measure. Lewit, (26, 27) and later Seifert (35) expressed a similar opinion in the German Democratic Republic.

Case Studies

V.S., 10-month-old male child

Congenital torticollis after suction-belljar delivery. Post-natal haemotoma of the sternocleidic mastoid on the right side.

In spite of intensive therapeutic gymnastics, no improvment in the torticollis. A clear-cut asymmetry had developed in the skull and face. Crawling, let alone sitting, was impossible. The orthopedic institute treating the patient diagnosed cerebral disturbances of movement.

Our x-ray findings: Moderate degree of inferior location of the Atlas with kyphotic position of the HWS and dislocation of the occiput (al) on the right side across from C 1 and C 2.

No clear blockage could be felt manually. Targeted manual impulse treatment (C 1/C 2 from the left with counter-support of the occiput (al).) In the course of the next 12 months, the first clear improvement in posture and motor responses, confirmed by colleagues collaborating in the treatment.

The second treatment was after four months. The parents reported that the child had literally made a great leap forward after each treatment.

Later reports from the parents and treating doctors confirmed unanimously that both motor responses and the previously retarded mental and linguistic development were now proceeding normally, that the facial asymmetry was completely gone and that the accompanying therapeutic gymnastics could be stopped after the second treatment.

Summary: Congenital torticollis with increasing asymmetry of the face and skull, disturbed postural and kinesiological development, disturbed mental and especially linguistic development; ongoing therapeutic gymnastics without significant improvement. Normalization in every respect after two impulse (thrust) treatment, including the asymmetry in face and skull.

R.R., 1½-year-old male child, normal birth

Early recurring tonsillitis. Frequent enteritis. Conjunctivitis resistant to therapy.

The child was strikingly often afflicted with colds, sniffles, earaches, increasing disturbance of sleep.

The child seemed quite literally to be afraid of sleeping, and by implication, of the horizontal position.

He refused to go to bed and ran around until he occasionally collapsed with fatigue.

At the age of $1^1/_2$ during another cold, the first cerebral spasm, which then was repeated several times. Since this time, especially restless sleep.

The child could not maintain a sleeping position for long, woke up screaming at night. His neck could not be touched without strong resistance from the child as well as painful cries.

As an infant, he had fallen several times from the diaper table. Fourteen days before the first spasm, he had fallen on the back of his head from a height of 1.5 meters (approximately five feet).

Manual and x-ray information: Extended HWS with kyphosis between C 2 and C 3. Blockage of the Atlas in the ventral flexion position and right-side dislocation.

First manual impulse treatment of the Atlas. Immediately thereafter the child spontaneously asked to be put to bed. He slept for the first time completely calm until the next morning.

His previously disturbed appetite became completely normal.

It was apparent that the child could now walk more surefootedly and did not fall as much as before, even though this problem had earlier been considered unchangeable.

The inflammation of the connecting membrane vanished completely.

Another fall on his head three months later, this time from a baby carriage. Two weeks later nausea and another spasm when turned over on the left side. In the pediatric clinic, a diagnosis of fever induced seizures was made.

Four weeks later, renewed impulse treatment of the Atlas, thereafter three spasms. After that normal development.

Fourteen months later during childish rough-housing, during which the head was held far back for a rather long time, the child that evening briefly lost consciousness, vomited, and experienced a seizure.

After treatment of the Atlas, three days later, undisturbed development.

Summary: Recurrent rhinitis, bronchitis, tonsillitis, enteritis, persistent conjunctivitis, instance of antalgue. Restless sleep with crying out at night, unmotivated central seizures, cerebral spasms, disturbed motor responses with frequent falls, and disturbance of the appetite and overall ability to thrive.

7-month-old male infant, normal birth

Asymmetric development of the skull since the eighth week of life, also, to an increasing degree, of the face. The child always lies on the right side only despite all efforts to put it to sleep in a different position or to move it to a different position while it is asleep. Orthopedic suspicion of incipient scoliosis and dysphasia of the hip joint. Maintenance in a plaster cast planned but rejected by parents.

Findings: On the right side, clearly flattened skull, clearcut asymmetry of the face, asymmetrically developed thigh flexures, distortion of the ilio-sacral joint.

Manually: Blockage of the Atlas.

X-ray: Right dislocational position.

After manual impulse treatment with the agreement of the treating orthopedist, immediate disappearance of ilio-sacral joint distortion. Three days later, the report of the overjoyed mother that the child is now sleeping completely restfully, moreover, in any and all positions. At the time of the next visit three weeks later, symmetrically developed thigh flexures.

Two months after the first treatment, the second atlantal manipulation takes place.

No further developmental problems. The skull becomes more and more symmetrical. Facial asymmetry no longer noticeable.

Summary: One-sided compulsive sleep position, increasing asymmetry of the skull and face, infantile scoliosis, hip dysphasia, distortion of the ilio-sacral joint.

These few case studies are presented from more than 1,000 small patients treated successfully, almost without exception.

Symptoms and Pathogenesis of the Clinical Picture

The clinical picture presents three characteristic groups of symptoms:

1. Disturbance of motor responses, both in postural-tonic and kinesiological-phasic portion.
2. A brain-stem component net central disturbance of negative regulatory systems.
3. Inclination to infections in the throat, nose, and ear region.

1. Disturbance of Motor Responses

According to Votja, disturbed postural activity is the common term of every pathological motor response development.

Now the central motor responses develop first and foremost from reflectoristic motor events. The tonic neck reflexes play a determining role in this process, both positively and negatively. If they are undisturbed, the transition to centrally directed motor activity takes place from the sixth to eighth month without a problem.

If they are disturbed—most often by functional damage in the atlanto-occipital joint—a one sided over- or under-valued reflexive response dominates and frustrates (and diminishes) the encephalization of motor responses.

Gesell (13), Bobath (1), Votja (43) have observed, as did Buchmann (4,5), that reflexive control in the case of primary cerebral damage maintains dominance over tonic neck reflexes and frustrates the building of central motor control, so that "certain head positions and movements force characteristic positions of the extremities in such children." (4)

The central nervous system has a deficient adaptibility to the changes in the position of the head and the body position. The spinal level of coordination comes under the influence of pathologic differences (stimuli?) led into the central nervous system or those which are normal but are processed in a pathological manner.

On the other hand, a disturbance of function fed pathologically from the periphery of the atlanto-occipital joint in a reflexive way can cause in secondary fashion a condition in the central area which can hardly be distinguished from a primary centrogenic disturbance, and may even exceed the effect of an originally central disturbance.

For the sake of differential diagnosis, the manual test treatment of the atlanto-occipital joint is decisive. These disturbances take place in the brain-stem within the reticular structure.

2. Brain Stem Component

The most frequent symptoms of this motor response brain-stem component are: Torticollis with one-sided compulsive position, with increasingly asymmetry of the skull. Delayed postural developed and upright position, disturbed and asymmetrical kinesiological motor response, infantile scoliosis, functional impairment of the hip joints, low to high grade hip dysplasia, ilio-sacral distortions, also so-called growing pains.

The vegetative brain-stem component in the clinical picture of this syndrome is therefore more self-evident than unexpected, for it is in the reticular apparatus as "the most important subcortical association mechanism" (32) that the capability for responses of all systems is directed; it is here that a surplus of pathological afferents finally released undirected and overshooting reactions. The direct neural connection between the atlanto-occipital joint(s) and the brain-stem region originally hypothetically postulated by us in 1953 has since then been frequently confirmed by experiments, thus the connection to the vestibular and abducent core region, especially the reticular formation (7,10,21,22,24,29,38).

Table 1. Relational disturbances of the head joints in the x-ray picture and manually diagnosed blockages. 1. Healthy persons (180). 2. Children with C.D.S. syndrome (100). 3. Infants with C.D.S. syndrome (75).

	No.	C 1 lateral-isation	C 1-Rot.	C 2-Rot.	Blocked Nerves
1. Healthy adults without problems	45	6 13%	0	15 33%	0
Fleeting problems	38	15 40%	4 11%	16 42%	0
Treated problems	97	32 33%	48 49%	54 55%	C 0/C 1 or C 0/C 1 and C 1/C 2 combination
2. Sick children (C.D.S.)	100	88 88%	23 23%	54 54%	fast 100% C 0/C 1
3. Infants (C.D.S.)	75	75	0	0	

The incomplete degree of maturity of the child's central nervous system with its sensitive plasticity explains the occasionally massive, at first sight unsystematic vegetative brain stem symptoms: Overall poor thriving, absence of appetite, circulatory disturbances, as well as those of digestion and equilibrium, nausea and vomiting, swift exhaustibility, restlessness to the point of psycho-motor attacks, disturbance of concentration initiative and the ability to learn, delayed and slow speech, inexplicable fever paroxysms, cerebral spasms and, in the age of articulation, head and neck aches.

3. The Susceptibility to Infection in the Throat, Nose, Ear and Bronchial Region

The inclination to recurrent otitis, tonsillitis, sinusitis, lasting rhinitis and recurrent bronchitis.

Lewit (27) found among primarily youthful patients with chronic tonsillitis that 92 percent had an atlanto-occipital joint blockage, primarily between the occiput (al) and the Atlas. These blockages may be triggered by the first case of tonsillitis, maintain, however, their own inclination to recur. After the removal of the blockage, recurrence is absent. (Lewit-the same observations by us.)

Mohn has reported to us that no tonsillectomy was needed after the systematically administered treatment of functional atlanto-occipital joint disturbances.

Diagnosis

The diagnosis results from:

Anamnesia: mechanism of delivery, birth trauma, early childhood trauma, typical postural, kinesiological post-natal development (especially torticollis).

Clincial Picture with many vegetative variants.

Manual Diagnostic:

X-ray Evaluations according to our criteria.

Last but not least, *the first test treatment.*

Anamnesia

Birth trauma, early childhood trauma. Birth trauma in the narrower sense is less frequent than originally assumed by us. Vacuum extraction does not seem unproblematic, likewise a much later administered intervention (c-section) after the little head has been lodged in the pelvic entrance, possibly in an extreme position. Post-natal investigations, especially computertomographics ones, have shaken the view that normal birth is a problem-free event. In the majority of newborn children, microparenchymic injuries of the brain-segments near the ventricle have been found. Other investigators more often confirmed a distortion of the head-neck connection (6, 11, 25, 28, 35, 44).

Post-natal Developmental Disturbances of the Motor System

Torticollis, disturbance of the typical position reflexes, especially in the modifications, according to Votja (43) and Rubis (35).

Clinical Picture

The clinical picture with many variants, including functional, i.e. secondary morphological deformations of the skeleton.

Manual Diagnosis

A. Massive pain and flight reactions during palpation, almost exclusively of the Atlas cross continuations, mostly differentiated sideways.

B. Muscular fixation and blockage in the area of the A-O head joints among infants and small children exclusively between the occiput and the Atlas. With young infants (our youngest patients were four weeks old) it is almost impossible to confirm a blockage. We have observed cases without any blockage in which only an x-ray confirmed relational disturbance between occiput and Atlas was present.

Table 2. Categories of At-Risk Children

1. Primary Children At Risk—Primary immediate cerebral damage pre-, con- and post-natal.
2. Secondary Children At Risk—Indirect reflexogenic brain stem disturbance during pre-, con- or post-natal traumatization of atlanto-occipital joints with persistent disturbances of relation and coordination.

X-ray Findings

X-ray finding of course produced only with our analytical functional recording technique along with evaluation on two standard levels, is for us less important for diagnosis than for the selection of the manual technique regarding point of contact and the direction of impulse. It is an absolute requirement.

Carrying out the x-ray examination is not very simple and demands a good deal of patience, experience and collaboration between parents, assistant, and occasionally the personal cooperating doctor.

Therapy

The therapy based exclusively on the x-ray findings, providing that there is no contraindication. It consists of a directed manual impulse application at the cross continuation of the Atlas in reclining position with the head fixed in place. The younger the child is, the gentler our impulse. We are again and again astonished at how even the lightest tap with the index finger gradually and uninterruptedly often, however suddenly, returns the condition to normal. (cf. Tables 3 & 4)

Exercises have proven themselves to be outstanding according to Votja (induced reflex creeping and reflex turning around).

The effect improves dramatically, however, when existing A-O joint disturbances are removed manually (4,5). This has been confirmed time and time again by our collaborating orthopedic colleagues Knopke and Hamm.

With cerebral spasms parents must be advised, however, that after the treatment a transient, crisis-like worsening may result. The family doctor or pediatrician should be informed of this. We cannot say anything about the frequency of this syndrome. It would have to be determined through field studies in pediatric and orthopedic practices. The syndrome is, however, assuredly much more frequent than could even have been suspected by us up to now. According to Mohr (30), based on reports from Borsche (3), only about 14% to 20% of all children are in a state of vegetative equilibrium.

Table 3. Treatment effect of manual Atlas treatment of a group of 29 children with C.D.S. syndrome with professional orthopedic pre- and post-examination. Average age 3.2 months (0.5 to 8 months).

Mode of Birth	
Vacuum extraction	5
Pelvic end positions	3
Section (C)	2
Premature	3
Twin Birth	1
Skeletal Disturbances	
Skull Asymmetry	13
Hip dysplasm	10
"C" Scoliosis	24
"S" Scoliosis	4
Head Position	
Torticollis	29
Kinesiological Disturbances	12

After one-time treatment of the Atlas with orthopedic post-examination on average after 6.3 months.

Results: In 16 children a complete normalization, in eight children far-reaching normalization of HWS and head mobility. The previously present skull asymmetrics were completely or almost completely removed in all children that were accessible to a lengthy observation.

There is a strong suspicion that among the 80% disturbed children there are many with the Atlas blockage syndrome. According to Frymann (11), there were among 1,250 infants chosen non-selectively examination five days post-partum, 211 suffered from nervousness, vomitting, muscular hypertonus to opistotonus, tremors, and insomnia.

During the manual examination of the skull, an increased strain was found in 95 percent of this group. If this strain was removed, an immediate calming often resulted, the crying stopped, the musculature relaxed, the children fell asleep.

Chagnon and Blery (6) emphasize that occipito-cervical lesions in children are still underestimated, least of all because of diagnostic inadequacies.

Seifert (35) found among 1,093 newborns, 298 children with a-o blockages significantly connected with the development of a "C- scoliosis."

We were able to do comparative investigations between healthy adults, those with mild and more severe vertebral disturbances and children with C.D.S. syndrome; equally large groups were involved (cf Table 3).

In keeping with this, C.D.S. syndrome in infants and small children is essentially an Atlas blockage syndrome.

Table 4.

Mode of Birth	
Twins	1
Naval Twisting	1
Section	4
Vacuum	2
Pelvic End Position	1
Skeletal Disturbances	
Skull Asymmetry	13
Hip Dysplasis	10
"C" Scoliosis	24
Left Side	21
Right Side	3
Kinesiological Disturbances	12
Head Position	
Torticollis	33
Number of Treatments	
Once	30
Twice with full success	1
Twice with partial success	1

Summary and Conclusion

We must identify two groups of children at risk (Table 2) according to today's state of knowledge: a. The primary, immediate cerebral damage with disturbed vegetative-postural reactability, either on the basis of a pre- or congenital trauma or through post-natal damage to the central nervous system: primary group of children at risk. Here parental, inter-cranial bleeding with periventricular parenchymic injuries play a role previously underestimated in its proportions. [CT examinations by Ludwig, et al (28)].

b. The secondary, indirect reflexcogenic disturbances of the brain-stem as a result of congenital or post-natal traumatization of head joints with lasting disturbance of relations and coordination: secondary children at-risk.

Conclusions for practice

Surveillance of infants should involve the observations of motor development and the manual control of a-o joints. This should be obligatory in difficult births, especially with congenital torticollis.

With developmental disturbances of every kind the atlanto-occipital joints should be examined and in each case be treated manually in a qualified manner. The success of this treatment eclipses every other attempt at treatment, including especially the use of medications and demands the directed reflex therapy in a decisive way according to Vojta (cf Table 3).

In the interim, we have been able to examine a further group of 33 children together with our colleague Mr. Knopke and treat them.

The average age was 3.06 months (3 weeks to 14 months). With increasing experience the children are given manual treatment earlier. The prospects are thus significantly improved and the costs of treatments are substantially reduced.

REFERENCES (Chapter XIV)

1. Bobath K. Bobath B (1955) Tonic reflexes and righting reflexing in the diagnosis and assessment of cerebral palsy. *Cereb Palsy Rev* 16:410
2. Bobath K. Bobath B (1956) The diagnosis of cerebral palsy in infancy. *Arch Dis Child* 31:4084
3. Borsche A (1970/76) Vegetative Regulationsstorungen im Kindesalter. Hess Arzteblatt 2 und ZAM 1976 (Zit n Mohr)
4. Buchmann J (1979) Motorische Entwicklung und Wirbelsaulenfunktionsstorungen, Bd 6. Congr FIMM *(Baden-Baden)

5. Buchmann J (1980) Motorische Entwicklung und Wirbelsaulenfunktionsstorungen. Maschinenschriftliches Manuskript
6. Chagnon S. Blery M (1982) Entroses et luxations du rachis cervical chez l'enfant. *J Radiol* 63:465-470
7. Choen LS.(1961) Role of eye and neck proprioceptive mechanisms in body orientation and motor coordination. *J Neurophysiol* 24:1-11
8. Ewerbeck H. Friedberg V (1965) Die Ubergangssitorungen des Neugeborenen und die Bekampfund der perinatalen Mortalitat. Thieme, Stuttgart
9. Flehmig J (1979) Normale Entwicklung des Sauglings und ihre Abweichungen. Thieme, Stuttgart
10. Fredrickson JM, Schwarz D, Kornhuber H H (1966) Convergence and interaction of vestibular and deep somatic afferents upon neurons in the vestibular nuclei of cats. *Acta Otolaryngol* 61:168-188
11. Frymann V (1966) Relation of disturbances of cranio-sacral mechanisms to symptomatology of the newborn. *JAOA* 65:1059
12. Gesell A (1945) *The embryology of behavior.* Harper and Row, New York
13. Gesell A (1954) The ontogenesis of infant behavior. IN: Carmichael (ed) *Manual child psychol.* Wiley & Sons, New York
14. Gesell A, Ames L B (1960) Tonic neck reflex and symmetro-tonic behaviour. *J Paediatr* 36:165-176
15. Grau H (1978) Analysis of cerebral defective states acquired in early life. *Neuroradiology* 16
16. Gutmann G (1953) Die obere HWS im Krankheitsgeschehen. *Neuralmedizin* 1
17. Gutmann G (1968) Das cervical-diencehalstatische Syndrom des Kleinkindes. *Manuelle Medizin* 6:112-119
18. Gutmann G, Biedermann H (1984) Die Halswirbelsaule. Allgemeine funktionelle Pathologie und klinische Syndrome. Fischer, Stuttgart New York
19. Haller U, Wille L (1983) Diagnostik intracranieller Blutungen bei Neugeborenen Springer. Berlin Heidelberg New York
20. Hikosaka O, Maeda M (1973) Cervical effects on abducens motoneurons and their interaction with vestibulo-ocular reflex. *Exp Brain Res* 18:512-530
21. Hulse M (1980) Die cervicale Gleichgewichtsstorung. Habilitationsschrift, Mannheim
22. Hulse M (1980) Differential diagnostic criteria for distinguishing proprioceptive cervical nystagmus from a vascular cervical one. *HNO* 28:390
23. Hulse M (1983) Die zervikalen Gleichgewichtsstorungen. Springer, Berlin Heidelberg New York
24. Kornhuber H H, Frederickson J M (1970) Gegenwartige klinische und experimentelle Ergebrisse der vestibularen and oculomotori schen Mechanismen. *Int J Neurol* 23
25. Kurrek H (1982) Die mikrozirkuatorische Belastung des menschilichen Gehirns bei der Geburt. Vortrag Phys Inst Univ Munster
26. Lewit K (1976) Kopfgelenkblockierungen und chronische Tonsillitis. *Manuelle Medizin* 14:106-109
27. Lewit K (1977) Manuelle Medizin im Rahmen der medizinischen Rehabilitation. Urban & Schwarzenberg. Munchen
28. Ludwig B, Brand M, Brockerhoff P (1980) Post partum CT- examinations

of the heads of full-term infants. *Neuroradiology* 20:145-54
29. Maeda M (1970) Neck influences on the vestibulo-ocular reflex arc and the vestibulocerebellum. *Progr Brain Res* 50:551- 559.
30. Mohr U (1977/79) Kopfgelenkblockierungen beim Keinking (cervical-diencephal-statistches Syndrom nach Gutmann). *Manuelle Medizin* 15:45 und in: Neumann HD, Wolff HD (Hrsg) Theoretische Fortschritte und praktische Erfahrungen der Manuellen Medizin. Kondordia, Buhl
31. Monnier M (1963) Vegetatives nervensystem, Bd 1 und 2. Hippokrates, Stuggart
32. Monnier M (1963) Vegetatives Nervensystem. Physiologie und Pathophysiologie, Bd 1a und 23. Hippokrates, Stuttgart
33. Muller D (1973) Die subakuten Massenverschiebungen des Gehirns unter der Geburt. VEB Thieme, Leipzig
34. Muller-Kuppers M (1969) Das leicht hirngeschadigte Kind. Hippocrates, Stuttgart
35. Seifert J (1975) Die Kopfgelenksblockierung des Neugeborenen. In: Lewit K, Gutmann G (Hrsg) Rehabilitacia, Bd 8. Prague, Bratislawa, S 53
36. Saling E (1979) Geburts- und Perinatalmedizin. *Dtsch Arzteblatt* 42
37. Schwartz P (1964) Geburtsschaden bei Neugeborenen. Fischer, Jena
38. Stejskal L (1972) Postural reflexes in theory and Moto-Reeducation Rada Matemat a Picronich *Ved Rocnik* 82:6-104
39. Stejskal L (1974) Funktionelle Pathologie des Bewegungssystems, Bd 4. Cong FIMM (Prag)
40. Stejskal L (1975) Five suggestions for manipulative treatment based upon a study of postural reflexes. *Rehabilitcia* 8:10-171
41. Vojta V (1965) Die Fruhdiagnostik des spastischen infantilen Syndroms. *Beitr Orthop Traumatol* 12:543-545
42. Vojta V (1968) Feflexkriechen und seine Bedeutung fur kraken-gymnastische Fruhbehandlung. *Z Kinderheilkd* 104
43. Vojta V (1974) Die cerebralen Bewegungsstorungen im Sauglingsalter. Fruhdiagnose und Fruhtherapie. Enke, Stuttgard
44. Yatres P O (1962) Perinatal injury to the neck and extracranial cerebral arteries. In: Jacob H (ed) *Int Congr Neuropathol*, vol 4. Thieme, Stuttgart

AUTHOR'S COMMENTS

How long must these truths be hidden? Hidden by the scientific pomposity of allopathic arrogance and their dominate paradigm of disease treatment therapeutics, rather than cause detection and correction. How long yet will the "cause within" be ignored by the collective majority of the health care community?

Dr. Gutmann reported on his findings first in 1953, next in 1968, then in 1984 and this report came out in 1987. He has repeatedly reported that bacterial infections of youth can be caused by vertebral subluxations. That musculoskeletal problems such as torticollis and scoliosis can be caused by subluxations and that adjustic correction of same resolves the problems. He describes the articular fixation between occiput and Atlas so clearly demonstrated by Dr. Gonstead and reported in Dr. Douglas Cox's paper reproduced in this text. Dr. Gutmann speaks to the necessity for specificity in the adjustment, and the need for cervical x-ray analysis in children; he mentions the seizures that children have when they have sustained atlanto occipital axial subluxations. The very first patient that I cared for in practice was an epileptic boy that responded beautifully to chiropractic care, and throughout my many years of practice I have seen many cases of epilepsy resolved chiropractically.

Gray's Anatomy mentions the synovial membranes of the odontoid, atlanto articulations. They exist between the odontoid and transverse ligament and the odontoid and the fovea dentis of the anterior arch of Atlas. In dealing with atlanto-axial-occipital subluxations chiropractors achieve excellent results in reducing the symptoms of the so-called occipital headache. This excruciating form of cranial headache can be so severe that at times it can cause loss of consciousness, or the so-called 'blacking out'; occipital headache is also common in rheumatoid arthritis. Should the Atlas Axis subluxations disrelationship become such that the odontoid articulations malposition is dramatic enough to stress its synovial membranes, then the resultant edema in this area could cause a reduction in size of the neural canal in the area of the medulla oblongata. Such encroachment in this area could result in pressure directly upon the meninges and medulla oblongata causing the symptoms afore mentioned. The complexities of the occipital-atlanto-axial articulations and their synovial membranes have not been completely investigated chiropractically. It is possible that soft tissue encroachment (due to edema produced by the stress of the malposition of the subluxation) is the major cause of neural canal encroachment in the upper cervical subluxation. Medical surgery[42], "Complete Odontoid Resectomy," has revealed that a swollen mass of articular tissue surrounding the odontoid can press directly upon the medulla oblongata.[42] Chiropractic's precise vertebral position analysis can point out the vertebral subluxation that causes this capsular swelling. The swelling of these tissues, encroaching upon the neural canal could produce the neurological symptoms so effectively reduced by chiropractic adjustment. One has only to relate to the many cases of epilepsy that have been corrected under chiropractic care as an example. As stated before, I personally have had considerable successful results in the management of epileptic children with chiropractic adjustic technics.

THE ATLANTO-ODONTIOD ARTICULATION (From Above Down)

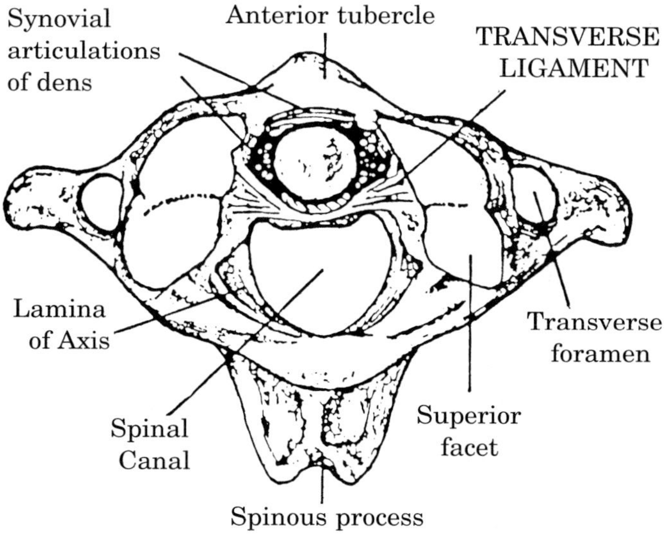

(Ill. XIV-6) On this illustration, taken from CLINICAL BIOMECHANICS[19], by R. C. Schafer D.C., you can see how swelling of the synovial membranes that surround the odontoid would cause a protrusion of the transverse ligament and encroachment upon the spinal canal.

A rotational subluxation between the Atlas and Axis vertebrae certainly, in and of itself, compromises the shape of the neural-canal. Add to that the swollen capsular membranes around the odontoid due to the subluxation and the dimensions of the neuro-canal are most certainly compromised.

Now I have spoken about the atlanto axial occipital subluxations throughout this text. The papers quoted and authors quoted, have addressed this important area of the spinal column. But, what about the subluxations below Axis? Just what are the foraminal encroachment factors that exist throughout the spine when it becomes subluxated? (Ill. XIV-7, below)

In 1994 Dr. Sid Williams* asked me to deliver an address in Recife, Brazil, to the WHO Workshop on "Low Back Pain." The paper I wrote for this conference was published in The Chiropractic Research Journal, CRJ, Vol. 3, #2, 1996.[43] CRJ is the research periodical of Life University and School of Chiropractic. It is with their kind permission that I reprint my entire paper. The foraminal encroachment factors that exist in spinal subluxations, and particularly in disc block subluxation, (Ill. XIV-7) are complex. This paper addressed these factors in the lumbar spine. The author contends that subluxations throughout the entire spine essentially involve the same physiological mechanisms in respect to neurological impairment.

DISC BLOCK SUBLUXATION, L 4

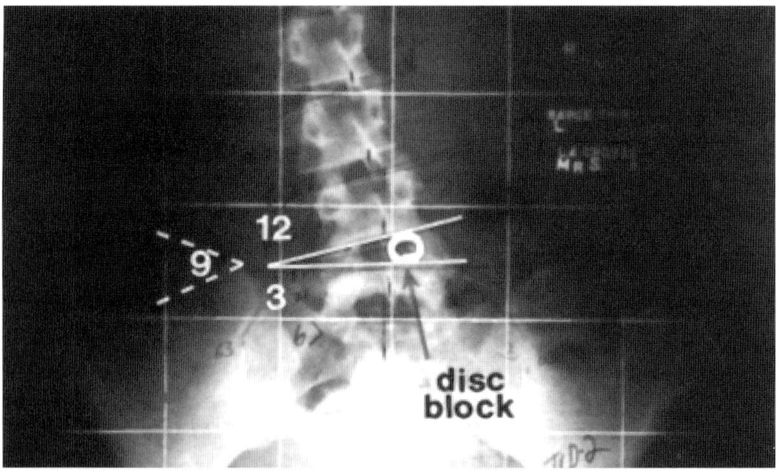

(Ill. XIV-7) The author holds that the disc block subluxation of Torticollis and Tortipelvis are essentially the same.

* President, Life University, Marietta, Georgia.

The Chiropractic Vertebral Subluxation and its Relationship to Vertebrogenic Lumbar Pain, Cruralgia and Sciatic Syndromes[43]

Fredrick H. E. Barge, D.C., Ph.C.

Editor's Note: The following is the text of a presentation delivered by Dr. Barge at a World Health Organization workshop entitled: "WHO - Education on Low Back Pain." The WHO workshop was one part of the Panamerican League Against Rheumatism (PAN-LAR) conference held in Recife, Brazil, on September 19, 1994.

Abstract

The identity of a singular vertebral subluxation, termed the disc block subluxation, has been established by the author. Its identity and analysis is taught in leading chiropractic colleges in the U.S.A. This subluxation is associated with cruralgia and the sciatic syndromes often termed sciatic rheumatism. Facet separation, swollen articular membranes, narrowing and lowering of the height of the foramen, biochemical products of inflammation, and turgidity within the foramen are all involved in the neuroforaminal encroachment factors of the disc block subluxation; these factors result in the symptoms of backache and differing types of radiculalgia associated with cruralgia and sciatic syndromes. This paper will explore the mechanical misalignment and neuroforaminal encroachment factors inherent in this subluxation.

Introduction

Pain syndromes associated with lumbar nerve root encroachment referred to as cruralgia, radiculalgia, sciatica, sciatic rheumatism, etc., have commonly responded rewardingly to chiropractic vertebral adjustment. Chiropractic science holds that biomechanical aspects of the vertebral subluxation complex result in nerve root encroachment and are often responsible for the aforementioned pain syndromes.

In the vertebral subluxation, the structural alignment of the vertebral articular surfaces are altered such that the zygapophyseal joints lose their juxtaposition, altering the contours of the intervertebral foraminal margins. Such articular misalignment is termed subluxation by chiropractors; chiropractic science contends that nerve root encroachment is involved in all such vertebral subluxations. The traditional chiropractic definition of the vertebral subluxation has always held forth a neuronal disturbance. Except for this factor, the definition varies little from that of White and Panjabi (1):

> A subluxation may be defined as a partial dislocation. It is any pathological situation in which there is not a normal physiological juxtaposition of the articular surfaces of a joint. Such situations should be reliably demonstrable radiographically.

The Chiropractic Definition of Subluxation, according to Stephenson (2).

> A subluxation is the condition of a vertebra that has lost its proper juxtaposition with the one above or the one below, or both; to an extent less than a luxation; which impinges nerves and interferes with the transmission of mental impulses.

The art of palpation of the vertebral articulations and processes has been a significant part of the art of chiropractic since its inception. Palpation of the facet joints in the lumbar spine elicits pain from the subluxated facet; often too, a trigger point of pain can be found on the lateral side of the multifidus spinae musculature adjacent to the disturbed facet. Palpation of the subluxated facet will often times not only elicit pain at the point of palpation but telegraph pain into the affected limb. Fenesson in his book *Low Back Pain* (3) describes this phenomenon thus:

> A clinical finding associated with facet dysfunction is acute tenderness to pressure over the affected facet. Sometimes this pressure will not only reproduce pain within the back but also aggravate extension of the pain into a lower extremity. It is further speculated that the facet dysfunction may occur from derangement and instability of the facet joint, resulting from overriding secondary to a collapsed degenerated intervertebral disc.

Notice how Fenesson describes the facet misalignment (subluxation) as an "overriding secondary to a collapsed degenerative intervertebral disc." When a disc collapses to one side it produces a lateral disc wedge between the vertebrae and lowers the foraminal height on the closed side of the disc wedge. This causes overriding of the facets on the same side (Fig. 1). Ruth Jackson, M.D. also refers to the facet overriding in like subluxations of the cervical spine (4).

Sir Sidney Sunderland in his book, *Nerve and Nerve Injuries* (5), describes this disc lesion subluxation in like manner:

> Narrowing of the lumbar intervertebral distance, whatever the cause, results in the subluxation of the apophyseal joints in which the facet of the vertebra above is displaced inferiorly across the surface of the facet of the vertebra below (Fig. 1). As a result of this displacement the medial branch of the lumbar dorsal ramus, which is fixed in this region is involved in two ways:
> 1. inflammatory swelling of the joint reduces the lumen of the tunnel containing the neurovascular bundle (Fig. 2);
> 2. the inferior articular pedicle comes to press directly on the nerve.

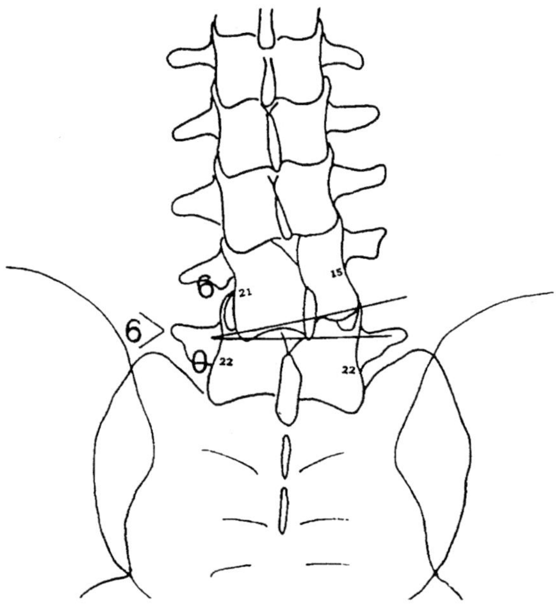

(Figure 1) The sketch illustrates the "disc block subluxation." As viewed from the posterior, the disc between L 4 & L 5 has collapsed on the left and bulged to the right, creating a disc wedge. The facet of 4th lumbar overrides the facet of 5th lumbar, lowering the height of the intervertebral foramina on the closed side of the disc wedge. A left rotatory scoliosis has formed above the 4th lumbar compensating for the inferiority created by the subluxation.

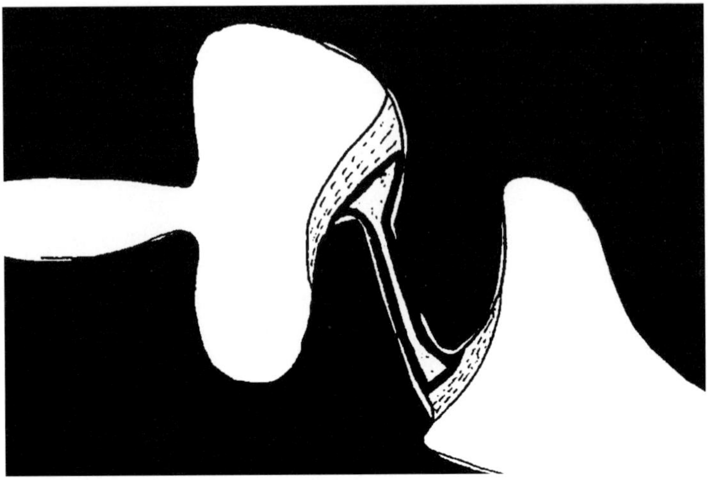

FIBROUS CAPSULAR LIGAMENT

(Figure 2) The capsular ligament is illustrated in the schematic sketch of the facet joint and the intervertebral foramen. It forms the major portion of the posterior foraminal wall. Swelling of this ligament encroaches upon the intraforaminal space.

From the last two quotes and others it can be seen that medical authorities today tend to agree on the biomechanical aspects of the vertebral subluxation complex. Since 1962, I have written extensively on the vertebral subluxation related to low back and leg pain syndromes. My text *Tortipelvis* (16) published in 1976 is devoted to this subject and is used as a curricular text in leading chiropractic colleges. I now draw from this text to describe this vertebra subluxation.

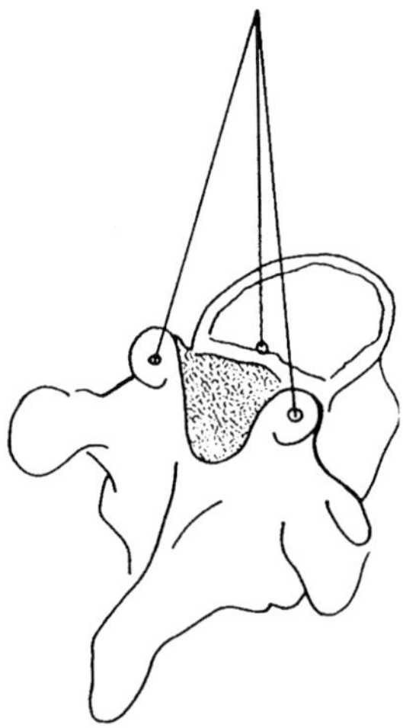

(Figure 3) The "Tripod Theory" of weight bearing in the lordotic regions of the spine has been propounded by the author. (15,16)

The spine in its development, normally establishes a significant lumbar lordotic curve. The sheer force of the erect upright stance and the actual weight of the upper body is born by the lumbar facets and the posterior aspect of the lumbar vertebral bodies (15,16) (Fig. 3). Farfan made this observation (6):

> Because in man there is a permanent lordosis, the lower lumbar joints are always subjected to a shearing force even in the relaxed upright stance. For this reason the apophyseal joints of the lower two or three segments have developed a reorientation which supports the shear when the posterior ligamentous system is relaxed.

The discs in the lordotic spine bear little weight (Fig. 4), they function mainly to prevent excessive flexion and give shape and stability to the lumbar spine. When the lumbar curve becomes flattened (kyphosis) (Fig. 5), the discs then bear an increased load and essentially become shock absorbers, a function they were not intended to bear. Normally, the shock absorber of the human lumbar spine is the lumbar lordotic curve itself. This curve absorbs the stress of compression by its leaf spring-like configuration. Thus gravitational forces applied down against this curve actually increase the curve rather than putting increased pressure upon the discs (Fig. 4). In the kyphotic lumbar spine the discs are afforded no such protection; directly proportionate to the degree of lumbar kyphosis, they come to bear the burden placed upon them by the upright posture (Fig. 5). The weight carried upon the discs in the kyphotic lumbar spine, reduces the pressure of the shear force from the zygapophyses. As a result there is more laxity in the facet joint articulations making them prone to subluxation (Fig. 5). Actually, the entire sigmoid curve of the human spine has been purposely engineered biologically to act like a shock absorber. Cyriax (7) put it this way:

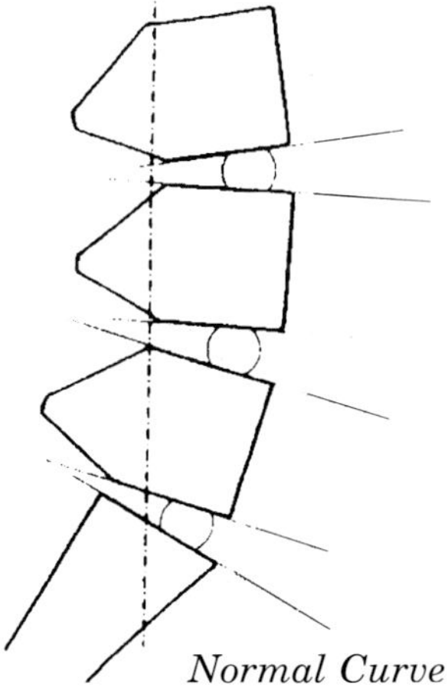

Normal Curve

(Figure 4) In the normal lordotic curve of the human lumbar spine the discs bear little weight. Gravitational force applied against the leaf spring configuration of this curve would tend to increase the curve, thus the curve itself is the shock absorber of the lumbar spine and not the discs.

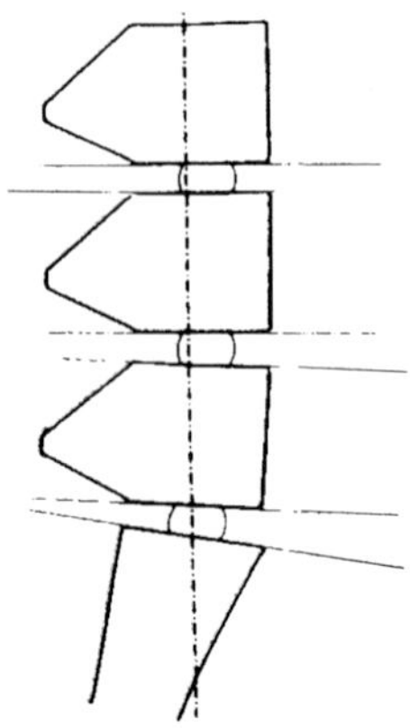

(Figure 5) The flattening of the normal lumbar lordotic curve (lumbar kyphosis) puts an increasing load upon the vertebral discs, a burden they are not intended to bear. The gravitational plumb line in the kyphotic lumbar spine comes down upon the discs not the facets. In consequence the normally high interfacet force is diminished, the joints become lax and prone to subluxation.

Abnormal Curve (Kyphosis)

The other advantage of the spinal curves is that they act as shock absorbers, a sudden vertical stress being in part converted into movement increasing the curves.

In patients with a flat spinal column, the intervertebral disc has no such protection, and it is noticeable that patients with a lumbar spine devoid of anterior convexity are more apt to suffer from backache than those with a normal degree of lordosis.

From these observations it can be seen that the development of a normal lumbar lordotic curve in children is an important factor in producing a spinal contour that is meant to provide protection for the vertebral joints and the discs. When this curve is absent the jolts, jars, and strains of every-day activities can cause a shift of a fragment of the nucleus pulposus to an unfavorable position. If the sequestered fragment moves laterally it may cause the superior vertebra to subluxate and incline to one side (disc wedge) causing overriding of the facet of the superior vertebra over its articular mate below on the same side (Fig. 1).

When the fragment of the nucleus shifts from its normal central position in the intervertebral space, it commonly causes the acute disc block subluxation of tortipelvis (16) and subsequently, the acute locked back described by Schmorl and Junghanns (11) (often erroneously referred to as the antalgic position).

In the acute phase of this subluxation, musculoskeletal symptoms predominate. Ernest Weitz, M.D. (17) puts this most succinctly when he states: "At the outset of symptoms, there is a remarkable absence of neurological signs in the presence of acute musculoskeletal findings."

In this case, the patient usually lists to one side (and/or forward) and presents with a severe lumbar backache. As the list is subsiding or is gone, the patient often begins to exhibit the symptoms and signs of radiculitis; again I return to the words of Dr. Weitz, (17): "Later on as the acute list subsides, radicular signs and symptoms appear."

It is apparent to this author that the subluxation must remain in its locked position for a goodly period of time to sufficiently insult the intervertebral foramen. Finally, the inflammatory process of the swollen capsular membranes narrow the already compromised intraforaminal space, impinge upon the nerve and elicit the symptoms of nerve root compression. If the subluxation corrects itself spontaneously there will be no radicular problems, but if the acute list subsides through the production of a scoliotic curve (as frequently happens) and the disc block subluxation remains unchanged, then the symptomatology addressed in this paper becomes apparent. The vertebral incline of the disc block subluxation initiates a rotational factor first succinctly described by H. B. Logan, D.C., who states that: "The body of a freely movable vertebra will rotate towards its low side". (8) This adds a rotational element to the subluxation so that one facet not only overrides the other but facet separation, or distraction, takes place resulting in what the author refers to as an "open facet."

As the body of the vertebra rotates towards its low side the spinous process moves in the opposite direction (Fig. 6). This rotation is limited due to the facet compression on the side of spinous process deviation. When the vertebra rotates beyond its physiologically permitted limits, the Axis of vertebral rotation changes from its central location in the posterior disc space or neural canal, to the compressed facet which acts like a pivot. Thus the contralateral facet separates (opens) causing injury to the capsular ligament. (Fig. 6) Ravichandran, quoting Farfan, pointed this out in a paper entitled *Spinous Process Deviation* (9):

> Deviation from the midline of the spinous process of a lumbar vertebra has long been regarded as a normal variation. Farfan pointed out that his deviation was associated with apophyseal injuries, leading to compression of the articular facet on the side of deviation, with distraction of the contralateral facet.

Typical Disc Block Subluxation 3rd Lumbar (A.P. View)

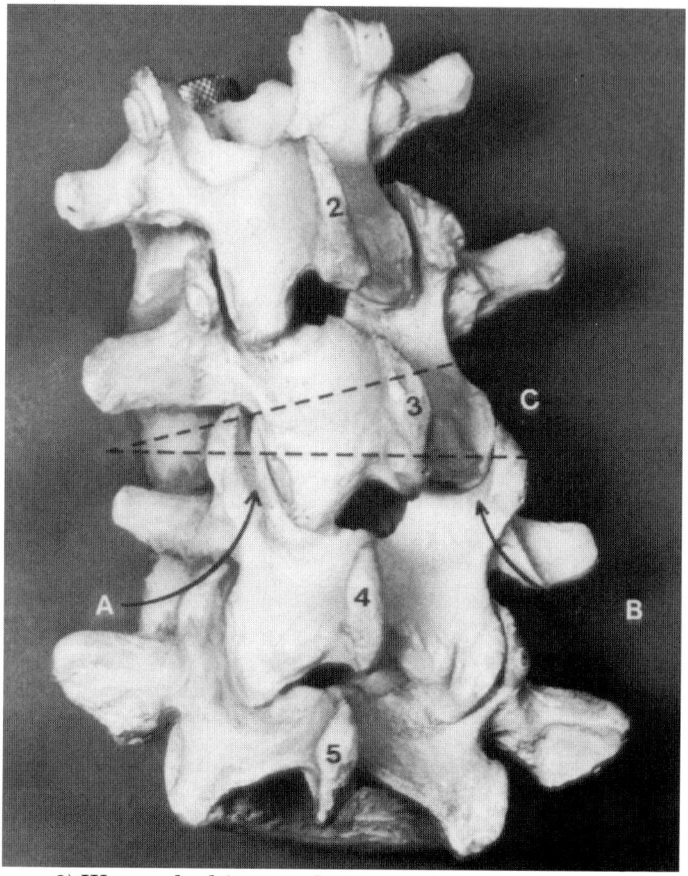

(Figure 6) We are looking at the posterior aspect of the lumbar spine L 2 through L 5. Responding to the inferiority created by the disc wedge between L 3 and L 4, the vertebral body of L 3 has rotated to the left. The body rotation of L 3 is away from the open side of the disc wedge (C) in relation to L 4. Facet (A) "opens" and its capsular ligament is palpably swollen and tender. Facet (B) is not "open," its surfaces are articulating one sliding up upon the other.

Kirkaldy-Willis also observed this occurrence on C.T. scan and he too, describes the facet separation as an "open facet" (10).

The combination of facet separation (open facet) and facet overriding compromises the normal dimension of the intervertebral foramen (Figures 7 & 8). Considering these factors let us now describe the aspects of neuroforaminal encroachment caused by the disc block subluxation. The term “disc block” is used by the author to describe the disc lesion involvement in this subluxation, as the sequestered portion of the disc “blocks” the vertebral subluxation from spontaneous correction (16). Schmorl and Junghanns have referred to this subluxation as a “vertebral locking” (11).

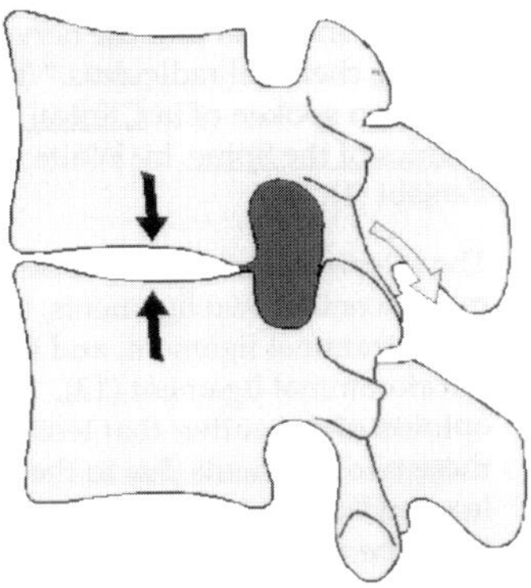

(Figure 7) The narrowing of the intervertebral space (black arrows) on the closed side of the disc wedge lowers the height of the foramen. This also results in overriding of the facets (white arrow).

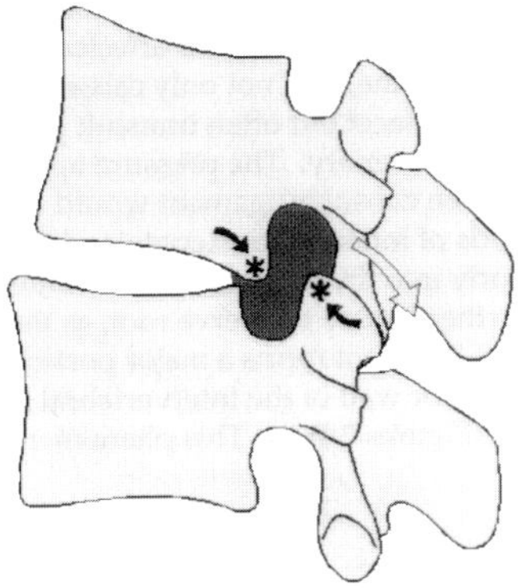

(Figure 8) The inferior articular pedicle (Sunderland) and the posterior inferior aspect of the vertebral body Logan (black arrows) approximate due to the lowering of the intervertebral distance and vertebral body rotation.

The causes of neuroforaminal encroachment:

1. The height of the foramen is lowered on the closed side of the disc wedge (Fig. 7).
2. The subsequent overriding of the facets brings the inferior articular pedicle into contact with the nerve, as observed by Sunderland (5) (Figs. 7 & 8).
3. Rotation of the vertebra to its inferior side approximates the inferior articular pedicle and the posterior inferior border of the body of the vertebra above, as observed by Logan (8) (Fig. 6).
4. Inflammatory swelling of the capsular ligament of the subluxated facet presses directly on the nerve as observed by Sunderland (5) (Fig. 9).
5. Biochemical products of inflammation irritate the

nerve, this has been recently verified by the work of Mituo Hasue, M.D. (12): "Inflammatogenic materials may leak from the degenerative disc and facet into the nerve root, causing chemical radiculitis." This has also been spoken of in *Clinical Biomehanics of the Spine,* by White and Panjabi (1).

6. The intervertebral foramina commonly contain two ligaments, the transforaminal ligament, and the intraforaminal ligament (13). It is the opinion of the author that tension on these two ligaments due to the subluxated "open" facet can cause turgidity in the foramen, and produce further insult to the neurovascular bundle by causing increased intraforaminal pressure.

These multiple factors cause the neuroforaminal encroachment of the lumbar vertebral subluxation complex that is involved in radiculalgia, cruralgia, and sciatic rheumatism syndromes. As Fenesson (3) pointed out, palpation of the affected facet (facet syndrome) will not only cause pain in the affected facet but often transmit pain into the lower extremity. The pressure applied to the swollen capsular ligament would extend the fluids of inflammation contained therein anteriorly into the intervertebral foramen and further irritate the nerve root, as the capsular ligament forms a major portion of the posterior wall of the intervertebral foramina (Figs. 2 & 9). This phenomenon has been termed the "door bell syndrome"—you press here, it rings there.

The author's hypothesis that turgidity is involved in the nerve root irritation would also explain the spontaneous relief often elicited when the vertebral segment is adjusted into an improved position. The relief of turgidity would certainly respond more rapidly than the inflammatory process and thus produce a degree of immediate relief.

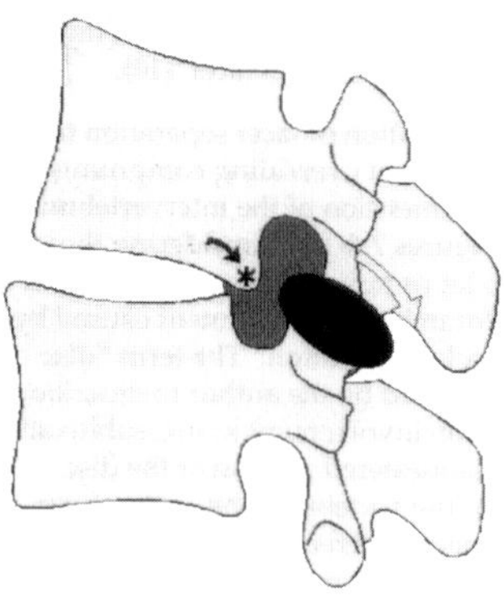

(Figure 9) The swollen articular membranes of the capsular ligament (black) further encroach upon the contents of the intraforaminal space.

X-Ray Analysis Of The Lumbar Subluxation

Subluxation in the lumbar spine exhibits three components: rotational misalignment, disc wedging and retropositioning. Methods have been developed to quantify the amount of subluxation by taking precise measurements from x-rays of the spine.

Rotational Misalignment

The rotational involvement of the lumbar vertebral subluxation was thoroughly analyzed by H. B. Logan, D.C. in the 1930s. On the A.P. radiograph, Logan would dot the junction of the lamina and the inferior tips of the lateral borders of the vertebral bodies. Measuring from the junction of the lamina to the inferior borders of the vertebral bodies, the wide side would be the side of vertebral body rotation (Fig. 10). Because the inferior tips of the vertebral bodies are often involved in pathology such as exostotic spurring, this author became dissatisfied with these points of reference and in 1959 began using the centers of the concavities of the lateral borders of the vertebral bodies (Fig. 11). The same procedure was reported by Russell in 1990 (14): "In the Bunnell method, the distance of the spinous process relative to the width of the body is used in a regression equation to calculate rotation."

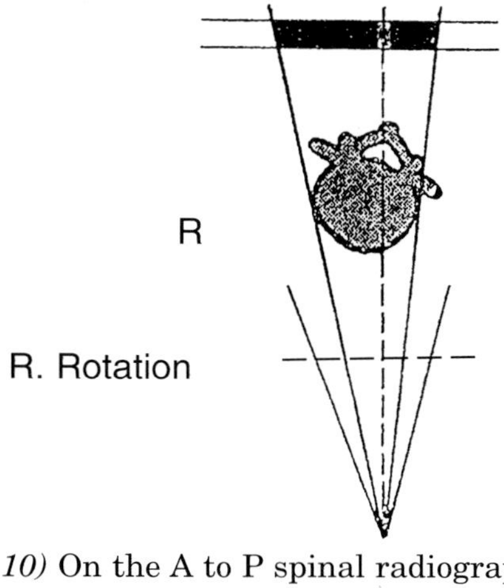

(Figure 10) On the A to P spinal radiograph, the x-ray's central ray projects a wider image of the vertebra on the side of vertebral body rotation. The schematic above illustrates right vertebral body rotation.

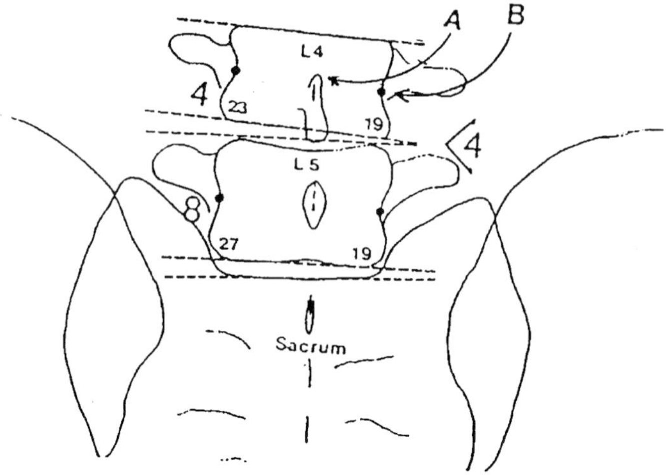

(Figure 11)

1. In the Barge method of determining vertebral rotation, the junction of the lamina (A) and the center of the concavities of the lateral vertebral body borders (B) are used as reference points to measure vertebral rotation.

2. Vertebral body wedge lines are used to determine intervertebral disc wedging as developed by C. S. Gonstead, D.C.

3. Logan held that when rotational differences between vertebral body rotations exceeded 3mm, foraminal encroachment occurred. On Figure 11, the rotational disparity between L 4 & L 5 would open the facet on the viewer's right, the foraminal encroachment would be on the same side.

Comparing four methods of determining vertebral rotation (14), the Bunnell method was found to be the most satisfactory. As Logan, Barge and Bunnell methods are quite similar, it can be seen that this method of determining vertebral rotation has become relatively well established in both the medical and chiropractic professions.

Disc Wedge

Dr. Clarence Gonstead, D.C., a graduate of The Palmer School of Chiropractic in 1923, developed what today is accepted throughout the chiropractic profession as an accurate method of determining the disc wedge involvement of the vertebral subluxation. Using a gliding parallel ruler, the inferior and superior body borders of the vertebrae are marked by drawing a line across them (Fig. 11). The ruler is glided up from one vertebra to the other (with vertebral body wedging taken into consideration) and disc wedging marked via plane lines across inferior and superior vertebral margins (Fig. 11).

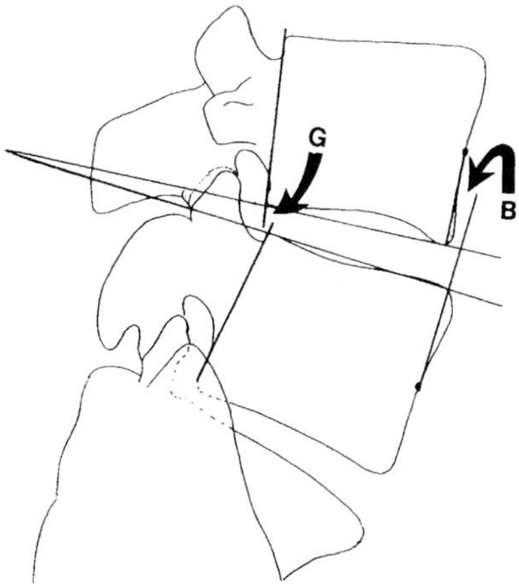

(Figure 12) George's (G) lines should cross or meet in the intervertebral space. In the Barge method (B) the space between the two lines drawn respectively perpendicular to the two body plane lines, should be approximately three millimeters. Utilizing these two guidelines retrolisthesis can be analyzed.

Retropositioning

Retropositioning of a lumbar vertebra can also add to the open facet factor of the vertebral subluxation. George's lines have long been used in this determination in the cervical and lumbar spine. In the George method (Fig. 12-G), the posterior body margins of the vertebra are delineated with a line drawn across each posterior vertebral body border. The lines should cross or meet in the intervertebral space, if they do not, a degree of retrolisthesis is denoted. The author also has developed an anterior guideline (Fig. 12-B). The centers of the concavities of the anterior vertebral body borders are marked. Utilizing plane lines drawn across the superior and inferior body borders of the vertebrae, a perpendicular line is dropped down from the center of the concavity of the superior vertebra to the inferior body plane line of the same vertebra. Then a line is drawn up from the inferior vertebra, perpendicular to its superior body plane line, up and through this superior plane line and the inferior plane line of the vertebra above. Where the line drawn up from the inferior vertebra intersects the inferior plane line of the superior vertebra a space is formed (Fig. 12-B). The author has found that if the disc wedge is within its normal range, this space should be approximately one to three mm. Utilizing this method, plus George's line, retropositioning can readily be measured.

Foraminal Encroachment Factor

Reducing the subluxation to numbers allows the calculation of the foraminal encroachment factor (FEF). This factor depends on the measurement of the factors of disc wedge, rotation and retropositioning. Giving a factor of one for every degree of disc wedge over three would numerically quantify the foraminal lowering inherent on the narrow side of the disc wedge. Let us say that beyond 3mm of rotation would be considered rotational encroachment (6). So if a lumbar vertebra differed in rotation from its articular mate by 5mm, that would be an FEF component of two (5mm-3mm). Suppose also that on the lateral film both George's and Barge's lines indicate a one millimeter retropositioning. The retropositioning factor would be added to the rotational and disc wedge components to produce a total foraminal encroachment fact or, FEF .

Radiographic Patient Placement

With the foregoing three methods of x-ray analysis employed, subluxations can be located, analyzed and quantified throughout the human spine. The correction and/or reduction of the subluxations can also be analyzed radiographically. Consistent and accurate radiographic patient placement are necessities for the analysis of the vertebral subluxation and its correction. The following is a method employed at the author's clinic:

> To insure consistent patient placement for x-ray analysis of the rotational and disc wedge factors of the vertebral subluxation, all x-rays are taken at a five degree incline. The patient stands before the vertical radiographic bucky on a platform attached to the base of the bucky. The patient is first reclined on the bucky to 45 degrees and then brought back up to five degrees. The tube is tilted to maintain perpendicular alignment of the central ray to the bucky. Gravitational force places the patient against the bucky in a consistent and repeatable manner, thus eliminating the distortions of faulty patient placement.

This radiographic procedure has been used by the author for the past decade and it has been found to be reliable and accurate. Furthermore, with the use of this procedure, consistent and repeatable patient placement makes the analysis of subluxation correction reliable. (14,16).

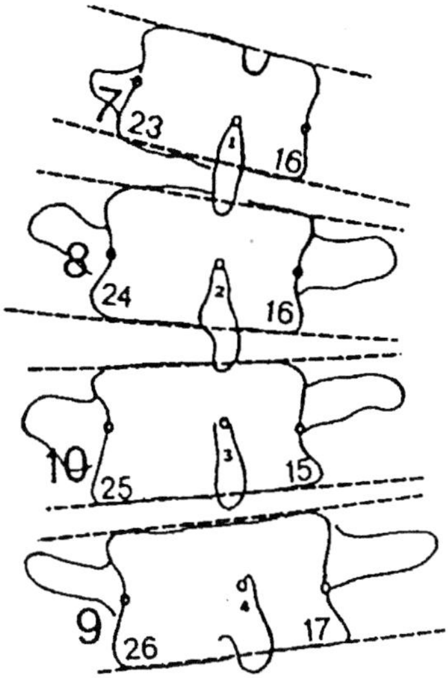

(Figure 13) In the usual compensatory lumbar scoliotic curve, the disc wedges are open to the convexity of the lateral curve. The vertebral body rotations are also toward the convexity of the curve.

Clinical Findings

From the foregoing discussion on radiographic analysis of the vertebral subluxation and patient radiographic placement, we can see a reasonable hypothesis emerging for determining the location of the neuronal disturbance caused by the facet subluxation of the lumbar vertebral subluxation complex. For example, radicular leg pain is commonly found on the side of vertebral incline (closed disc wedge) and on the side of facet separation (open facet). Both of these involvements of the disc block subluxation are commonly found on the convexity of a lateral lumbar scoliotic curve (Fig. 1).

It should be noted here that in the usual compensatory lumbar scoliotic curve, the disc wedge lines diverge towards the convexity of the curve (Fig. 13). In other words, the disc wedges are closed to the concavity of the curve and open to the convexity of the curve.

The disc block subluxation reveals itself by producing a disc wedge open to the concavity of the scoliotic curve at the base of the curve (Fig. 14). The body of the vertebra immediately above the disc wedge will be rotated away from the open side of the disc wedge in relationship to the vertebral body below. The "open facet" would thus be on the closed side of the disc wedge (Fig. 14). However, this is not to say that rotatory disrelationship alone cannot be responsible for facet separation. When rotation exceeds the normal physiological range of movement, a facet will separate (open) on the side of the body rotation of the excessively rotated vertebra. This, of course, is a relative rotational disrelationship between two vertebra. The facet separates on the side of relative body rotation of the superior vertebra in the subluxation.

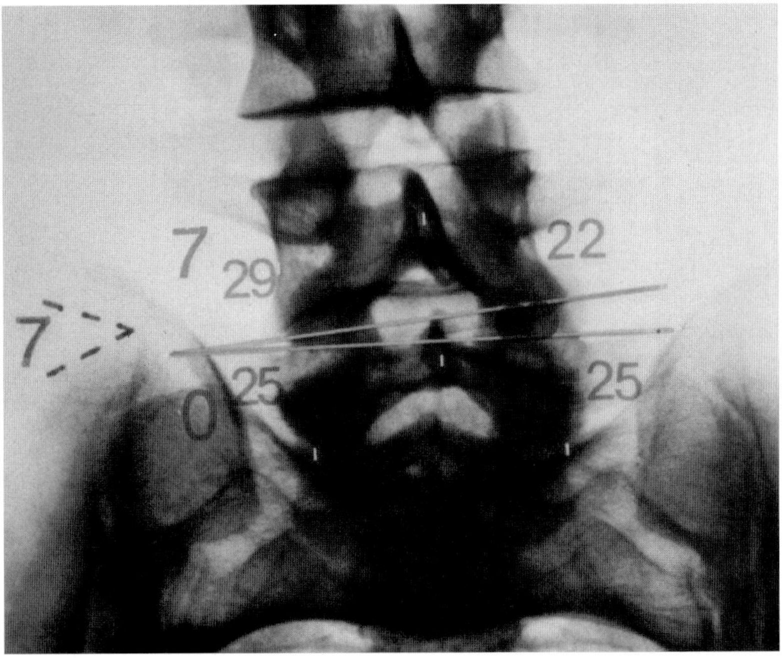

(Figure 14) Viewed from the posterior the disc block subluxation of L 4 produces an inferiority that initiates an accommodating left scoliotic curve. The author has called this type of scoliosis "the sciatic scoliosis" for its common associationship with sciatic rheumatism. The analysis of the subluxation reveals a body rotation of L 4 of 7mm towards the **closed** side of the disc wedge, the **open** side of the disc wedge is toward the concavity of the scoliotic curve. In relation to L 5 the spinous process of

L 4 has moved right, thus the facet is compressed on the right and the contralateral facet opens. In the typical disc block subluxation the **open** facet is on the side of the **closed** disc wedge.

The discussion of the disc block subluxation and the purely rotational subluxation does not however, explain the leg pain syndrome that manifests itself on the side of the concavity of a lateral lumbar curve with no unusual rotational disparity and no "open facet" (Such a scoliotic curve is seen on Fig. 13). Like most neuromuscular skeletal pain syndromes, the victims of such occurrences do not succumb to the problem, so post mortem studies are not available. This leaves us with only reasoned theoretical discussion and x-ray film analysis gleaned from observation and experience, to guide us in determining the cause of the problem.

This author has now practiced four decades as a chiropractor; I followed in the footsteps of my father who graduated from The Palmer School of Chiropractic in 1923. Early on my father told me that leg pain elicited on the concavity of a lateral lumbar scoliotic curve was usually an easily responding case. He said, "simply place a heel lift in the patient's shoe on the side opposite the leg pain (convex side of the curve, the pain free leg) and the pain would be relieved." My father would use our city's phone book (then only 1/2-inch thick) to test a patient for this phenomenon. After placing the phone book under the heel of the patient on the pain-free side he would ask the patient if it gave him/her relief of the pain? Patients would often exclaim with astonishment, yes! He would then place a heel lift in the patient's shoe. I dubbed this test, the "phone book test" but quickly made 1/2-inch boards to use for the test, as the phone book would get quite ragged with such abuse.

To explain this phenomenon, I would say this. As "the medial branch of the lumbar dorsal ramus is fixed in this region" (5), possible tethering takes place causing stretch stress to the nerve as it is drawn down across the inferior foraminal border (or the foraminal ligaments) by the lateral bend of the scoliosis (16). Such stretch stress would be quite spontaneously relieved by raising the spine on its convex side; this is exactly what happens in the placing of a heel lift on the side opposite the leg pain. Pre and post x-rays of patients using lifts thus, and receiving chiropractic adjustments to reduce the vertebral rotations concomitant to lateral scoliosis, have shown a decrease in rotations and cobb angulations of the lateral curve (15,16). Such leg pain syndromes respond dramatically to chiropractic vertebral adjustments.

It should be noted here that heel lifts should not be used to simply compensate for an anatomical short leg. The spine does not rest upon the acetabulums, its base is the sacrum. This author has often found that the sacrum is level regardless of "short leg," and at times it is actually low on the side opposite the anatomical short leg. This is such a universal occurrence that the placing of heel lifts by the criteria of anatomical short leg alone is fraught with error. The sacrum and the pelvis commonly accommodate to the anatomical short leg if not too great in deficiency. (15)

CARE AND PREVENTION

The prevention of disease should take precedence over the treatment of disease and it is to our youth that we must look in preventing the spinal aberrations that lead to low back and leg pain problems. The old adage "as a tree is bent so shall it grow" certainly applies to the spine. Development of a good lordotic lumbar contour can do much to prevent lumbar kyphosis, lateral deviation (scoliosis), vertebral rotation, disc wedging, disc degeneration and vertebral subluxation (15). Babies should be encouraged to creep. The use of walkers and playpens should be discouraged as they lead to early walking by infants and thus developmental lumbar kyphosis (15,16). Creeping nurtures the already existing thoracic kyphotic curve and helps in the development of the lumbar and cervical lordotic curves. Once established, the curves should continue to be nurtured throughout adult life as they will help prevent the stooped posture and old age. Flexion exercises should be greatly reduced in all physical education regimens, especially for children, as such exercises are damaging to the lumbar spine and discs and hinder the development of normal lumbar, pelvic and cervical spinal contours (16). Cyriax in his book *Orthopaedic Medicine* made this observation (7):

> It is to the gymnasts who teach at schools that we must look first for a reversal of policy. No endeavor must be made to persuade children to bend down and touch the floor. Those who can, well and good; those who cannot must not force their trunks, nor have them forced, towards flexion. Lessons on how to sit and lift maintaining the lordosis should become part of gymnastic school training everywhere. Once such postures become second nature, they can be carried on into working life indefinitely.

CONCLUSION

The use of chiropractic x-ray analysis methods can determine abnormal spinal contours that predispose the spine to the occurrence of the vertebral subluxations that initiate nerve root irritation and resultant back and leg pain syndromes. The identity of the disc block subluxation should be suspect in all leg pain symptomatology. Chiropractic spinal adjustments (specific manipulations) can reduce vertebral subluxations, enhance normal spinal contours and relieve nerve root compression.

The use of heel lifts can be useful in controlling leg pain. Lifts are applied appropriately when they are used to support lateral curvatures, reduce disc wedges and stabilize subluxations. The use of sacral base x-rays to determine the actual level of the sacrum is invaluable in determining the need for heel lifts (15).

Finally, the chiropractic intervertebral subluxation is a determinable cause of the neuroforaminal disturbances that lead to a multitude of radicular leg pain syndromes. X-ray analysis and palpation for the open facet can reliably identify the level and side of the vertebral foraminal involvement. Corrective spinal adjustment (specific manipulation) should be the first consideration before more radical forms of treatment, i.e. drugs and surgery, are resorted to.

REFERENCES
(The Chiropractic Vertebral Subluxation)

1. White AA, Panjabi M. Clinical Biomechanics of the Spine, Lippincott Co., 504,288,1978.
2. Stephenson, Chiropractic Textbook, Palmer College of Chiropractic, Davenport, Iowa, p2,1927.
3. Fenesson B, Low Back Pain 2nd Edition, Lippincott, p563,1980.
4. Jackson R, The Cervical Syndrome, 3rd Edition, Charles C. Thomas, Publisher, 1987.
5. Sunderland S, Nerve and Nerve Injuries, Churchill Livingston, p1029,1978.
6. Farfan HF, The Biomechanical Advantage of Lordosis and Hip Extention for Upright Activity, Spine, Vol.3, No. 4,1978.
7. Cyriax J, Orthopaedic Medicine, the Textbook of Orthopaedic Medicine, Bailliere Tindall, Publisher, 1984.
8. Logan, HB, Logan Basic Methods, 1950, Logan College of Chiropractic, St.Louis, Missouri.
9. Ravichandran G, Spinous Process Deviation, Spine, Vol.8, No.3,1983.
10. Kirkaldy-Willis, WH, Managing Low Back Pain, Williams & Wilkens, Baltimore, Hong Kong, London, Sydney, 2nd Edition, 1988.
11. Schmorl and Junghanns, The Human Spine in Health and Disease, 2nd American Edition, 1971, Grune and Stratton, New York and London,221.

12. Hasue M, Pain and the Nerve Root, Spine, Vol.18(14),1993.
13. Bachop W, Transforaminal Ligaments and The Straight Leg Raising Test of Laseque. Twelfth Annual Biomechanics conference on the spine, University of Colorado, Boulder, Colorado, Dec.5-6,1981.
14. Russell GG, Raso VJ, Hill D, McIvor J, A Comparison of Four Computerized Methods for Measuring Vertebral Rotation, Spine 15(1),1990.
15. Barge FHE, Scoliosis, 2nd Edition 1986, Barge Chiropractic Clinic.
16. Barge FHE, Tortipelvis, 4th Edition 1986, Barge Chiropractic Clinic.
17. Weitz EM, The Lateral Bending Sign, Spine, Vol.6, No.4, July/August, 1981.

Subluxations exist throughout the spine and early detection and correction in children can prevent most chronic spinal curvatures. The neuroforaminal encroachment factors spoke of in the paper I have just quoted can cause physiological disturbances that lead to the symptomatology that we, today, label as disease. Disease starts out first as malfunction and malfunction has its causes.

Final "THOTS"

After 43 years of active practice and over three decades of serving this profession as a writer, educator and lecturer, it concerns me that our great truths still seem to be hidden away, doomed as yet to obscurity. With the pervasive influence of the economics of drug development and production, the sale of drugs and vaccines, the therapeutic paradigm of medicine driven by the myth of the germ theory of disease continues on. Hopefully, in the next millennium, the horrors produced by drugs, needless surgery, and genetic tampering, will bring forth an era of enlightenment that will reveal the basic truths that chiropractic has espoused for over 100 years..

"When truth and error have fair play the former is always an overmatch for the latter."

Benjamin Franklin

Chiropractic must continue to insist on "fair play" and a level playing field with medicine. Outcome assessment will prove once and for all the truth of the chiropractic principle. As I reflect now on the theories of D. D. and B. J. Palmer, as I reflect on the myriad of so-called "diseases" I have personally seen respond to chiropractic care. It is apparent to me that the human spine is of major importance in respect to the overall health of all, as D. D. Palmer would say, vertebrata. The list of "diseases" that respond to the adjustments of infants reported in the paper by Dr. Gutmann are quite profound. Congenital Torticollis, retarded mental and linguistic development, facial asymmetry; infectious conditions such as rhinitis, bronchitis, tonsillitis, enteritis, conjunctivitis, and a myriad of other symptomatologies - infant scoliosis, hip dysphasia, vomiting, sleeplessness, muscular hypertonicity, seizures, tremors and more. All these conditions, often called diseases, were resolved in infants through the upper cervical adjustment. What about adults? Could chiropractic claims of the past and the present soon be coming into the light of the public's collective understanding? Is it just possible that disease starts first as malfunction caused by spinal subluxations and the resultant nerve interference inherent in all vertebral subluxations? These questions will only be answered as time evolves and the principles that have been brought forth by the chiropractic profession are increasingly made known.

B. J. Palmer held that "mental impulses" were interfered with by occipital/atlanto/axial subluxations. By "mental impulses" he meant more than just nerve interference, he was speaking of the "brain cell to tissue cell" coordinate responses necessary to produce the normal function of the human body called homeostasis. Such interference to coordinate physiological function could certainly be caused by brain stem pressures on neural centers located in the brain stem of the occipital/atlanto/axial area of the spine as held forth by B. J. Palmer. Add to this the subluxations that can occur at any level of the human spine and you can begin to see that Hippocrates admonition was correct.

"Look well to the spine for the cause of disease."

D. D. Palmer stated:

"The science of chiropractic has modified our views concerning life, death, health, and disease. WE no longer believe that disease is an entity, something foreign to the body, which may enter from without, and with which we have to grasp, struggle, fight and conquer, or submit and succumb to its ravages. Disease is a disturbed condition, not a thing of enmity. Disease is an abnormal performance of certain functions; the abnormal activity has its causes."

Yes, "abnormal activity has its causes."

Chiropractors and chiropractic have long withstood the abuse of the medical professions castigation; medicine scoffed at the principles brought forth by chiropractic. Spencer said:

"There is a principle which is a bar against all information, which is proof against all argument, and which cannot fail to keep a man in everlasting ignorance. That principle is condemnation before investigation."

Yes, "condemnation before investigation" has certainly been used well against the chiropractic profession. Darwin said it so succinctly:

"Great is the power of steady misrepresentation."

Will chiropractic be able to overcome the heavy cloud of misrepresentation that has been laid upon it? This writer thinks so. In my lifetime of chiropractic practice that has not only included a high volume individualistic practice; but also bringing 17 chiropractors into direct practice with me and observing their results. By developing three chiropractic clinics and engaging in numerous research projects into the many aspects of the vertebral subluxation. By extensive writing, reading, and the publishing of nine books on the philosophy, science and art of chiropractic, I too hold that the major cause of disease is bodily malfunction and the major cause of that malfunction is the vertebral subluxation. I will continually strive to bring forth these truths as did the members of my family before me and as I hope those that now follow will continue to do. The indications of this are good.

As the vast army of chiropractors grow and the failing paradigm of the Descartesian biomedical model continues on its inevitable slide to oblivion; we see the beginning of the emergence of a new post modern world in healing. In this new enlightenment the adjustment of the vertebral subluxation will take its rightful place as a primary consideration in the care of all vertebrata. Chiropractic adjustic technics will improve, analysis will be ameliorated, specificity will be paramount and the Palmer's contribution to the welfare of man in health and disease will be recorded as a major leap of perception rendered well in advance of its time.

This book has expressed my knowledge gained through practice and research into the acute disc block subluxation of torticollis. Prevention of spinal distortions is covered in my text

VOL. III SCOLIOSIS. The acute disc block subluxation of tortipelvis is well addressed in VOL. I by the same name. It is time now to lay the pen aside on this my final text on this singular subluxation of the cervical spine. Time and future research will determine its veracity. As a final comment I must say this, it is to the children that we must pay particular attention, we must detect and correct the small causes from which diseases come - **subluxations**. As the great medical physician, Dr. Charles Mayo, said:

"It is unfortunate that so few appreciate from what small causes disease come."

and he also said:

"That which can be foreseen can be prevented."

Yes, the maintenance of health should take precedence over the treatment of disease, and the correction of subluxations in youth maintains the coordinate physiological functionating that produces health.

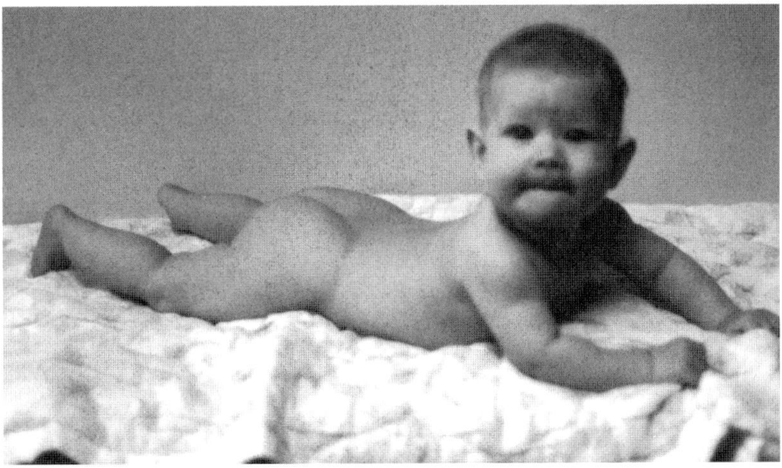

(Ill. XIV-8) And, as my granddaughter, Amanda, above purses her lips tightly closed, I now close this text.

"Enuf" Said,

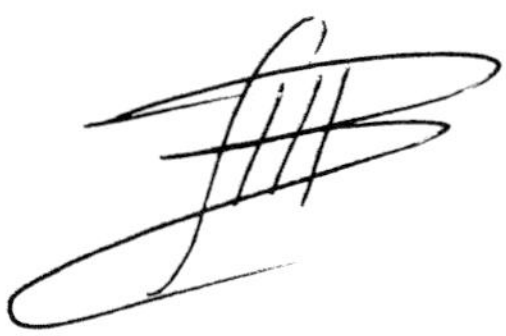

Notes

BIBLIOGRAPHY

1 THE SCIENCE, ART AND PHILOSOPHY OF CHIROPRACTIC, D. D. Palmer 1910, contact Palmer College of Chiropractic, Davenport, Iowa.

2 CHIROPRACTIC SYMPTOMATOLOGY, James N. Firth D.C., Ph.C., 1919, contact Palmer College of Chiropractic, Davenport, Iowa.

3 CAMPBELL'S OPERATIVE ORTHOPAEDICS, 1956, C.V. Mosby Co.

4 THE PRINCIPLES AND PRACTICE OF MEDICINE, William Osler M.D., 1892, 95, 98 D. Appleton & Co., Appleton.

5 THE HOME HAND-BOOK OF DOMESTIC HYGIENE AND RATIONAL MEDICINE, J. H. Kellog M.D. 1896, Modern Medicine Publishing Co., Battle Creek, Michigan.

6 THE PRACTITIONERS MANUAL, Charles W. Allen M.D. 1898, William Wood and Co., New York.

7 THE DISEASES OF INFANCY AND CHILDHOOD, L. Emmet Holt M.D. 1901, D. Appleton & Co., New York.

8 THE DIAGNOSTICS OF INTERNAL MEDICINE, Glenworth Reeve Butler A.M., M.D. 1902, D. Appleton & Co., New York.

9 DIFFERENTIAL DIAGNOSIS AND TREATMENT OF DISEASE, Augustus Caille M.D., 1907, D. Appleton & Co., New York & London.

10 TEXT BOOK OF PEDIATRICS, Waldo E. Nelson M.D.D.Sc., 8th Edition 1964 W. B. Saunder Company Philadelphia, London.

11 PRINCIPLES AND PRACTICE OF SPINAL ADJUSTMENT, Forrestor, D.C. 1915, National School of Chiropractic, Chicago.

12 FUNDAMENTALS OF INTERNAL MEDICINE, Wallace Mason Yater, 1944, D. Appleton, Century Co. New York, London.

13 THE SPINE, A RADIOLOGICAL TEXT AND ATLAS, Bernard Epstein M.D. 1962 Loa & Febiger, Philadelphia.

14 MUSCULOSKELETAL DISORDER, Robert D. D'Ambrosia M.D. 1977, J.B. Lippincott Co., Philadelphia, Toronto.

15 CLINICAL BIOMECHANICS OF THE SPINE, White and Panjabi, 1978, J.B. Lippincott Co., Philadelphia, Toronto.

16 TORTIPELVIS, VOL. I, 1976, 4th Edition 1982, F. H. Barge, D.C., Ph.C., Barge Chiropractic Publishing, Inc., LaCrosse, WI.

17 BACKACHE, ITS EVOLUTION AND CONSERVATIVE TREATMENT, 1982, David P. Evans M.D., University Park Press, Baltimore.

18 TORTICOLLIS, Vol. II, 1979, F. H. Barge, D.C., Ph.C., Barge Chiropractic Publishing, Inc., LaCrosse, WI.

19 CLINICAL BIOMECHANICS, R.C. Shafer, D.C., 1983, Williams & Wilkens, Baltimore/London.

20 LOGAN BASIC METHODS, Hugh B. Logan D.C., 1950, Logan Chiropractic College Chesterfield, MO.

21 SCOLIOSIS, Vol. III, 2nd Expanded Edition 1996, F. H. Barge, D.C., Ph.C., Barge Chiropractic Publishing, Inc., LaCrosse, WI.

22 JOURNAL OF CLINICAL CHIROPRACTIC PEDIATRICS, Vol.2, No.2, Oct. 1997, International Chiropractors Association, Arlington, Virginia.

23 FUNDAMENTALS OF CHIROPRACTIC TECHNIQUES, 1983, Otto C. Reinert, D.C., Marion Press Inc., Chesterfield, MO. Contact Logan College of Chiropractic, Chesterfield, MO.

24 A METHOD OF CHIROPRACTIC ANALYSIS AND PROCEDURE, 1958, W. Frederic Keck D.C., Ph.C., Bronx, New York.

25 ARE YOU THE DOCTOR, DOCTOR?, Vol. IV, 1st Edition 1984, 3rd Edition 1989, F. H. Barge, D.C., Ph.C., Barge Chiropractic Publishing Inc., LaCrosse, WI.

26 THE NEURODYNAMICS OF THE VERTEBRAL SUBLUXATION, A.E. Homewood LL.B. D.C. N.D. 1981, Copyright by the Author.

27 CARVER'S CHIROPRACTIC ANALYSIS 1915-1922, Willard LL.B.D.C. (out of print).

28 SPINE, Vol. 18, No. 12, 1993, Paper, "A Possible Cause of Scoliosis Maquire, Madigan, Wallace, Leppanen and Draper, pages 1621-1626, Lippincott-Raven, Philadelphia PA.

29 SPINE, THE INTERNATIONAL JOURNAL FOR THE STUDY OF THE SPINE, Vol.2, No.3, Sept. 1977, Paper, pages 179, 180. Harper & Row, Hagerstown, MD, published today by Lippincott-Raven, Philadelphia PA.

30 SUCCESS EXPRESS, Vol. 7, No. 1, Spring 1984, Paper, "The Role of Cervical Joint Dysfunction In Balance and Coordination," Timothy G. Gerhart D.C.

31 SPINE, Vol. 19, No. 11, 1994; Paper, "The Relationship Between Pes Cavus and Idiopathic Scoliosis," Carpentero, Entrenas, Gonzales, Garcia and Mesa; Lippincott-Raven, Philadelphia, PA.

32 A TEXTBOOK OF PATHOLOGY, Structure and Function in Disease; William Boyd, C.C., M.D. Lea & Febiger - Philadelphia, page 1389.

33 CHIROPRACTIC AND PREGNANCY, 1994, Joan Fallon D.C., published by International Chiropractors Association.

34 THE ROLE OF THE CHIROPRACTIC ADJUSTMENT IN THE CARE AND TREATMENT OF 322 CHILDREN WITH OTITIS MEDIA. Paper, Joan Fallon D.C., Oct. 1997, Journal of Clinical Chiropractic Pediatrics, International Chiropractors Association Council on Chiropractic Pediatrics, Arlington, Virginia.

35 CHIROPRACTIC CARE OF THE NEWBORN WITH CONGENITAL TORTICOLLIS. Paper, Joan Fallon D.C., Peter Fysh, D.C., Journal of Clinical Chiropractic Pediatrics, Vol. 2, No. 1, Jan. 1997, International Chiropractors Association, Council on Chiropractic Pediatrics, Arlington, Virginia.

36 RARE STUDY OF SIAMESE TWINS IN THE SOVIET, MASHA & DASHA; Article, LIFE Magazine, April 1966.

37 THE MOST INTIMATE BOND; Article, TIME Magazine, March 25, 1996.

38 THE BIGNESS OF THE FELLOW WITHIN; Vol. XXII, 1949, page 403, B. J. Palmer D.C., Ph.C., Published by The Palmer School of Chiropractic, Davenport Iowa.

39 THE CONDYLE SUBLUXATION IN INFANTS; Paper, Douglas B. Cox, D.C., I.C.A. REVIEW, International Chiropractors Association, March/April 1991.

40 VOICE; Chiropractic Journal of the Kentucky Association of Chiropractors, 1988 (?), Vol. 4, No. 4, article, Marcia Segura D.C.

41 BLOCKED ATLANTO NERVE SYNDROME IN INFANTS AND SMALL CHILDREN; Paper 1987, Manuelle Medizin, Gutmann, Springer - Verlag, Germany.

42 BRAIN STEM COMPRESSION IN RHEUMATOID ARTHRITIS; Paper, Dec. 12, 1977, Vol. 238, No. 24, JAMA, by Robert C. Davidson M.D., John R. Horn M.D., James H. Herndon M.D., Oliver D. Grin M.D.

43 THE CHIROPRACTIC VERTEBRAL SUBLUXATION AND ITS RELATIONSHIP TO VERTEBROGENIC LUMBAR PAIN CRURALGIA AND SCIATIC SYNDROMES; Paper, 1994, F. H. Barge, D.C., Ph.C., The Chiropractic Research Journal, Vol. 3, No. 2, 1996, Life University and School of Chiropractic, Marietta, Georgia.

Notes

INDEX OF ILLUSTRATIONS

Notes

INDEX

B

C

J

K

L

O

P

S

U

V

Notes

THE BOOKS OF
Fred H. Barge, D.C., Ph.C

Tortipelvis, Vol. I 4th Edition
Dr. Barge's first published book has been a required curricular text since 1976 in leading chiropractic colleges. The analysis and adjustic correction of the classic low back disc syndrome subluxation.

Torticollis, Vol. II 2nd Edition
OUT OF PRINT
The analysis and adjustic correction of "Wry Neck," the disc syndrome subluxation of the cervical spine. Torticollis is not muscle spasm, it is a subluxation and adjustment provides correction.

Scoliosis, Vol. III Expanded 2nd Edition
The detection, analysis, control, reduction and correction of the four basic causes of "Idiopathic" scoliosis through chiropractic methods. Contains over 350 pages, fully illustrated, including a chapter on "heel lifts!"

Are You the Doctor, Doctor? Vol. IV 3rd Edition
The philosophy of successful practice, this text is a "Cookbook" on the art of good, ethical, and responsible doctoring. Dr. J. Clay Thompson stated: "Once you start reading this book you cannot put it down."

Life Without Fear, Vol. V
Pure, traditional, Palmer Chiropractic Philosophy. From D.D. & B.J. Palmer through the present teachings of modern chiropractic authors, Dr. B clearly explains the sound philosophical tenets of chiropractic.

One Cause, One Cure, VOl. VI
For as long as man has existed on the face of the earth he has searched for THE CAUSE. The cause of disease, of health, success, failure; and the answer has been there all the time. The "Big Idea" explained.

Giant vs. Pygmy + "Thots", Vol. VII
Giant vs. Pygmy is a B.J. Palmer classic; herein he speaks of the metaphysical concepts of chiropractic. This book contains an exact copy of B.J.'s book plus the interpretations and additional "Thots" of Dr. B.

It Is As Simple As That & More, VOl. VIII

B.J. Palmer's most popular lay lecture interpreted by Dr. B. This book also contains two of B.J. Palmer's and three of Dr. Barge's most popular patient explanatory brochures, chiropractic's "33 Principles," "The Nine Primary Functions" and much more.

Wryneck, Vol. IX

Dr. Barge's completely revised and augmented treatise on the cause and correction of Torticollis. With contributions of other noted chiropractic authors on pediatric adjusting and a chapter on Upper Cervical Specific Technic, this text promises to be a classic in chiropractic literature.

Old Dad Chiro

Written by Vern Gielow and copyrighted by Dr. Barge, the only thoroughly documented book ever written on The Life and Times of D.D. Palmer. (Soft Bound)

Dr. Barge's Other Writings

AUDIO TAPES AND BROCHURES

Comprehensive - multiple page

"Tortipelvis"
"Deterioration/Degeneration"
"Torticollis"
"Chiropractic Care"
"Scoliosis"
"Healing Takes Time"

Concise - bi-fold

"Bedwetting"
"Common Cold"
"Child Care"
"Senior Years"
"Immunization"
"Cause of Disease"

"Pregnancy"
"High Blood Pressure"
"Hemorrhoids"
"Asthma & Children"
"Ear Infection"
"Heart Burn"

Audio Tapes

Series I
THE LIFE WITHOUT FEAR
The Beginning-Tape 1
The Palmer Paradigm-Tape 2
Why-Tape 3

Series II
"THOTS"
Simple Isn't It-Tape 1
A Founder's Day Message -Tape 2